D1285140

Substance Use Disorders

3rd Edition

By

Audrey Darville
PhD, APRN, CTTS, FAANP

Peggy El-Mallakh
PhD, RN, PMH APRN-BC

Dianna Inman
DNP, RN, APRN, CPNP-PC, PMHS, PMHNP-BC

Upon successful completion of this course, continuing education hours will be awarded as follows:
Nurses: 30 Contact Hours*

*Western Schools is accredited as a provider of continuing nursing education by the American Nurses Credentialing Center's Commission on Accreditation.

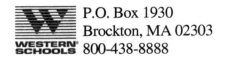

P.O. Box 1930
Brockton, MA 02303
800-438-8888

ABOUT THE AUTHORS

Audrey Darville, PhD, APRN, CTTS, FAANP, is an associate professor in the College of Nursing at the University of Kentucky. She has been a practicing family nurse practitioner since 1998. Currently the tobacco treatment specialist with the University of Kentucky Health Care System, she is also director of the BREATHE Tobacco Treatment Specialist online training program. As a Certified Tobacco Treatment Specialist, Audrey works with inpatients, outpatients, and employees to provide group and intensive individual tobacco dependence treatment. She is president of the Association for the Treatment of Tobacco Use and Dependence. She was honored as the Kentucky Nurse Practitioner of the Year in 2014 and inducted as a Fellow in the American Academy of Nurse Practitioners in 2016.

Audrey Darville has disclosed that she has no significant financial or other conflicts of interest pertaining to this course book.

Peggy El-Mallakh, PhD, RN, PMH APRN-BC, has degrees from the Central Connecticut State University in 1982, a Master of Science in Nursing from the University of Kentucky College of Nursing in 1998, and a Doctor of Philosophy in Nursing from the University of Kentucky College of Nursing in 2005. She is currently an associate professor at the University of Kentucky College of Nursing, where she serves as the co-coordinator of the Psychiatric-Mental Health Nurse Practitioner Program. Her research interests include training undergraduate and graduate nursing students in the use of a Screening, Brief Intervention, and Referral to Treatment Intervention to address substance use disorders in outpatient settings. She also conducts research on medical illness management and health promotion among people diagnosed with schizophrenia, the use of evidence-based practices in community mental health treatment settings, and evaluation of Doctor of Nursing Practice Programs. Dr. El-Mallakh is active in the American Psychiatric Nurses Association and the National Organization for Nurse Practitioner Faculties.

Peggy El-Mallakh has disclosed that she has no significant financial or other conflicts of interest pertaining to this course book.

Dianna Inman, DNP, APRN, CPNP-PC, PMHS, PMHNP-BC, received a Bachelor of Science in Nursing from East Carolina University, a Master of Science in the Pediatric Nurse Practitioner Track at Virginia Commonwealth University, and Doctor of Nursing Practice at Arizona State University. She is certified as a pediatric nurse practitioner, pediatric primary care mental health specialist, and psychiatric mental health nurse practitioner. Dr. Inman is actively involved in practice in developmental/behavioral pediatrics and school-based mental health. She is an assistant professor of nursing at the University of Kentucky and teaches in the Doctor of Nursing Practice Program. Dr. Inman has presented nationally on substance use. She received funding from the Substance Abuse Mental Health Services Administration to teach healthcare providers and students how to screen, provide brief intervention, and know when to refer patients for substance use problems. Dr. Inman is actively involved in the National Association of Pediatric Nurse Practitioners and Association of Psychiatric Nurse Practitioners.

Dianna Inman has disclosed that she has no significant financial or other conflicts of interest pertaining to this course book.

ISBN: 978-1-68041-394-6

FP0218CR

ABOUT THE PEER REVIEWERS

Dana Murphy-Parker, MS, CRNP, PMHNP-BC, CARN-AP, FIAAN, is co-director of the Psychiatric/Mental Health Nurse Practitioner Program at Drexel University College of Nursing and Health Professions and the immediate past-president of the International Nurses Society on Addictions. Ms. Murphy-Parker has lead in encouraging nurses and nurse practitioners to use the evidence-based knowledge available for treating persons with opioid use disorders during this public health crisis. In 2017, Ms. Murphy-Parker was inducted as a Fellow in the International Academy of Addictions Nursing and is in the Doctor of Nursing Practice (DNP) Program at Widener University.

> **Dana Murphy-Parker** has disclosed that she has no significant financial or other conflicts of interest pertaining to this course book.

Roseann Regan, PhD, APRN, BC, received her Bachelors of Science (Nursing) from the University of Pennsylvania, a Master of Science (Advanced Practice) from the University of Delaware, and a Doctor of Philosophy in Nursing from Widener University in Pennsylvania. Currently an assistant professor of nursing at Gwynedd Mercy University and an adjunct professor at Drexel University, Dr. Regan has taught behavioral health nursing, adult health nursing, evidence-based practice, and research. She has taught or mentored both masters and doctoral nursing students and has served as a DNP Project Committee member. Dr. Regan is certified in psychiatric-mental health nursing and has clinical and teaching experience in both behavioral health and adult health nursing. She is a board member of Iota Kappa Chapter of Sigma Theta Tau International and a member of the National League of Nursing, the Psychiatric Nurses Association, and the Simulation Consortium of the Tristate (PA, NJ, DE) Area.

> **Roseann Regan** has disclosed that she has no significant financial or other conflicts of interest pertaining to this course book.

Heather Frye, APRN, PMHNP-BC, MSN, MBA, is an assistant clinical professor and co-track director of the Psychiatric-Mental Health Nurse Practitioner Program in the College of Nursing and Health Professions at Drexel University. Mrs. Frye is an American Nurses Credentialing Center board certified adult-psychiatric mental health nurse practitioner and holds a dual Master Degree in Nursing - Leadership, and Business Administration - Healthcare. Her area of expertise is focused in the specialty of addiction and co-occurring disorders, and she maintains her clinical practice in a residential co-occurring treatment program.

> **Heather Frye** has disclosed that she has no significant financial or other conflicts of interest pertaining to this course book.

Nurse Planner: Marcie Scott, MSN, RN

> The planner who worked on this continuing education activity has disclosed that she has no significant financial or other conflicts of interest pertaining to this course book.

Copy Editor: Graphic World, Inc.
Indexer: Dianne Schneider

COURSE INSTRUCTIONS
IMPORTANT: Read these instructions *BEFORE* proceeding!

HOW TO EARN CONTINUING EDUCATION CREDIT

To successfully complete this course you must:
1) Read the entire course
2) Pass the final exam with a score of 75% or higher*
3) Complete the course evaluation

You have three attempts to pass the exam. If you take the exam online, and fail to receive a passing grade, select "Retake Exam."
If you submit the exam by mail or fax and you fail to receive a passing grade, you will be notified by mail and receive an additional answer sheet.

Final exams must be received at Western Schools before the **Complete By** date located at the top of the FasTrax answer sheet enclosed with your course.

Note: The **Complete By** date is either 1 year from the date of purchase, or the expiration date assigned to the course, whichever date comes first.

HOW TO SUBMIT THE FINAL EXAM AND COURSE EVALUATION

ONLINE: BEST OPTION!

For instant grading, regardless of course format purchased, submit your exam online at **www.westernschools.com/my-courses**. Benefits of submitting exam answers online:

➢ Save time and postage
➢ Access grade results instantly and retake the exam immediately, if needed
➢ Identify and review questions answered incorrectly
➢ Access certificate of completion instantly

Note: If you have not yet registered on Western Schools' website, you will need to register and then call customer service at 800-618-1670 to request your courses be made available to you online.

Mail or Fax: To submit your exam and evaluation answers by mail or fax, fill out the FasTrax answer sheet, which is pre-printed with your name, address, and course title. If you are completing more than one course, be sure to record your answers on the correct corresponding answer sheet.

Complete the FasTrax Answer Sheet using blue or black ink only. If you make an error use correction fluid. If the exam has fewer than 100 questions, leave any remaining answer circles blank. Respond to the evaluation questions under the heading "Evaluation," found on the right-hand side of the FasTrax answer sheet. See the FasTrax Exam Grading & Certificate Issue Options enclosed with your course order for further instructions.

CHANGE OF ADDRESS?

Contact our customer service department at 800-618-1670, or customerservice@westernschools.com, if your postal or email address changes prior to completing this course.

WESTERN SCHOOLS GUARANTEES YOUR SATISFACTION

If any continuing education course fails to meet your expectations, or if you are not satisfied for any reason, you may return the course materials for an exchange or a refund (excluding shipping and handling) within 30 days, provided that you have not already received continuing education credit for the course. Software, video, and audio courses must be returned unopened. Textbooks must not be written in or marked up in any other way.

Thank you for using Western Schools to fulfill your continuing education needs!

WESTERN SCHOOLS
P.O. Box 1930, Brockton, MA 02303
800-618-1670 • www.westernschools.com

WESTERN SCHOOLS
COURSE EVALUATION

SUBSTANCE USE DISORDERS

INSTRUCTIONS: Using the scale below, please respond to the following evaluation statements. All responses should be recorded in the right-hand column of the FasTrax answer sheet, in the section marked "Evaluation." Be sure to fill in each corresponding answer circle completely using blue or black ink. Leave any remaining answer circles blank.

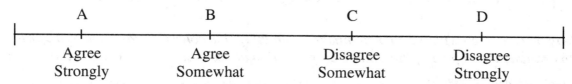

A	B	C	D
Agree Strongly	Agree Somewhat	Disagree Somewhat	Disagree Strongly

OUTCOMES: After completing this course, I am able to:

1. Describe trends in the epidemiology of substance use in the United States.
2. Identify principles of preventing substance use disorders.
3. Describe the components of an assessment for substance use disorders.
4. Distinguish among the various substances linked to substance use disorders.
5. Identify the clinical effects of various substances on the body.
6. Describe the psychosocial issues for patients with substance use disorders.
7. Summarize the treatment approaches for patients with a substance use disorder.
8. Review the scope of substance use among healthcare professionals.

COURSE CONTENT

9. The course content was presented in a well-organized and clearly written manner.
10. The course content was presented in a fair, unbiased, and balanced manner.
11. The course content presented current developments in the field.
12. The course was relevant to my professional practice or interests.
13. The final examination was at an appropriate level for the content of the course.
14. The course expanded my knowledge and enhanced my skills related to the subject matter.
15. I intend to apply the knowledge and skills I've learned to my practice.

    A. Yes   B. Unsure   C. No   D. Not Applicable

CUSTOMER SERVICE

The following section addresses your experience in interacting with Western Schools. Use the scale below to respond to the statements in this section.

    A. Yes   B. No   C. Not Applicable

16. Western Schools staff was responsive to my request for disability accommodations.
17. The Western Schools website was informative and easy to navigate.
18. The process of ordering was easy and efficient.
19. Western Schools staff was knowledgeable and helpful in addressing my questions or problems.

continued on next page

ATTESTATION

20. I certify that I have read the course materials and personally completed the final examination based on the material presented. Mark "A" for Agree and "B" for Disagree.

COURSE RATING

21. My overall rating for this course is

    A. Poor   B. Below Average   C. Average   D. Good   E. Excellent

You may be contacted within 3 to 6 months of completing this course to participate in a brief survey to evaluate the impact of this course on your clinical practice and patient/client outcomes.

Note: To provide additional feedback regarding this course and Western Schools services, or to suggest new course topics, use the space provided on the Important Information form found on the back of the FasTrax instruction sheet included with your course.

CONTENTS

FIGURES AND TABLES

PRETEST

1. Begin this course by taking the pretest. Circle the answers to the questions on this page, or write the answers on a separate sheet of paper. Do not log answers to the pretest questions on the FasTrax test sheet included with the course.

2. Compare your answers to the PRETEST KEY located at the end of the pretest. The pretest key indicates the chapter where the content of that question is discussed. Make note of the questions you missed, so that you can focus on those areas as you complete the course.

3. Complete the course by reading the chapters and completing the exam questions at the end of each chapter. Answers to the exam questions should be logged on the FasTrax test sheet included with the course.

Note: Choose the one option that BEST answers each question.

1. Binge alcohol use is defined as
   a. any use of alcohol in the previous 30 days.
   b. drinking eight or more drinks in a weekend.
   c. having five or more drinks (men) or four or more drinks (women) on the same occasion on at least 1 day
   d. drinking resulting in a blood alcohol concentration level of 0.05 g/dL.

2. Recurrent substance use in situations in which it is physically hazardous is known as
   a. impaired control.
   b. social impairment.
   c. risky use.
   d. tolerance.

3. The Family Check-Up is an example of a prevention program that targets an at-risk subgroup within a larger population. This type of program is considered
   a. universal.
   b. selective.
   c. indicated.
   d. primary.

4. Which is a model used to determine readiness for change?
   a. CAGE
   b. SBIRT
   c. AUDIT
   d. Motivational interviewing

5. Screening and treatment of mild substance use disorders are shifting from
   a. specialty care to primary care.
   b. acute care to specialty care.
   c. outpatient care to inpatient care.
   d. long-term care facilities to inpatient care.

6. Tobacco use disorder is best defined as a
   a. dangerous and deadly habit.
   b. problematic pattern of use leading to impairment or distress.
   c. personal choice in health care.
   d. severe respiratory syndrome leading to acute distress.

7. Caffeine content is not required to be listed as an ingredient in some energy drinks because

    a. energy drinks can be marketed as "dietary supplements," which are not regulated by the U.S. Food and Drug Administration.

    b. the amount of caffeine in energy drinks is negligible.

    c. caffeine intake is harmless in patients who consume energy drinks.

    d. manufacturers are not required to list caffeine as an ingredient in products consumed by children and adolescents.

8. According to the changes in the *Diagnostic and Statistical Manual of Mental Disorders,* fifth edition, individuals who drink alcohol beyond the recommended limits and meet certain criteria are classified as having a(n)

    a. addiction disorder.

    b. alcohol use disorder.

    c. substance use disorder.

    d. mental health disorder.

9. Marijuana use is most prevalent in patients belonging to which age group?

    a. 12 to 17 years

    b. 18 to 25 years

    c. 26 to 40 years

    d. Over 40 years

10. Methamphetamine differs from amphetamine in that methamphetamine

    a. is derived from a plant.

    b. has medical use as a local anesthetic in many surgeries.

    c. is evacuated from the body within 1 hour.

    d. causes a high that lasts significantly longer than that of amphetamine.

11. Which substance, when used in combination with heroin, results in a significantly increased risk of death?

    a. Alcohol

    b. Alprazolam

    c. Methadone

    d. Fentanyl

12. Abrupt discontinuation of high doses of benzodiazepines after long-term use can cause

    a. convulsive status epilepticus and death.

    b. sedation and catatonia.

    c. muscle pain and bradycardia.

    d. psychomotor retardation and weight gain.

13. The peak effect of inhalant intoxication occurs

    a. 30 seconds after inhalant use.

    b. 2 minutes after inhalant use.

    c. 4 minutes after inhalant use.

    d. 10 minutes after inhalant use.

14. A hallucinogen commonly used by young adults during "raves" is

    a. peyote.

    b. lysergic acid diethylamide.

    c. ketamine.

    d. MDMA (Ecstasy).

15. The use of synthetic designer drugs is increasingly popular because they

    a. have fewer adverse effects compared with drugs in their natural forms.

    b. have less risk of addiction compared with drugs in their natural forms.

    c. are less costly than drugs in their natural forms.

    d. are not detected with most drug-screening methods.

16. Most individuals who misuse anabolic steroids are

   a. athletes.

   b. recreational weightlifters.

   c. part of the general population.

   d. older adults.

17. A campaign on the effects of substance use on the developing fetus best targets

   a. older adults.

   b. early adolescents.

   c. reproductive-age women.

   d. men.

18. Which of the following people is at the highest risk for developing infective endocarditis?

   a. An 18-year-old who injected heroin using a clean needle from a needle exchange program

   b. A 64-year-old who has snorted cocaine for 30 years

   c. A 24-year-old who injected methamphetamine with a group of friends

   d. A 45-year-old with an alcohol use disorder and severe malnutrition

19. Impaired practice by a healthcare professional is best defined as

   a. the direct effects of alcohol and other substances on the delivery of patient care.

   b. the inability to provide care that is consistent with the legal and ethical standards of one's profession.

   c. a substance use disorder that jeopardizes the quality and safety of patient care.

   d. a trend of persistently poor clinical outcomes related to the influence of illegal substances.

PRETEST KEY

1.	C	Chapter 1	Page 4
2.	C	Chapter 1	Page 5
3.	B	Chapter 2	Page 17
4.	D	Chapter 3	Page 46
5.	A	Chapter 4	Page 56
6.	B	Chapter 5	Page 80
7.	A	Chapter 6	Page 104
8.	B	Chapter 7	Page 116
9.	B	Chapter 8	Page 148
10.	D	Chapter 9	Page 161
11.	D	Chapter 10	Page 185
12.	A	Chapter 11	Page 212
13.	C	Chapter 12	Page 225
14.	C	Chapter 13	Page 241
15.	C	Chapter 14	Page 252
16.	B	Chapter 15	Page 269
17.	C	Chapter 16	Page 274
18.	C	Chapter 17	Page 298
19.	B	Chapter 18	Page 309

INTRODUCTION

LEARNING OUTCOMES

After completing this course, the learner will be able to:

1. Describe trends in the epidemiology of substance use in the United States.

2. Identify principles of preventing substance use disorders.

3. Describe the components of an assessment for substance use disorders.

4. Distinguish among the various substances linked to substance use disorders.

5. Identify the clinical effects of various substances on the body.

6. Describe the psychosocial issues for patients with substance use disorders.

7. Summarize the treatment approaches for patients with a substance use disorder.

8. Review the scope of substance use among healthcare professionals.

Substance use disorders are a major public health problem with a wide range of negative effects on the mental, physical, and social well-being of individuals. Mental health problems co-occurring with substance use disorders include depressive, anxiety, and psychotic disorders, as well as organic brain syndromes (American Psychiatric Association [APA], 2013). Physical health problems associated with substance use disorders include cardiovascular disorders, HIV/AIDS, cancer, hepatitis, and pulmonary disorders (National Institute on Drug Abuse [NIDA], 2017a). The societal costs of substance use disorders are considerable. These costs are directly or indirectly related to high crime rates, increased rates of legal involvement, incarceration, lost work productivity, drug-related emergency room use (NIDA, 2017c), unstable families and chaotic family interactions, child abuse and neglect, and parental involvement with child welfare services (National Council on Child Abuse and Family Violence, 2016). Illicit drug use in the United States increased between 2007 and 2013, especially among teenagers and young adults (NIDA, 2015).

Various legal, political, and social factors influence substance use trends and treatment. For example, changes specific to marijuana use are evident in recent state efforts to legalize marijuana for recreational and medical use, increased potency of marijuana, increased availability of synthetic marijuana, and decreased perceptions of harm related to marijuana use among adolescents (NIDA, 2017b). Additional trends include increased use of electronic cigarettes, identification of newly emerging misused substances, increasing rates of heroin and polysubstance use, and societal "normalization" of substance use promoted by social media (e.g., Facebook, YouTube) and industry marketing (Barry, Hiilamo, & Glantz, 2014). The evolving trends in substance use in the United States present considerable challenges to healthcare workers who are faced with the dilemma of promoting abstinence during increasingly relaxed social norms and complexities of use.

The content of the course focuses on the epidemiology of addiction, sociocultural influences, commonly used substances, and current standards of treatment and nursing care for patients with substance use disorders. Prevention practices, patient assessment, and therapeutic modalities, including pharmacologic, psychological, group, and nontraditional therapies, are described. Twelve types of substances are described, including their biochemistry and effects on the human body. This course uses terminology for substance-related and addictive disorders defined by the *Diagnostic and Statistical Manual of Mental Disorders,* 5th edition (APA, 2013).

Because nurses have an increasingly complex role in providing care to patients with substance use disorders, there is a demonstrated need for content to increase their knowledge of trends in the epidemiology of substance use disorders and the effect of these trends on the delivery of high-quality patient care. The overall purpose of this course is to provide nursing professionals with a comprehensive overview of substance use disorders and the addiction process, including the knowledge and skills necessary to comprehensively assess and care for patients with substance use disorders, the epidemiology and prevalence of these disorders, evidence-based strategies to prevent and treat substance use problems, and resources to further develop professional skills in providing care for patients with substance use disorders.

References

American Psychiatric Association. (2013). *Diagnostic and statistical manual of mental disorders* (5th ed.). Washington, DC: Author.

Barry, R. A., Hiilamo, H., & Glantz, S. A. (2014). Waiting for the opportune moment: The tobacco industry and marijuana legalization. *The Milbank Quarterly, 92*(2), 207-242.

National Council on Child Abuse and Family Violence. (2016). *Parental substance abuse a major factor in child abuse and neglect.* Retrieved from https://www.childwelfare.gov/pubPDFs/parentalsubabuse.pdf

National Institute on Drug Abuse. (2015). *Drug and alcohol use in college-age adults in 2014.* Retrieved from https://www.drugabuse.gov/related-topics/trends-statistics/infographics/drug-alcohol-use-in-college-age-adults-in-2014

National Institute on Drug Abuse. (2017a). *Health consequences of drug misuse.* Retrieved from https://www.drugabuse.gov/related-topics/medical-consequences-drug-abuse

National Institute on Drug Abuse. (2017b). *Monitoring the Future Survey: High school and youth trends.* Retrieved from https://www.drugabuse.gov/publications/drugfacts/high-school-youth-trends

National Institute on Drug Abuse. (2017c). *Overdose death rates.* Retrieved from https://www.drugabuse.gov/related-topics/trends-statistics/overdose-death-rates

CHAPTER 1

THE EPIDEMIOLOGY
AND BIOLOGICAL BASIS
OF SUBSTANCE USE

LEARNING OUTCOME

After completing this chapter, the learner will be able to describe the epidemiology of substance misuse and substance use disorders in the United States.

CHAPTER OBJECTIVES

After completing this chapter, the learner will be able to:

1. Discuss methods for collecting epidemiological data on substance use and misuse patterns.

2. Define epidemiological trends of substance use and misuse in various populations.

3. Identify the diagnostic categories of substance use disorders.

4. Explain the neurobiology of substance use and drug addiction.

INTRODUCTION

Epidemiology is the basic science of disease prevention focusing on an approach to understanding disease and developing the basis for interventions designed to modify and improve its natural history. It also plays major roles in developing and evaluating public policy related to health and to social and legal issues. The field is concerned with the critical issue of how to distinguish people who have a disease from those who do not, including the environmental conditions uniquely associated with the affected populations (Gordis, 2014).

The distinct difference between the work of healthcare professionals (i.e., nurses and other clinicians) and the work of epidemiologists in this area is the focus of their efforts. Healthcare professionals are concerned with individuals, whereas epidemiologists gather data on the health of a population within an environmental context. Epidemiologists are often concerned with incidence rates (the rates at which people without a disease develop the disease during a specific time) and prevalence rates (the rates of individuals in a population with a disease at a given time). The data gathered through the efforts of epidemiologists are used to plan prevention and treatment services. Substance use epidemiology investigates patterns, trends, and risk factors for substance use. Areas of interest include behavioral, developmental, environmental, and social/cultural factors that can either promote or protect against risky substance use (National Institute on Drug Abuse [NIDA], 2017).

This chapter will compare the various methods of collecting data and monitoring substance misuse; briefly discuss epidemiological trends of substance misuse in the United States; discuss the value and uses of epidemiological data in the drug addiction field; define the criteria used to diagnose substance use disorders; and describe the neurobiological effects of substance misuse.

MONITORING SUBSTANCE USE

There are two approaches to monitoring substance use and misuse: collecting existing data to determine drug use patterns within drug-using populations (surveillance) and using surveys to estimate the incidence and prevalence of use within a general population. Surveillance collects information from existing or archival data systems that reflect the consequences of substance use, such as substance use disorder treatment facilities, arrest reports for adults and adolescents, hospital emergency department visits, hospital discharge information, mortality information, and infectious disease reports (Substance Abuse and Mental Health Services Administration [SAMHSA], 2014). Surveys are snapshots of substance use in a defined population.

Surveillance

The National Drug Early Warning System (NDEWS) is an example of surveillance. Established in 2014 and supported through a cooperative agreement with the University of Maryland, it consists of a national network of scientists, government and public health officials, and law enforcement representatives who identify and monitor emerging trends in drug use. The NDEWS assists with local research on emerging drug issues and shares information on trends, such as rates of use and overdoses in specific regions of the United States. Collection of information by NDEWS involves

innovative strategies, such as scanning social and news media, for identification and monitoring of emerging drug problems. Access the NDEWS site at https://www.drugabuse.gov/related-topics/trends-statistics/national-drug-early-warning-system-ndews.

National Surveys

Three surveys are used to monitor substance use trends in the general population: Monitoring the Future (MTF) survey, Youth Risk Behavior Surveillance System (YRBSS), and National Survey on Drug Use and Health (NSDUH). See Table 1-1 for summaries of these surveys. These surveys offer researchers, planners, and practitioners an understanding of the substance use trends in the United States. They also provide comparisons among various ethnic and racial groups.

MTF is an ongoing study of drug, alcohol, and cigarette use, along with attitudes about use, among adolescents in the United States. It began in 1975 and is conducted by the University of Michigan's Institute for Social Research. Each year 50,000 8th grade, 10th grade, and 12th grade students are surveyed (12th graders since 1975 and 8th and 10th graders since 1991). The study focuses on the recent trends in the use of licit and illicit drugs, as well as the trends in the levels of perceived risk and personal disapproval associated with each drug (Johnston, O'Malley, Bachman, & Schulenberg, 2012a, 2012b, 2013). In addition, annual follow-up questionnaires are mailed to a sample of each graduating class for a number of years after their initial participation.

NSDUH is sponsored by SAMHSA. It is the primary source of information on illicit drug use by those in the United States aged 12 and older. It was initiated in 1971 and is currently conducted annually. This report provides national estimates of use, number of users, and other measures related to the use of illicit drugs, alco-

TABLE 1-1: THREE NATIONAL SURVEYS FOR MONITORING TRENDS IN SUBSTANCE USE	
Name of Survey	**Description**
Monitoring the Future	This is an ongoing study of the behaviors, attitudes, and values of secondary school students, college students, and adults up to 50 years of age in the United States. Each year 50,000 8th grade, 10th grade, and 12th grade students are surveyed (12th graders since 1975 and 8th and 10th graders since 1991). The study focuses on the recent trends in the use of licit and illicit drugs, as well as the trends in the levels of perceived risk and personal disapproval associated with each drug.
National Survey on Drug Use and Health	This is the primary source of information on illicit drug use in the U.S. population aged 12 years and older. This report, conducted annually, provides national estimates of use, number of users, and other measures related to use of illicit drugs, alcohol, and cigarettes and other forms of tobacco by population. It includes national estimates of trends in the initiation of substance use, as well as the extent of drug dependence and treatment in the United States.
Youth Risk Behavior Surveillance System	This survey monitors six categories of priority health-risk behaviors among children in grades 9 through 12. It tracks behaviors that contribute to unintentional and intentional injuries; tobacco use; alcohol and other drug use; sexual behaviors that contribute to unintended pregnancy and sexually transmitted diseases (including HIV infection); unhealthy dietary behaviors; and physical inactivity (including being overweight).

Note. Adapted from:

The Regents of the University of Michigan. (2017). *Monitoring the future: A continuing study of American youth.* Retrieved from http://www.monitoring thefuture.org

Substance Abuse and Mental Health Services Administration. (2016a). *Population data/NSDUH.* Retrieved from https://www.samhsa.gov/data/population-data-nsduh

Centers for Disease Control and Prevention. (2016a). *Youth Risk Behavior Surveillance System (YRBSS).* Retrieved from https://www.cdc.gov/healthy youth/data/yrbs/index.htm

hol, and cigarettes and other forms of tobacco by population. It includes national estimates of trends in substance use initiation, as well as both the prevalence of substance use disorders and statistics about treatment rates. The primary objectives of the NSDUH are to collect timely data on the magnitude and patterns of alcohol, tobacco, and illegal substance use and misuse; assess the consequences of substance use and misuse; and identify those groups at high risk for substance use and misuse. A scientific random sample of households throughout the United States is used. A professional field representative visits each household. Because the survey is based on a random sample, each selected individual represents approximately 3,000 other U.S. residents (SAMHSA, 2016b).

YRBSS is a means of monitoring health-risk behaviors among youth and young adults. It includes a national school-based Centers for Disease Control and Prevention (CDC) survey for students in grades 9 through 12. The YRBSS monitors six categories of priority health-risk behaviors among youth and young adults:

1. Behaviors that contribute to unintentional and intentional injuries

2. Tobacco use

3. Alcohol and other drug use

4. Sexual behaviors that contribute to unintended pregnancy and sexually transmitted diseases

5. Unhealthy dietary behaviors

6. Physical inactivity, including being overweight

(CDC, 2016b)

These surveys also monitor measures related to youth substance misuse prevention. The NSDUH, for example, includes items addressing attitudes about drug use, perceptions related to harm of use, perceived availability of drugs, and perceived parental disapproval of substance use. When perceptions of harm decrease, or a change of attitudes resulting in a more positive view about drug use occurs, concern about the efforts to counteract these changes arises. Conversely, an increase in perceived risks of using a substance is positive and has been shown to be associated with subsequent decreases in the use of certain substances. For example, 30-day use of cigarettes among 12th graders was 37% in 1997, which decreased to 11% in 2016. During that same period, perception of risks from smoking and disapproval of smoking increased in this age group (Johnston, O'Malley, Miech, Bachman, & Schulenberg, 2017).

Each of these data sets has a set of biases. For example, in the national surveys, one has to look at whether the surveys are randomly chosen and the completion rates of those participating. The primary issue to consider overall is whether the data are representative of the country. Whether national data should be used in local planning is a common concern. In many cases, national data may not provide the information necessary to meet local needs; however, local surveys could be conducted to obtain information that is more specific. In these cases, national data should not be used to make decisions about states or communities that are not average in population distributions (in terms of, for example, race and ethnicity). In addition, the NSDUH reports on a select number of age groups – ages 12 to 17, ages 18 to 25, and ages 26 and older – which limits the tracking of substance misuse trends in middle-age and elderly adults.

There are also differences in national survey results. These differences usually occur because of differences in sampling designs and weighting procedures used to make the sampling data nationally representative. Knowledge of the different sources of data and the potential biases is critical in making the best use of the data for planning. In analyzing data, keep in mind that select groups of individuals may be missing. For example, by the time students get to the 12th grade, many have dropped out of school. Therefore, the MTF will have an inherent bias in this respect.

EPIDEMIOLOGICAL TRENDS IN SUBSTANCE USE

Nationally representative surveys provide researchers, planners, and practitioners with an understanding of the substance use and misuse trends in the United States. NSDUH surveys in 2014 found that about 27 million people in the United States reported illicit drug use in the previous month (Center for Behavioral Health Statistics and Quality [CBHSQ], 2015). In addition, illicit drug use in the United States is increasing; overall rates of use in all age groups were 10.2% in 2014, compared with 9.2% in 2012 (CBHSQ, 2015).

Trends in use differ, depending on the substance. Alcohol is, by far, the most commonly used psychoactive drug in all U.S. age groups, with 138.3 million Americans age 12 and over reporting alcohol use in 2015, representing almost 52% of the population. The NSDUH also reports on binge drinking and heavy alcohol use. Binge drinking is defined as drinking five or more drinks (men) or four or more drinks (women) on the same occasion on at least 1 day in the past 30 days. In 2015, about 66.7 million people age 12 and over reported binge alcohol drinking in the previous 30 days, representing about 25% of the population. Binge drinking was highest in the 18-25 age group, with 39% of people in this age group reporting binge drinking during 2015. Heavy alcohol use is defined as five or more drinks on the same occasion on 5 or more days in the previous 30 days. In 2015, about 17.3 million people age 12 or older reported heavy alcohol use, and this was highest in the 18-25 group, at 10.9%.

Past month cigarette use was also high in the US population in 2015, although rates have decreased since 2012, with 19.4% of the population age 12 and over reporting past month use in 2015, compared to 22.1% in 2012 (see Table 1-2). Despite these decreases, cigarette use remains a concern due to evidence that tobacco use is the leading cause of preventable deaths in the US (CBHSQ, 2016). About 52.0 million people in the US report current cigarette use, and 30.2 million of these are daily smokers, representing about 58.1% of the U.S. smoking population.

Another commonly used drug in the US is marijuana. Overall, 22.2 million Americans reported marijuana use in the previous month, and marijuana use has increased in the 18 to 25 and the 26 and older age groups. In the 18 to 25 age group, past month use of marijuana was 19.8% in 2015, compared to 19.6% in 2014 and 18.7% in 2012. Past month marijuana use in the 26 and older group was 6.5% in 2015, compared to 6.6% in 2014 and 5.3% in 2012 (CBHSQ, 2016).

Past month cocaine use in people age 12 and over was 0.7% in 2015, compared to 0.6% in 2014 and 2012. The highest rates of cocaine use in 2015 were reported in the 18-25 age group, at 1.7%. Past month heroin use was reported at 0.1% of those 12 and older in 2015, with the highest use in the 18-25 age group, at 0.3% (CBHSQ, 2016).

DIAGNOSIS OF SUBSTANCE-RELATED DISORDERS

Diagnosis of substance-related disorders is guided by the *Diagnostic and Statistical Manual of Mental Disorders,* fifth edition *(DSM-5;* American Psychiatric Association [APA], 2013). The *DSM-5* classifies substance-related and addictive disorders into two categories: substance use disorders and substance-induced disorders.

Substance use disorders are defined as "a cluster of cognitive, behavioral and psychological symptoms" (APA, 2013, p. 483) seen in individuals who continue to use substances despite significant problems associated with substance use.

Substance use disorder diagnostic criteria used by the *DSM-5* consist of four broad categories of symptoms:

1. Impaired control, defined as the inability to control use

2. Social impairment, defined as failure to fulfill role expectations because of use

3. Risky use, defined as recurrent use in situations in which it is physically hazardous

4. Pharmacological criteria, defined as the presence of tolerance and withdrawal

(APA, 2013)

The severity of substance use disorders is classified as mild, moderate, or severe based on the number of symptoms related to substance use present in a patient (APA, 2013; CBHSQ, 2015). Mild is the presence of two or three symptoms associated with a specific substance. Moderate is the presence of four to five symptoms. Severe is the presence of six or more symptoms associated with the use of a specific substance.

TABLE 1-2: PAST MONTH ILLICIT DRUG USE FOR SELECT DRUGS AMONG PEOPLE AGE 12 OR OLDER, PERCENTAGE BY AGE GROUP, IN YEARS 2012-2015

	2012	2013	2014	2015
Past Month Marijuana Use				
12 and older	7.3	7.5	8.4	8.3
12 to 17	7.2	7.1	7.4	7.0
18 to 25	18.7	19.1	19.6	19.8
26 and older	5.3	5.6	6.6	6.5
Past Month Cigarette Use				
12 and older	22.1	21.3	20.8	19.4
12 to 17	6.6	5.6	4.9	4.2
18 to 25	31.8	30.6	28.4	26.7
26 and older	22.4	21.6	21.5	20.0
Daily Cigarette Use Among Past Month Smokers				
12 and older	60.7	59.6	58.8	58.1
12 to 17	22.0	19.4	24.1	20.0
18 to 25	45.2	43.1	43.0	42.0
26 and older	66.0	64.9	63.3	62.7
Past Month Cocaine Use				
12 and older	0.6	0.6	0.6	0.7
12 to 17	0.1	0.2	0.2	0.2
18 to 25	1.1	1.1	1.4	1.7
26 and older	0.6	0.5	0.5	0.6
Past Month Heroin Use				
12 and older	0.3	0.1	0.2	0.1
12 to 17	Not reported	0.1	0.1	0.0
18 to 25	0.	0.3	0.2	0.3
26 and older	0.1	0.1	0.2	0.1
Past Month Alcohol Use				
12 and older	52.1	52.2	52.7	51.7
12 to 17	12.9	11.6	11.5	9.6
18 to 25	60.2	59.6	59.6	58.3
26 and older	55.6	55.9	56.5	55.6

Note. Adapted from Center for Behavioral Health Statistics and Quality. (2016). *Behavioral health trends in the United States: Results from the 2014 National Survey on Drug Use and Health.* (HHS Publication No. [SMA] 16-4984, NSDUH Series H-50). Retrieved from http://www.samhsa.gov/data/

Substance-induced disorders are classified as intoxication, withdrawal, and other substance-induced or medication-induced mental disorders. Intoxication includes problematic behavioral changes attributed to the physiological effects of substances. For example, in alcohol intoxication, these behavioral changes include impaired judgment, mood lability, and belligerence (APA, 2013). Withdrawal is the behavioral, physiological, and cognitive symptoms that result from cessation or reduced substance use following chronic and prolonged use. Substance-induced or medication-induced disorders refer to a variety of central nervous system syndromes that occur during substance use, including depression, psychosis, or delirium.

NEUROBIOLOGY OF SUBSTANCE USE

Substance use directly or indirectly interferes with the normal physiological actions of a neurotransmitter known as dopamine. Dopamine regulates brain functioning, particularly the brain's perceptions of reward, motivation, and pleasure. The brain's "reward system" (NIDA, 2014, p. 5) is located in the limbic system, which regulates the ability to feel pleasure and experience emotions and motivation. The limbic system is linked to the brain's pre-frontal cortex, the area of the brain that controls thought, decision making, and planning. In addition, the basal ganglia regulate the pleasurable effects of drugs and the formation of "habitual" substance use (HHS, 2016, p. 5). Drugs of abuse cause excessive release of dopamine into the neural circuits of these areas of the brain, which produces the pleasurable sensations associated with drugs of abuse. The pleasurable stimulation of these areas of the brain due to substance use is a reward and a positive reinforcer for continued use. Eventually, repeated use depletes the dopamine stores in the neurons, which reduces the ability of the drug to produce a pleasurable response. The addictive substances hijack the brain's reward systems, and the user gradually increases substance use to prevent negative physiologic responses to dopamine depletion, such as depression. At this point, the user is unable to control substance use.

In the past, addiction was considered a moral weakness or character flaw, but neurobiologic research provides evidence that it is a "brain disease" (Volkow, Koob & McClellan, 2016, p. 363). Addiction is a severe substance use disorder (HHS, 2016). The model for addiction includes 3 stages: the binge/intoxication stage; the withdrawal/negative affect stage, and the preoccupation/anticipation stage.

The binge or intoxication stage is the "feeling good" stage (Volkow et al., p. 365). In this stage, substance use results in a pleasurable sensation or euphoria, which activates the reward system and serves as a positive reinforcement that increases the likelihood of continued use. Substance use during this stage causes dysregulation of dopamine in the basal ganglia area of the brain, which is responsible for both the pleasurable effects of substance use and the development of substance use as a brain disorder (HHS, 2016). Substance use during this stage is often driven by impulsivity, which is the inability to delay gratification and to act without consideration of the potential harmful consequences of an action (HHS, 2016).

The withdrawal/negative affect stage is the "feeling reduced excitement" stage (Volkow et al., 2016, p. 365). The user experiences a negative emotional state and physical symptoms when substance use stops (HHS, 2016). This stage is characterized by a gradual transition from "controlled, occasional misuse to chronic use, which is difficult to control" (HHS, 2016, p. 2-2). Withdrawal symptoms depend on the substance that is used. For example, alcohol withdrawal symptoms include anxiety, tremors, diaphoresis, nausea, elevated vital signs, and seizures, while opiate withdrawal symptoms can include flu-like symptoms, pupil dilation, bone or joint aches, piloerection (goosebumps) and abdominal cramps. The pleasurable effects of substance use are reduced because of dysregulation of dopamine in the extended amygdala, which diminishes the action of the brain's reward system (HHS, 2016). The extended amygdala and its subregions also regulate the fight-or-flight response to stress and negative emotions, such as anxiety and irritability. A phenomenon known as tolerance develops during this stage in which increasing amounts of the substances are used to produce the original desired effect (National Institute on Drug Abuse [NIDA], 2016b). Over time, negative emotions – such as depression, irritability, anxiety, and stress – occur in the absence of substance use. These unpleasant responses serve as a negative reinforcement, and therefore use of the substance continues primarily to avoid these negative emotional responses.

The preoccupation, or anticipation, stage is the "desiring drug" stage (Volkow et al., 2016, p. 365). In this stage, substance use becomes compulsive, regardless of the harmful effects resulting from use. According to *Facing Addiction in America: The Surgeon General's Report on Alcohol, Drugs, and Health* (HHS, 2016), compulsive use, despite the harmful and negative consequences, indicates a loss of control over substance use, which is the key feature of addiction. People who engage in compulsive behaviors view the behaviors as wrong and harmful, yet they are unable to stop the behaviors. During this stage of the addiction cycle, dopamine dysregulation occurs in the prefrontal cortex, which is part of the reward system, and controls planning, decision making, attention, and behavioral and emotional regulation.

Dysregulated dopamine function in the prefrontal cortex has been described as impairment of a go-stop system (HHS, 2016). In this model of substance use, the go system in the prefrontal cortex is overactivated, which promotes the chronic, continued use of substances. Simultaneously, the stop system of the prefrontal cortex is underactivated, which promotes compulsive substance use. The substance user becomes preoccupied with substance use and devotes much mental effort to plans for obtaining substances for further use. Craving, in which the substance user experiences increased urges or desire for substance use (NIDA, 2016b), can also occur during this stage. Cravings are particularly strong when triggers occur, which are situations or emotions that the user associates with use.

Not everyone who uses substances experiences a transition from use to addiction. Genetics and environmental factors can increase vulnerability for developing substance use disorders. Genetic factors account for 40% to 60% of vulnerability to addiction, mainly because of variations in the expression of genes associated with response to substance use (NIDA, 2014; Volkow & Warren, 2015). Environmental factors also increase risk of substance addiction. These factors include low socioeconomic status, peer pressure, parental substance use, and lack of parental oversight in teens (NIDA, 2014). Adverse childhood events – such as abuse, neglect, and chaotic home environments – also contribute to increased risk of substance addiction (NIDA, 2014). Age at first use is an additional risk factor for developing substance use problems. Research has suggested that people who start to use alcohol before the age of 15 are 6 times more likely to develop an alcohol use disorder later in life, compared with those who start to use alcohol at or after the age of 21 (CDC, 2016c).

SUMMARY

Epidemiology is a tool that helps public health officials and others to monitor the trends of substance use in the United States. Data are derived from researchers, practitioners, self-reports by substance users, and recorded events, such as impaired driving arrests. The two most commonly used surveys that provide data about substance use among youth are secondary school-based surveys (MTF and YRBSS). Some data are also available from the NSDUH study, which monitors households with individuals aged 12 years and older. The value of epidemiological data to local areas varies; however, it is generally agreed that the prevailing problems among young people can be identified with national data. The *DSM-5* (APA, 2013) distinguishes substance-related and addictive disorders as substance use disorders or substance-induced disorders. are patterns of substance use characterized by impairments in ability to control use, social impairment, risky use, pharmacologic criteria, such as withdrawal and tolerance (APA, 2013). Research has provided increasing evidence that addiction is a "brain disease" that causes dysregulation in the actions of dopamine in each of the stages of the addiction cycle: the binge, or intoxication stage; the withdrawal, or negative affect stage; and the preoccupation, or anticipation stage. Substance-induced disorders refer to the toxic effects of substances on the brain, which often mimic mental health conditions (Volkow et al., 2016).

EXAM QUESTIONS

CHAPTER 1
Questions 1–5

Note: Choose the one option that BEST answers each question.

1. The Monitoring the Future study is a

   a. primary source of information on illicit drug use in the United States.

   b. network of scientists, government regulators, and law enforcement representatives who monitor trends in current substance use.

   c. survey of drug, alcohol, and cigarette use among adolescents in the United States.

   d. national school-based Centers for Disease Control and Prevention survey for students in grades 9 through 12.

2. The most commonly used psychoactive drug in all age groups in the United States is

   a. alcohol.

   b. marijuana.

   c. stimulants.

   d. heroin.

3. The problematic behavioral changes attributed to the physiological effects of substances are known collectively as

   a. substance use.

   b. intoxication.

   c. withdrawal.

   d. tolerance.

4. Substance use directly or indirectly interferes with the functioning of which neurotransmitter?

   a. Acetylcholine

   b. Norepinephrine

   c. Serotonin

   d. Dopamine

5. The first stage in the addiction cycle is

   a. binge, or intoxication.

   b. craving.

   c. preoccupation, or anticipation.

   d. withdrawal, or negative affect.

REFERENCES

American Psychiatric Association. (2013). *Diagnostic and statistical manual of mental disorders* (5th ed.). Arlington, VA: Author.

Center for Behavioral Health Statistics and Quality. (2016). *Behavioral health trends in the United States: Results from the 2014 National Survey on Drug Use and Health.* (HHS Publication No. [SMA] 16-4984, NSDUH Series H-50). Retrieved from http://www.samhsa.gov/data

Centers for Disease Control and Prevention. (2016a). *Youth Risk Behavior Surveillance System (YRBSS).* Retrieved from https://www.cdc.gov/healthyyouth/data/yrbs/index.htm

Centers for Disease Control and Prevention. (2016b). *Youth risk behavior surveillance system.* Retrieved from https://www.cdc.gov/healthyyouth/data/yrbs/index.htm

Centers for Disease Control and Prevention. (2016c). *Fact sheets: Underage drinking.* Retrieved from http://www.cdc.gov/alcohol/fact-sheets/underage-drinking.htm

Gordis, L. (2014). *Epidemiology* (5th ed.). Philadelphia, PA: Elsevier Saunders.

Johnston, L. D., O'Malley, P. M., Bachman, J. G., & Schulenberg, J. E. (2012a). *Monitoring the Future national survey results on drug use, 1975-2011. Volume I: Secondary school students.* Ann Arbor: Institute for Social Research, University of Michigan.

Johnston, L. D., O'Malley, P. M., Bachman, J. G., & Schulenberg, J. E. (2012b). *Monitoring the Future national survey results on drug use, 1975-2011. Volume II: College students and adults ages 19-50.* Ann Arbor: Institute for Social Research, University of Michigan.

Johnston, L. D., O'Malley, P. M., Bachman, J. G., & Schulenberg, J. E. (2013). *Monitoring the Future national results on drug use: 2012 overview, key findings on adolescent drug use.* Ann Arbor: Institute for Social Research, University of Michigan.

Johnston, L. D., O'Malley, P. M., Miech, R. A., Bachman, J. G., & Schulenberg, J. E. (2017). *Monitoring the Future national survey results on drug use, 1975-2016: Overview, key findings on adolescent drug use.* Ann Arbor: Institute for Social Research, The University of Michigan.

National Institute on Drug Abuse (2014). *Drugs, brains and behavior: Drugs and the brain.* Accessed 05/13/2017 at https://www.drugabuse.gov/publications/drugs-brains-behavior-science-addiction/drugs-brain

National Institute on Drug Abuse. (2016a). *National Drug Early Warning System (NDEWS).* Retrieved from https://www.drugabuse.gov/related-topics/trends-statistics/national-drug-early-warning-system-ndews

National Institute on Drug Abuse. (2016b). *The science of drug abuse and addiction: The basics.* Retrieved from https://www.drugabuse.gov/publications/media-guide/science-drug-abuse-addiction-basics

National Institute on Drug Abuse (2017). *Epidemiologic Research Branch.* Accessed 05/13/2017 at https://www.drugabuse.gov/about-nida/organization/divisions/division-epidemiology-services-prevention-research-despr/epidemiology-research-branch-erb

Substance Abuse and Mental Health Services Administration. (2014). *SAMHSA's major data collections.* Retrieved from https://www.samhsa.gov/samhsa-data-outcomes-quality/major-data-collections

Substance Abuse and Mental Health Services Administration. (2016a). *Population data/ NSDUH.* Retrieved from https://www.samhsa.gov/data/population-data-nsduh

Substance Abuse and Mental Health Services Administration. (2016b). *Population data: NSDUH.* Retrieved from https://www.samhsa.gov/data/population-data-nsduh

The Regents of the University of Michigan. (2017). *Monitoring the future: A continuing study of American youth.* Retrieved from http://www.monitoringthefuture.org

U.S. Department of Health and Human Services, Office of the Surgeon General. (2016). *Facing addiction in America: The Surgeon General's report on alcohol, drugs, and health.* Washington, DC: Author. Retrieved from https://www.surgeongeneral.gov/library/reports/index.html

Volkow, N. D., & Baler, R. (2015). Drug addiction: The neurobiology of behavior gone awry. In A. J. Herron & T. K. Brennan (Eds.). *The ASAM essentials of addiction medicine* (2nd Edition), pp. 9-14. Philadelphia: Wolters Kluwer.

Volkow, N. D., Koob, G. F., & McClellan, A. T. (2016). Neurobiologic advances from the brain disease model of addiction. *The New England Journal of Medicine, 374*(4), 363-371.

CHAPTER 2

PREVENTION OF SUBSTANCE USE

LEARNING OUTCOME

After completing this chapter, the learner will be able to discuss the concepts and principles of preventing substance use and addiction.

CHAPTER OBJECTIVES

After completing this chapter, the learner will be able to:

1. Explain the levels of substance use prevention.

2. Identify risk and protective factors important in substance use prevention.

3. List the principles of prevention, including the four areas that prevention programs should address.

4. Discuss implementation of prevention programs, including their planning, impact, and future.

INTRODUCTION

Prevention is the key to reducing and eliminating substance use disorders. Healthy People 2020 is a national effort to develop comprehensive, evidence-based goals and objectives to achieve a healthier population over 10 years (Office of Disease Prevention and Health Promotion, 2016). A smaller set of Healthy People 2020 priority health issues, called leading health indicators (LHIs), has been identified. Substance misuse has been marked as a priority issue and included in the 2020 LHIs. The primary goal of the Healthy People 2020 substance misuse initiative is to "reduce substance abuse to protect the health, safety and quality of life for all, especially children" (Office of Disease Prevention and Health Promotion, 2016, p. 1).

Strategic plans have been developed to address substance use disorders nationally. The *National Drug Control Strategy* report (Office of National Drug Control Policy, 2015) identified seven core areas to address substance use disorders:

1. Preventing drug use in our communities

2. Seeking early intervention opportunities in health care

3. Integrating treatment for substance use disorders into health care and supporting recovery

4. Breaking the cycle of drug use, crime, and incarceration

5. Disrupting domestic drug trafficking and production

6. Strengthening international partnerships

7. Improving information systems to better address drug use and its consequences

These strategies are helpful in focusing our prevention efforts to address substance use. *Facing Addiction in America: The Surgeon General's Report on Alcohol, Drugs, and Health* (U.S. Department of Health and Human Services [HHS], 2016) stated, "it is critical to prevent substance misuse from starting and to identify those who have already begun to misuse substances and intervene early" (pp. 3-1).

CONCEPTUALIZATION OF PREVENTION

Prevention refers to those interventions that take place before the onset of a disorder. Models have been created to assist in conceptualizing such a complex topic as prevention. One approach is based on the work of the Commission on Chronic Illness. This approach introduces primary, secondary, and tertiary levels of prevention (*Chronic Illness in the United States,* 1957). This model is mentioned because of its presence in earlier works in the prevention literature. Another approach by the Institute of Medicine (IOM; Springer & Phillips, 2006) introduced a mental health spectrum model with universal, selective, and indicated categories. These two models differ most at their third prevention level. An IOM report clearly stated that prevention can occur only at the primary level, whereas secondary and tertiary prevention are considered good treatment practices rather than true prevention (Shea & Shern, 2011).

Levels of Prevention

The Commission on Chronic Illness, established in the 1940s, developed a prevention framework featuring primary, secondary, and tertiary levels of prevention. In primary prevention, efforts are focused on promotion of health and global elimination of alcohol abuse and its consequences through community programs (National Institute on Alcohol Abuse and Alcoholism [NIAAA], 2005). Secondary prevention uses approaches to help identify those at risk and provide intervention. Tertiary prevention focuses on addressing a problem after it develops.

Prevention Strategies

The IOM (Springer & Phillips, 2006) mental health spectrum model was later adapted and renamed the behavioral health continuum of care model (Substance Abuse and Mental Health Services Administration [SAMHSA], 2016c). This model recognizes the opportunity to address behavioral health problems and disorders, including substance use (see Figure 2-1).

The model depicts these variables:

- Promotion of health strategies enhances the environment and conditions that support the individual when challenges present. Promotion strategies help support the individual throughout the continuum of care.

- Prevention strategies are delivered before the onset of a disorder.

- Treatment services are delivered to the individual diagnosed with a mental health or substance use disorder. An example of a treatment service is counseling and medication-assisted treatment.

- Recovery services support the individual to live a productive life within the community, with emphasis on abstinence. Examples of a recovery service include transportation to appointments, employment, and support groups (spiritual, faith based, and peer).

Within this model, a prevention classification schema outlined by Gordon (1987) and discussed in an IOM report (Kellam & Langevin, 2003; Mrazek & Haggerty, 1994) included the categories of universal, selective, and indicated to better define prevention strategies.

Universal prevention strategies are delivered to everyone in the community. They usually address the root causes of risky behaviors to assist in changing the environment and often involve changes in policies or laws. These strategies are similar to or consistent with primary prevention. An example of a universal prevention

FIGURE 2-1: BEHAVIORAL HEALTH CONTINUUM MODEL

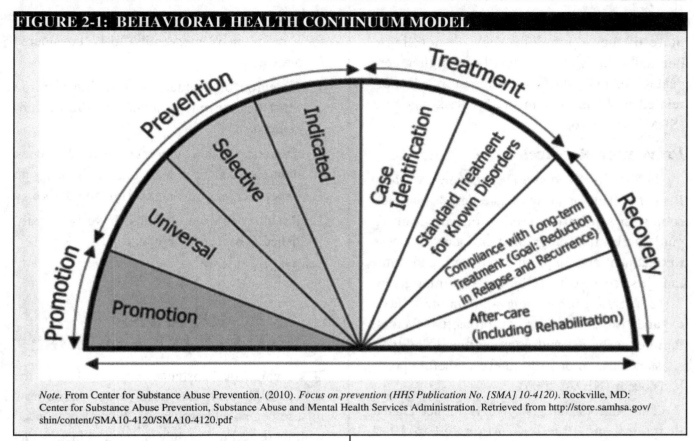

Note. From Center for Substance Abuse Prevention. (2010). *Focus on prevention (HHS Publication No. [SMA] 10-4120)*. Rockville, MD: Center for Substance Abuse Prevention, Substance Abuse and Mental Health Services Administration. Retrieved from http://store.samhsa.gov/shin/content/SMA10-4120/SMA10-4120.pdf

strategy is the Strengthening Families program for youth aged 10 to 14 and parents. This program is delivered to families in rural communities. It provides guidance on family management skills, communication, academic support, and parent-child relationships (Blueprints for Healthy Youth Development, 2017d).

Selective prevention strategies focus on individuals to empower them to make good choices. Selective strategies use approaches similar to secondary prevention. An example of a selective prevention program is the Family Check-Up in which families are assessed and determined to be at greater or lesser risk. Interventions are designed to meet their specific needs. The Family Check-Up is part of the Adolescent Transitions program, a three-tiered intervention program (Blueprints for Healthy Youth Development, 2017b).

Indicated prevention strategies are designed to prevent individuals with identified risk fac-

tors for substance use from progressing to the diagnosis of substance use disorder. Indicated prevention targets individuals who have a high probability of the development of the problem or show early signs of problem behavior, unlike the tertiary prevention focus of addressing an existing problem. An example of an indicated prevention strategy is the Project Towards No Drug Abuse, which focuses on students who have failed in school and are using drugs (Blueprints for Healthy Youth Development, 2017c; National Institute on Drug Abuse [NIDA], 2003). The program is a classroom-based high school substance use program to promote drug awareness and prevent teen drinking, smoking, marijuana use, and other hard drug use. The curriculum teaches students skills in self-control, communication, resource acquisition, and decision making (Lisha et al., 2012).

There are advantages to implementing universal programs over selective or indicated programs. Universal programs are likely to reach more of the population. They do not single out individuals at risk. Lastly, a higher percentage of individuals with misuse of alcohol-related problems fall in the low-risk category (SAMHSA, 2016a).

Prevention Research

In 2013, the *National Drug Control Strategy Report* called for an evidence-based approach rooted in scientific research on addiction to guide prevention programs that increase access to treatment and emphasize recovery and criminal justice reform (Obama Administration, 2013). Evidence-based approaches have expanded to focus on risks, protective factors, families, schools, and communities to address substance use in order to intervene before problems occur (NIDA, 2003).

The National Registry of Evidence-Based Programs and Practices originated in 1997 in SAMHSA's Center for Substance Abuse Prevention (CSAP) as part of the Model Programs initiative. More than 1,100 programs were reviewed, and more than 150 were designated as model, effective, or promising programs. SAMHSA expanded the system, and the new registry was launched in 2006. It provides ratings for each outcome targeted by the intervention registry.

Several characteristics of evidence-based prevention have been formulated: a reliance on theory, addressing risk and protective factors, and representation in settings of influence (such as schools, community, and media). SAMHSA continues to work to improve access to information on evaluated interventions to make available evidence-based interventions that can be implemented in the community. Programs are rated as effective, promising, and no effects.

Three minimum requirements must be met for a program or intervention to be considered for a review:

1. Research or evaluation of an intervention must be relevant to mental health or substance use.

2. Evidence-based outcomes must have been demonstrated in at least one study using an experimental or quasiexperimental design.

3. Results of the study must have been published in a peer review journal.

(SAMHSA, 2016d)

RISK AND PROTECTIVE FACTORS

Research on substance use disorders in the past 20 years has tried to determine how misuse begins and progresses. Factors associated with increased use of substances and factors that protect against the use or misuse of substances are important in designing preventive efforts.

Risk factors are characteristics at the biological, psychological, family, community, or cultural level that can precede the initiation of substance use and are associated with a higher likelihood of negative outcomes (SAMHSA, 2015). Protective factors are characteristics associated with a lower likelihood of negative outcomes or that reduce a risk factor's impact. Protective factors may be seen as decreasing one's likelihood of developing a substance use disorder (SAMHSA, 2015).

Risk factors can influence substance misuse in several ways. The more risk factors a patient has, the greater the likelihood that he or she will develop a substance use disorder. The protective factors can reduce risks; therefore, prevention programs should enhance protective factors and reverse risk factors (NIDA, 2003). An important goal of prevention is to reduce risk and enhance resiliency so that protective factors outweigh risk factors. The influence of risk and protective factors is different based on the patient's age. For instance, families have more of an influence with younger children, whereas peers have more of an influence on adolescents and young adults (SAMHSA, 2015).

Risk factors and protective factors exist within five domains, or settings:

1. Individual
2. Family
3. Peer
4. School
5. Community

(NIDA, 2003)

Table 2-1 contains a listing for all domain levels and shows how protective factors can eliminate or decrease risk factors.

Individual Domain

Individual risk factors include personality traits, attitudes favorable toward drug use, decision-making skills, personal efficacy, lack of knowledge and comprehension of the consequences of use, antisocial behavior or conduct, sensation-seeking behavior, and a lack of adult supervision. Research has shown that social and personal skill building can enhance individual capacities, influence attitudes, and promote positive behavior (CSAP, 2010). These interventions generally include information about the negative physical and psychological effects of substance use and consider race, ethnicity, age, and gender in their designs. Interventions must emphasize the immediate effects of use and social acceptance rather than the long-term effects of use. Such alternatives as sports programs, involvement in the arts, and community service can provide effective ways of reaching high-risk youth.

Examples of risk factors for adolescent and young adults for substance use include the following:

- Early initiation of substance use
- Early and persistent problem behavior
- Rebelliousness and favorable attitude toward substance use
- Peer substance use and genetic predictors

(HHS, 2016)

In contrast, examples of protective factors for the adolescent and young adult include self-efficacy, spirituality, resiliency, opportunities for positive social involvement, and recognition for positive behavior. Evidence-based programs for preventing substance misuse emphasize these protective factors.

When designing a program around protective factors, it is important to consider the following (SAMHSA, 2016a):

- Determine how the protective factors will be assessed.

TABLE 2-1: RISK AND PROTECTIVE FACTORS		
Domain	**Risk Factors**	**Protective Factors**
Individual	Early aggressive behavior	Self-control
Family	Lack of parental supervision	Parental monitoring
Peer	Substance use	Academic competence
School	Drug availability	Antidrug use policies
Community	Poverty	Strong neighborhood attachment

Note. From National Institute on Drug Abuse. (2003). *Preventing drug abuse among children and adolescents* (2nd ed.). Retrieved from http://www.drug abuse.gov/sites/default/files/redbook_0.pdf

- This information may not be readily available, so the first step is to collect the data. It is important to use reliable, valid, and standard measures of substance abuse and mental and behavioral health indicators and outcomes.

- SAMHSA's Center for the Application of Prevention Technologies has compiled a listing of valid measures (SAMHSA, 2012).

- Conduct a needs assessment.

- Figure out which protective factors to address first.

- Prioritize protective factors in the community and determine which evidence-based programs support these factors.

A growing body of evidence has found that social-emotional competencies – learned traits that individuals strive to master – influence future substance use and promote the well-being of the individual. These competencies include self-awareness, self-management, social awareness, relationship skills, and responsible decision making (Collaborative for Academic, Social, and Emotional Learning, 2015). Designing prevention programs around these competencies will enhance protective factors and reduce the probability of substance use, especially in adolescents.

Family Domain

Family risk factors include low parental investment, low family cohesion, parental conflict, poor parent-adolescent communication, low parental monitoring of children, ineffective parental management, and parental drug use. Research has shown that interventions targeting the entire family can be effective in preventing adolescent substance abuse. Some selected effective strategies include focusing on developing parenting skills beyond simply providing information about parenting; emphasizing family bonding; training parents to listen and interact in developmentally appropriate ways; and training parents to use positive and consistent discipline techniques and improve family communication through modeling, coaching, rehearsal, and role playing (CSAP, 2010).

One example of a parenting program that has outcome measures to support its effectiveness is the Incredible Years program. Incredible Years is a multifaceted evidence-based program that targets parents, children, and teachers (Incredible Years, 2013). SAMHSA has rated this program an effective program. (SAMHSA, 2016a). Children with high rates of aggressive behavioral problems who do not receive treatment have shown to be at great risk for developing substance abuse problems, becoming involved with deviant peer groups, dropping out of school, and engaging in delinquency and violence. The Incredible Years Program has shown to decrease aggression in children thus reducing or eliminating the trajectory of engaging high-risk substance use behaviors (Presnall, Webster-Stratton, & Constantino, 2014; Incredible Years, 2013).

Peer Domain

The risk factors associated with the peer domain include peer use, peer norms positive to use, and peer activities conducive to use. Preventive strategies that relate to peers are structured alternative activities, such as a sober prom, in settings antithetical to drug use and that incorporate social and personal skills building. Other strategies include involving youth in developing alternative programs and peer-led interventions (CSAP, 2010). A potential problem arises, however, when youth who display deviant behavior are included in these endeavors and change the culture of the group.

School Domain

School risk factors include a lack of commitment to education, poor grades, school failure, a lack of attachment to school, negative school climate, and lenient school policies. School protective factors include academic achievement, school bonding, educational aspirations, and educational commitments.

Research related to school-based approaches to prevention has found several important facts:

- Knowledge-oriented interventions alone do not produce measurable changes in behavior or attitudes and are considered the least effective educational strategy.

- Educational interventions that focus on correcting misconceptions about the prevalence of use can change attitudes favorable toward use. These are most effective when combined with other educational approaches, such as fostering social skills.

- Interventions that are peer led or include some peer-led component are more effective than adult-led or teacher-led approaches.

- Interactive approaches help engage youth.

- Booster sessions help youth retain skills.

- Parental involvement and school policies that communicate a commitment to substance abuse prevention are important as effective strategies.

(CSAP, 2010)

Prevention programs should be designed to intervene as early as preschool to address risk behaviors. The programs should target academic and social-emotional learning improvements to address such risk factors as early aggression and academic failure. In middle school and high school, such areas as communication, self-efficacy, resistance skills, antidrug attitudes, and peer relationships should be promoted to increase academic and social competence (NIDA, 2003). Prevention programs should be aimed at the general population.

Arthur and colleagues (2015) conducted a study to determine whether the levels of substance use and risk and protective factors predicted academic test score performance of students in middle school and whether prevention curricula could remove barriers. Schools that implemented prevention programs that addressed identified risk and protective factors had a positive effect on academic performance. An example of an evidence-based school program is Lifeskills Training. The curriculum is classroom based and teaches students self-management skills, social skills, and drug awareness and resistance skills (Blueprints for Healthy Youth Development, 2017a).

Community Domain

Community risk factors include a lack of bonding to social and community institutions, lack of awareness of community substance abuse problems, community norms favorable to use, and insufficient community resources to support prevention efforts. Community institutions include churches, Boys and Girls Club, YMCA, and workplaces (CSAP, 2010).

Researchers reported these findings:

- Controlling the environment around schools helps reinforce strong community norms.

- Mentoring programs can increase school attendance and create positive attitudes.

- Community service can increase positive attitudes toward others.

- Influencing increased worksite commitments to prevention efforts can be done by emphasizing decreased costs to employers.

- Communicating a clear policy can help change workplace norms.

- Coalitions are important in formulating and implementing approaches to preventing substance abuse.

Lastly, it is recommended that the most effective approach to reaching populations in multiple settings is to present consistent community-wide messages in each setting (NIDA, 2003).

Societal Influences Domain

Risk factors in the societal influences domain include norms tolerant of use, policies that enable use and misuse, a lack of enforcement of laws designed to prevent use and misuse, and inappropriate negative sanctions for use and abuse (CSAP, 2010). The preventive approaches to addressing the societal influences domain involve interventions targeted to populations.

Here are some findings from research of the societal influences domain:

- Community awareness and media efforts can be effective in changing perceptions.

- Mass media can influence community norms on substance use.

- Audience perceptions and capacities to understand media messages are based on gender, culture, and stage of cognitive development.

- Effective mass media messages are broadcast through multiple channels.

- Counter-advertising campaigns that disseminate information about the hazards of the product (e.g., tobacco) may help reduce sales.

- Beverage server training to enforce laws against service to intoxicated patrons is effective in changing selling and service principles.

- Increasing the price of alcohol and tobacco through excise taxes can be an effective strategy.

- Increasing the minimum purchase age for alcohol to 21 has been effective in decreasing alcohol use among youth.

(NIDA, 2003)

Interventions at the societal influences level are a systems approach directed at public health concerns. In the case of alcohol, policy change is an approach to addressing prevention. It involves producing such structural changes in the environment as regulation of legal drinking ages, alcohol outlets, and legal blood alcohol level for drinking and driving; advertising restrictions; and services for intoxicated persons and underage drinkers (HHS, 2016; Holder, 2000).

PRINCIPLES OF PREVENTION AND PREVENTION PROGRAMS

Prevention science is a relatively new discipline that integrates development research, community epidemiology, and preventive interventions. Principles of prevention are based on the assumption that if verifiable precursors are identified early and targeted and evidence-based interventions are implemented, there will be a decrease in the quantity and effect of risk factors. In addition, protective factors will be enhanced that can mediate or moderate exposure to risk or eliminate the likelihood that the problem will develop (Catalano et al., 2012).

Principles of Prevention

Research guides the development of prevention programs and principles of prevention, and has outlined 16 principles (NIDA, 2003). These 16 principles can be divided into four areas of prevention to include in prevention programs.

Area 1: Risk Factors and Protective Factors

- Principle 1: Enhance protective factors and reverse or reduce risk factors.

- Principle 2: Address all forms of substance use.

- Principle 3: Address the type of substance use problem.

- Principle 4: Tailor programs to address risks specific to the population.

Area 2: Family Programs

- Principle 5: Enhance family bonding and relationships.

- Principle 6: Intervene as early as preschool.

- Principle 7: Focus on improving academic and social-emotional learning for elementary school children.

- Principle 8: Focus on increasing academic and social competence for middle and high school students.

Area 3: Community Programs

- Principle 9: Aim to develop programs for general populations at key transition points.

- Principle 10: Recognize that combining two or more programs can be more effective.

- Principle 11: Reach populations in multiple settings.

Area 4: Prevention Program Delivery

- Principle 12: Retain core elements of the original research-based intervention.

- Principle 13. Ensure long-term delivery with repeated interventions.

- Principle 14: Provide teacher training on good classroom management practices.

- Principle 15: Employ interactive techniques.

- Principle 16: Remain cost effective.

Principle 12 emphasizes that the core elements (structure, content, and delivery) of an original research-based intervention should be retained in the actual implementation; programs should be long term with repeated interventions; and the most effective interventions use interactive techniques, such as peer discussion or parent role playing (NIDA, 2003). It is critical when adapting a program to fit the community that core elements remain intact to ensure effectiveness and fidelity (NIDA, 2003). Both fidelity of implementation and program adaptation are essential, resulting in the need to develop hybrid prevention programs that build in adaptation and maximize fidelity of program implementation and effectiveness.

Cultural adaptation involves a planned, organized, iterative, and collaborative process for modifications to programs that are culturally sensitive and includes individuals from the target population for whom the adaptation is being developed (Castro, Barrera, & Holleran Steiker, 2010). Cultural considerations are important in addressing not only overall prevention but also primary prevention and recovery from substance abuse.

Elements of a cultural competent prevention system include the following:

- Valuing diversity and awareness of diversity

- Understanding the dynamic of different attitudes

- Ability to institutionalize culture

- Cultural knowledge and adaptation to diversity

- Cultural self-assessment

(SAMHSA, 2016e)

When developing prevention programs, it is essential to be respectful, have knowledge of health beliefs and practices, and understand the cultural and linguistic needs of the community. Those delivering the services should be willing and have the skills to work within the context of the culture, draw on community-based values and customs, and work closely with knowledgeable people from the community (SAMHSA, 2016d).

Harm Reduction

Harm reduction is another approach to prevention. "Harm reduction is a pragmatic approach to reduce the harmful consequences of alcohol and drug use or their associated high-risk activities by incorporating several strategies that cut across the spectrum from safer use to managed use to abstinence" (Marlatt & Witkiewitz, 2010, p. 1). The overarching goal of harm reduction is to meet the individual where he or she is. It is based on the principle of acceptance and collaboration (Marlatt & Witkiewitz, 2010).

Harm reduction focuses on a range of strategies to target consequences of alcohol and drug use. This type of strategy includes making sterile syringes available to intravenous drug users to reduce the risks of associated health issues and reducing such social consequences as crime. Other examples include education regarding safer drug ingestion methods, complementary and alternative therapies, and safe places where users can consume drugs and alcohol. There is evidence that harm-reduction strategies can be effective in saving lives and affecting measures at a population level (Marlatt & Witkiewitz, 2010). However, there is some dispute surrounding harm-reduction strategies, especially from individuals and programs that emphasize abstinence from alcohol or drugs (Erickson, 2007).

A recent harm-reduction initiative supported by the HHS released the Opioid Overdose Toolkit (SAMHSA, 2016b). The toolkit includes information for first responders, prescribers, and patients on overdose prevention, treatment, and recovery. This toolkit includes information about the use of naloxone as a life-saving intervention in overdose reversal prevention. Some communities may be reluctant to implement harm-reduction programs or strategies for a variety of reasons: the perspective than an individual's underlying mental health issues are not addressed, the physical and financial resources required for implementation and sustainability, and the attention to other community challenges. However, many of these harm-reduction strategies have helped save lives.

Planning of Prevention Programs

Evidence-based interventions are programs and interventions supported by research through demonstration of efficacious outcomes. In planning for substance abuse prevention in the community, SAMHSA's strategic prevention framework (SPF) provides a guide to assist professionals and communities to address behaviors associated with substance misuse.

There are five steps of the SPF:

1. Assess need: What is the problem, and how can I learn more?
2. Build capacity: What do I have to work with?
3. Plan: What should I do, and how should I do it?
4. Implement: How can I put my plan into action?
5. Evaluate: Is my plan succeeding?

The two guiding principles of the SPF are cultural competence and sustainability of the program. In this model, cultural competence is described as the ability to interact effectively with members of diverse populations; sustainability is the process of achieving and maintaining long-term results. Culture must be considered at every step of the SPF. Culture is a term that goes beyond race and ethnicity. It also refers to such characteristics as age, gender, sexual orientation, disability, religion, income level, education, geographical location, and profession (SAMHSA, 2016f).

The planning process, which is a critical step in the SPF model, has four distinctive features:

1. Decisions are driven by data.
2. Assessment is ongoing.
3. Interventions are focused on population-level change.
4. Prevention efforts are planned for people of all ages. To be successful, this process requires a team approach.

Poor time management and futuristic planning can be detrimental when designing a prevention strategy or implementing an evidence-based prevention program. Sustaining outcomes that have positive results is often overlooked. The goal is to sustain prevention outcomes, not programs. It is critical that cost and sustainability be considered in the initial steps of the planning process (SAMHSA, 2016f).

Effectiveness of Prevention Programs

How effective is substance use prevention? Evaluating programs and efforts has become a part of evidenced-based policy. SAMHSA's Center for the Application of Prevention Technologies, which is supported through the CSAP, has a focused interest in evaluating effectiveness. Data-driven, evidence-informed prevention planning processes lead to more successful prevention outcomes. Prevention efforts and programs have shown improved outcomes and are effective across the life span. They are also cost effective. Evidence also supports communities' critical role in the planning process; when they were consulted early in the planning phase, outcomes improved (SAMHSA, 2016f). Communities that received grants that supported Drug-Free Communities from 2002 to 2012 showed positive outcomes. Alcohol, tobacco, and marijuana use declined significantly among middle and high school students (SAMHSA, 2016f) in communities that received the grant support to implement evidence-based programs. A review conducted for the surgeon general's report (HHS, 2016) found 42 of 600 programs were developed based on published research studies. These studies examined data across the life span, with the majority focusing on children, adolescents, and young adults.

The emerging area of prevention is Internet-based programs. An example of an internet based intervention is *I Hear What You Are Saying* (Schinke, Fang, & Cole, 2009a, 2009b). This evidence-based program involves nine 45-minute sessions to improve communication, establish family rules, and manage conflict. Specifically focused on mothers and daughters, the follow-up results of this program showed lower rates of substance use in an ethnically diverse population (HHS, 2016).

Family-based initiatives also identified in this report included the Strengthening Families program for youth aged 10 to 14 and parents as a universal program on substance use (Spoth, Trudeau, Guyll, & Shin, 2012), and Coping Power as an indicated intervention designed to target early aggression (Lochman & Wells, 2003). These programs have shown positive outcomes in preventing or delaying the initiation of substance use.

Future Directions of Prevention Programs

Significant developments in prevention have been made over the past three decades. It is critical that prevention programs address all forms of drug misuse, including legal substances (cigarettes or alcohol), illegal drugs, and the inappropriate use of legally obtained substances (inhalants, prescription medications, and over-the-counter drugs). Programs should also be targeted to the substance use disorders prevalent in the local community and to potential user populations (age, gender, and ethnicity).

Translating prevention science into community prevention systems is a priority in prevention research. This is not an easy process; it takes time and effort upfront to ensure the best results. It is imperative that the dissemination and implementation of evidence-based programs are improved by increasing awareness of such programs and by providing training to communities and individuals implementing these programs.

Operating systems have been developed to assist with broad-based implementation of evidence-based programs. An example of such a system is Promoting School-Community-University Partnership to Enhance Resilience. This system has shown long-term success in implementing prevention programs for substance use based on risk and protective factors (Spoth & Greenberg, 2011). Another system – developed by Hawkins et al. (2008) and adopted by SAMHSA to address the underuse of the effective prevention programs and policies – is Communities That Care, a coalition-based community prevention operating system. This system provides communities with consultation, training, and research-based tools. It is tailored to identify the risks and needs of each community. A study by Horn, Fagan, Hawkins, and Osterele (2014) demonstrated that this model was effective in reducing overall adolescent alcohol consumption in a certain community.

The NIAAA proposed in its strategic plan to develop and improve interventions to prevent alcohol misuse, alcohol use disorder, and alcohol-related consequences by formulating two goals:

1. Promote universal screening and brief intervention for alcohol and other substances.

2. Develop, evaluate, and promote effective interventions for preventing alcohol misuse, alcohol use disorder, and related consequences for individuals at all stages of life.

(NIAAA, 2016)

Workforce capacity is another area of prevention and substance misuse that needs to be addressed. Up-to-date information on substance use in curricula for nurses, teachers, social workers, and other persons in a care-provider role is needed. These professionals need knowledge of evidence-based prevention practices and how to practice within a team to address complex issues of substance use. A prevention program may operate on other modalities, such as a strength-based approach. In this approach, persons offering the opportunity for a significant positive interaction with a population benefit from specific education on implementa-tion strategies of evidenced-based prevention principles. Incorporating these skills may foster nurturing treatment approaches among professionals (Shea & Shern, 2011).

Significant progress has been made in the prevention of substance use. Research efforts moving forward need to continue to evaluate the effectiveness of new interventions and programs.

CASE STUDY 2-1

*G*rayson is a 17-year-old high school male student who started drinking alcohol when he was in the 8th grade. Substance use has been on the increase in his home community – especially in the high school where he and some of the other students have been drinking alcohol on weekends at parties. Recently, Grayson and his friends have been partying every weekend.

Grayson's grades are dropping, and he has lost interest in school and sports. Things are not going well at home with Grayson and his parents. He is constantly arguing with them, and when he is home, he stays in his room listening to music. His parents are unaware of Grayson's drinking problem. The students are getting alcohol from home when their parents leave to go out for the evening. The principal of the school overheard several students talking about getting drunk last weekend. Community leaders, some parents, and school personnel are all concerned that students at the high school are at risk for substance use.

The principal of the high school approaches the school nurse to help design a prevention program for alcohol use among the students. The principal is concerned that students are drinking outside of school. The school has a zero-tolerance policy for alcohol and drugs. The school nurse begins to plan an alcohol prevention plan for the students based on knowledge about prevention programs found by conducting research and contacting community resources.

Questions

1. What are the school nurse's first steps in designing a prevention program for this school?

2. The school nurse decides to implement an alcohol prevention program that targets those students already identified as using alcohol. What additional information does the nurse obtain from each student when planning an intervention for this group of students?

3. When considering modifying a program to fit the cultural norms of the school community, whom does the school nurse consult?

4. Based on the school nurse's knowledge of prevention strategies in the community, what level of prevention program does the nurse consider implementing?

Answers

1. When planning a prevention program, it is important to consider the type of program and the intended audience. The nurse's first steps include completing a needs assessment to identify the gap between the current and future state of the identified problem in the target population, and identifying stakeholders to assist in program development.

2. The nurse assesses the targeted students' protective factors instead of focusing only on risk factors of the group. The nurse also promotes social-emotional competency traits that have led to good outcomes in reducing substance use: self-awareness, self-management, social awareness, relationship skills, and responsible decision making. The nurse hopes that designing a prevention program around social-emotional competencies will enhance the students' protective factors and reduce the probability of substance use among the adolescent students.

3. It is important to include individuals from the target population and target community for whom the adaptation is being developed.

4. The nurse decides that a universal program is the best approach because it is delivered to everyone in the community, usually addresses the root causes of risky behaviors to assist in changing the environment, and often involves changes in policies or rules. The program could still include selective prevention strategies that empower all students to make good choices and indicate prevention strategies for those adolescents with identified risks.

SUMMARY

An understanding of risk and protective factors is critical in designing effective prevention strategies. Risk factors can influence the development of substance use disorders in several ways. The more risk factors a patient has, the greater the likelihood of that patient misusing drugs. How these factors relate to one another is also critical in designing efforts for preventing substance use disorders.

Prevention of substance use disorders extends beyond primary prevention efforts; it involves a multitude of strategies directed toward the needs of populations for decreasing substance use and addiction. Identifying risk factors and enhancing protective factors can reduce the risk of developing a substance use problem. Effective prevention programs include strategies to enhance protective factors. Comprehensive prevention efforts aligned with strategic principles lead to the greatest program efficacy. Various prevention programs – including universal, selective, and indicated programs – have been designed with positive outcomes. Evidence-based approaches offer tremendous promise in addressing the complex issues surrounding substance use. Models help guide the implementation of prevention programs and ensure that what is delivered is effective and culturally appropriate.

The time has never been better to address substance use. National, state, and local leaders have implemented substantial initiatives to improve health across the life span. Nurses have a unique opportunity to gain the skills and knowledge to lead teams in substance use disorder prevention.

EXAM QUESTIONS

CHAPTER 2
Questions 6–11

Note: Choose the one option that BEST answers each question.

6. The concept of prevention is focused on

    a. interventions before the onset of symptoms.
    b. harm reduction to reduce major health consequences.
    c. early identification of symptoms.
    d. treatment of dependence and relapse.

7. A prevention program that targets an individual who shows early signs of problem behavior is considered

    a. universal.
    b. selective.
    c. indicated.
    d. primary prevention.

8. The Substance Abuse and Mental Health Services Administration provides a review of prevention programs and rates them as effective,

    a. ineffective, or neutral.
    b. promising, or no effects.
    c. tailored, or comprehensive.
    d. successful, or sustainable.

9. Which is a risk factor for substance use among adolescents?

    a. Educational aspirations
    b. Early antidrug education
    c. Parental conflict
    d. Consistent discipline techniques

10. The four areas of prevention principles to address when planning a prevention program are risk and protective factors, family, community, and

    a. prevention program delivery.
    b. participation readiness.
    c. evaluator preparedness.
    d. cost.

11. When planning a prevention program, the first step in the planning process is to assess the

    a. cost.
    b. need.
    c. size of the community.
    d. risk factors.

REFERENCES

Arthur, M. W., Brown, E. C., Briney, J. S., Hawkins, J. D., Abbott, R. D., Catalano, R. F. ... Mueller, M. T. (2015). *Journal of School Health, 85*(8), 497-507.

Blueprints for Healthy Youth Development. (2017a). *Lifeskills training.* Retrieved from http://www.blueprintsprograms.com/fact sheet/lifeskills-training-lst

Blueprints for Healthy Youth Development. (2017b). *Positive family support – Family check-up.* Retrieved from http://www.blue printsprograms.com/factsheet/positive-family-support-family-check-up

Blueprints for Healthy Youth Development. (2017c). *Project Towards No Drug Abuse.* Retrieved from http://www.blueprintspro grams.com/factsheet/project-towards-no-drug-abuse

Blueprints for Healthy Youth Development. (2017d). *Strengthening families 10-14.* Retrieved from http://www.blueprintspro grams.com/factsheet/strengthening-families-10-14

Castro, F. G., Barrera, M., & Holleran Steiker, L. K. (2010). Issues and challenges in the design of culturally adapted evidence-based interventions. *Annual Review of Clinical Psychology, 6,* 213-239. doi:10.1146/annurev-clinpsy-033109-132032

Catalano, R. F., Fagan, A. A., Gavin, L. E., Greenberg, M. T., Irwin, C. E., Ross, D. A., & Shek, D. T. L. (2012). Worldwide application of prevention science in adolescent health. *Lancet, 379*(9826), 1653-1664. doi:10.1016/S0140-6736(12)60238-4

Center for Substance Abuse Prevention. (2010). *Focus on prevention* (HHS Publication No. [SMA] 10-4120). Rockville, MD: Center for Substance Abuse Prevention, Substance Abuse and Mental Health Services Administration. Retrieved from http://store.samhsa.gov/shin/content/SMA10-4120/SMA10-4120.pdf

Chronic Illness in the United States. Volume I: Prevention of chronic illness. (1957). *JAMA, 165*(11), 1513. doi:10.1001/jama.1957.0298 0290153030

Collaborative for Academic, Social, and Emotional Learning. (2015). *Core SEL competencies.* Retrieved from http://www.casel.org/core-competencies/

Erickson, C. (2007). *The science of addiction. From neurobiology to treatment.* New York: W. W. Norton.

Gordon, R. (1987). An operational classification of diseases prevention. In J. A. Steinberg & M. M. Silverman (Eds.), *Preventing mental disorders* (pp. 20-26). Rockville, MD: U.S. Department of Health and Human Services.

Hawkins, J. D., Catalano, R. F., Arthur, M. W., Egan, E., Brown, E. C., Abbott, R. D., & Murray, D. M. (2008). Testing communities that care: The rationale, design and behavioral baseline equivalence of the Community Youth Development Study. *Prevention Science, 9*(3), 178-190. doi:10.1007/s11121-008-0092-y

Holder, H. (2000). Prevention of alcohol problems in the 21st century: Challenges and opportunities. *The American Journal on Addictions, 10,* 1-15.

Horn, M., Fagan, A., Hawkins J., & Osterele, S. (2014). Effects of the Communities That Care system on cross-sectional profiles of adolescent substance use and delinquency. *American Journal of Preventive Medicine, 47*(2), 188-197. doi:10.1016/j.amepre.2014.04.004

The Incredible Years. (2013). The Incredible Years parents, teachers, and children training series. Retrieved from http://incredible years.com/

Kellam, S. G., & Langevin, D. S. (2003). A framework for understanding "evidence," in prevention research and programs. *Preventive Science, 4,* 137-153.

Lisha, N. E., Sun, P., Rohrbach, L. A., Spruijt-Metz, D., Unger, J. B., & Sussman, S. (2012). An evaluation of immediate outcomes and fidelity of a drug abuse prevention program in continuation high schools: Project Toward No Drug Abuse (TND). *Journal on Drug Education, 42*(1), 33-57.

Lochman, J. E., & Wells, K. C. (2003). Effectiveness of the Coping Power Program and of classroom intervention with aggressive children: Outcomes at a 1-year follow-up. *Behavior Therapy, 34*(4), 493-515.

Marlatt, G. A. & Witkiewitz, K. (2010). Update on harm-reduction policy and intervention research. *Annual Review of Clinical Psychology, 6,* 591-606.

Mrazek, P. J., & Haggerty, R. J. (Eds.). (1994). *Reducing risks for mental disorders: Frontiers for preventive intervention research. Institute of Medicine, Committee on Prevention of Mental Disorders.* Retrieved from https://www.nap.edu/read/2139/chapter/1

National Institute on Alcohol Abuse and Alcoholism. (2005). *Social work education for the treatment of alcohol use disorders. Module 3: Preventing alcohol abuse and dependence.* Retrieved from http://pubs.niaaa.nih.gov/publications/Social/Module3Prevention/mODULE3.HTML

National Institute on Alcohol Abuse and Alcoholism. (2016). *NIAAA draft strategic plan.* Retrieved from https://www.niaaa.nih.gov/about-niaaa/our-work/strategic-plan

National Institute on Drug Abuse. (2003). *Preventing drug abuse among children and adolescents* (2nd ed.). Retrieved from http://www.drugabuse.gov/sites/default/files/red book_0.pdf

Obama Administration. (2013, April). *National drug control strategy.* Retrieved from https://obamawhitehouse.archives.gov/ondcp/policy-and-research/ndcs

Office of Disease Prevention and Health Promotion. (2016). *Healthy People 2020: 2020 topics & objectives – Substance abuse.* Retrieved from https://www.healthypeople.gov/2020/topics-objectives/topic/substance-abuse

Office of National Drug Control Policy. (2015). *2015 national drug control strategy.* Retrieved from https://obamawhitehouse.archives.gov/ondcp/policy-and-research/ndcs

Presnall, N., Webster-Stratton, C., Constantino, J. (2014). Parent training: Equivalent improvement in externalizing behavior for children with and without familial risk. *Journal of the American Academy of Child and Adolescent Psychiatry, 53*(8), 879-887.

Schinke, S. P., Fang, L., & Cole, K. (2009a). Computer-delivered, parent-involvement intervention to prevent substance use among adolescent girls. *Preventive Medicine, 49*(5), 429-435.

Schinke, S. P., Fang, L., & Cole, K. (2009b). Preventing drug abuse among adolescent girls: 1-year outcomes of a computerized, mother-daughter program. *Addictive Behaviors, 34,* 1060-1064.

Shea, P., & Shern, D. (2011). *Primary prevention in behavioral health: Investing in our nation's future.* Alexandria, VA: National Association of State Mental Health Program Directors.

Spoth, R., & Greenberg, M. (2011). Impact challenges in community science-with-practice: Lessons from PROSPER on transformative practitioner-scientist partnerships and infrastructure development. *American Journal of Community Psychology, 48*(1-2), 106-119.

Spoth, R. L., Trudeau, L. S., Guyll, M., & Shin, C. (2012). Benefits of universal intervention effects on a youth protective shield 10 years after baseline. *Journal of Adolescent Health, 50*(4), 414-417. doi:10.1016/j.jadohealth.2011.06.010

Springer, F., & Phillips, J. L. (2006). The IOM Model: A tool for prevention planning and implementation. *Prevention Tactics, 8*(13), 1-7. Retrieved from http://www.cars-rp.org/publications/Prevention%20Tactics/PT8.13.06.pdf

Substance Abuse and Mental Health Services Administration. (2012). *An annotated bibliography of measurement compendia: Reliable, valid, and standard measures of substance abuse and other behavioral health indicators and outcomes of interest.* Retrieved from https://www.samhsa.gov/capt/sites/default/files/resources/bibliography-standard-measure.pdf

Substance Abuse and Mental Health Services Administration. (2015). *Risk and protective factors.* Retrieved from http://www.samhsa.gov/capt/practicing-effective-prevention/prevention-behavioral-health/risk-protective-factors

Substance Abuse and Mental Health Services Administration. (2016a). *National registry of evidence-based programs and practices.* Retrieved from http://www.samhsa.gov/nrepp

Substance Abuse and Mental Health Services Administration. (2016b). *Opioid prevention toolkit.* Retrieved from http://www.samhsa.gov/capt/tools-learning-resources/opioid-overdose-prevention-toolkit

Substance Abuse and Mental Health Services Administration. (2016c). *Prevention of substance abuse and mental illness.* Retrieved from http://www.samhsa.gov/prevention

Substance Abuse and Mental Health Substance Administration. (2016d). *Sources of data on substance use and misuse among boys and young men of color.* Retrieved from http://www.samhsa.gov/capt/tools-learning-resources/sources-data-substance-use-boys-young-men-color

Substance Abuse and Mental Health Substance Administration. (2016e). *Elements of a culturally competent prevention system.* Retrieved from https://www.samhsa.gov/capt/tools-learning-resources/elements-culturally-competent-prevention-system

Substance Abuse and Mental Health Substance Administration. (2016f). *Applying the Strategic Prevention Framework: Step 1: Assess Needs.* Retrieved from https://www. samhsa.gov/capt/applying-strategic-preven tion-framework/step1-assess-needs

U.S. Department of Health and Human Services, Office of the Surgeon General. (2016). *Facing addiction in America: The Surgeon General's report on alcohol, drugs, and health.* Washington, DC: Author. Retrieved from https://www.surgeongeneral. gov/library/reports/index.html

CHAPTER 3

ASSESSMENT OF SUBSTANCE USE DISORDERS

LEARNING OUTCOME

After completing this chapter, the learner will be able to describe the components of a comprehensive assessment for patients with substance use disorders.

CHAPTER OBJECTIVES

After completing this chapter, the learner will be able to:

1. Describe the goals of a comprehensive assessment for patients with substance use disorders.

2. Discuss screening methods for signs and symptoms of substance use disorders.

3. List laboratory tests for detection of substances.

4. Describe assessment strategies to determine a patient's readiness for change.

5. Identify key considerations for synthesizing substance use assessment data.

INTRODUCTION

All individuals should be screened for substance misuse and substance use disorders. This can be a challenging process because of many factors. These include the sheer number and identification of misused substances, the impact of comorbidities, patient engagement in the assessment and treatment process, and social stigma and biases often associated with using or even asking about substance use. It is critical to understand that substance use disorders are chronic processes subject to relapse and that assessment should be ongoing.

SUBSTANCE USE ASSESSMENT

Developing an appropriate treatment plan for a patient with a substance use disorder will depend on conducting an appropriate substance use assessment. The clinician will need to determine the type and severity of substance misuse, medical and psychiatric history of the patient, and individual circumstances and preferences (U.S. Department of Health and Human Services, 2016).

In addition to obtaining data from the patient's general medical history, physical examination, and laboratory testing, the goals of a comprehensive substance use assessment are to

- determine the presence and extent of substance use (mild, moderate, or severe);

- evaluate the individual's level of functioning both with and without substance use, such as cognitive capacity and social skills;

- identify the impact of substance use on the individual's medical, psychological, and social status, including relationships with family, peers, and workplace concerns;

- identify facilitators and barriers to treatment and recovery, including cultural considerations and degree of social support;

- establish a formal diagnosis based on evidence-based criteria, such as the *Diagnostic and Statistical Manual of Mental Disorders,* fifth edition *(DSM-5);*

- assess the individual's readiness to change his or her behavior and engage in the treatment process; and

- initiate decisions about the appropriate level of care using a collaborative approach.

(U.S. Department of Health and Human Services, 2016)

The assessment interview should ideally be completed by an addiction specialist, but it may be conducted by other healthcare professionals with adequate training. The International Nurses Society on Addictions, in collaboration with the American Nurses Association, has developed a scope and standards of practice for addictions nursing, and they offer certification for both registered nurses (certified addictions registered nurse) and advanced practice nurses (certified addictions registered nurse – advanced practice). Substance misuse is alarmingly common, and there is a need for clinicians in many healthcare settings to develop the skills to identify patients at risk through proper screening and to initiate treatment when indicated.

Substance use disorder is the generic term that will be used in this chapter to refer to problem use of nicotine; alcohol; and illicit, over-the-counter (OTC), or prescription drugs, and it includes substance dependence or abuse.

Risk and Protective Factors

According to the National Institute on Drug Abuse (NIDA, 2016b), risk and protective factors for developing substance use disorders have been identified in the literature across five domains:

1. Individual (early aggression versus self-control)
2. Family (lack of parental supervision versus parental control)
3. Peers (substance using versus academic focus)
4. School or workplace (access to drugs versus antiuse policies)
5. Community (poverty versus strong neighborhood attachment)

For youth, having peers who abuse substances presents the greatest risk (Van Ryzin, Fosco, & Dishion, 2012).

Signs and Symptoms of Addiction

Substance use and even acute intoxication can be challenging to identify at a glance. People who misuse substances encompass a wide range of demographic characteristics. Adopting a process of universal screening is needed. Signs and symptoms vary based on the effects of the substance being misused (which will be discussed in detail in subsequent chapters) and characteristics of the individual. "Red flag" signs associated with substance use disorders are listed in Table 3-1.

Specific inquiry must be made separately for each substance ever used and the drug primarily used. For OTC and prescribed drugs, direct questioning includes whether the use is other than what is recommended or prescribed. Individuals should be questioned about whether the medications were prescribed for them or someone else. Other questions include age at first use, duration, amount, and route (such as inhalation or intravenous).

TABLE 3-1: RED FLAGS FOR SUBSTANCE USE PROBLEMS

- Frequently missed appointments
- Frequent absences from school or work
- History of frequent injuries
- Subjective concerns, such as pain, difficulty sleeping, anxiety, or depression
- Frequent requests for medication refills with the potential for abuse (such as opioids)
- Frequent changes in medical providers
- Periods of memory loss
- Tremors
- Alcohol odor on breath or clothing
- Red eyes
- Nicotine stains
- Unsteady gait
- Dilated or pinpoint pupils
- Needle marks

Note. Western Schools, 2017.

Estimating the amount and pattern of use (monthly binge, daily, increasing use) of substances can be difficult. For example, practitioners can ask heroin users about the amount used and the associated cost to get a general sense of the frequency and heaviness of use. Information regarding what source of funds supports the substance use can be a marker of risk behaviors associated with addiction, which can include borrowing money from significant others, neglecting personal responsibilities to focus on obtaining and using substances, and engaging in such behaviors as stealing or prostitution. These characteristics of use are included in an assessment of the severity of the substance use disorder as outlined in the *DSM-5* and included in the summary of *DSM-5* substance use disorder diagnostic criteria in Table 3-2. If needles or other drug para-phernalia are employed, individuals are asked if these items are shared and, if reused, inquire if and how they are cleaned between uses.

Substance Use History Screening

The goal of screening is to identify patients at risk for substance use disorders. Periodic screening should be completed for all individuals presenting for care in various settings. Screening approaches are brief and applicable to diverse populations in a wide range of clinical settings. Standardized screening instruments, which are also brief and applicable to diverse populations across a range of clinical settings, promote consistency. Gender, age, and culture are also considered when using screening instruments. At present, there is no clear evidence as to what age screening should be universally implemented. Experimentation with alcohol and other substances begins during middle school for many adolescents, so screening during these years is generally recommended. Screening is deferred for patients who are acutely intoxicated because the information provided is unlikely to be reliable.

Screening and brief intervention (SBI) is an evidence-based approach recommended across a variety of settings and patient populations (Zgierska & Fleming, 2014). Initially focusing on identifying alcohol misuse, it has been studied and found to be effective with other substances. The NIDA has developed a quick screening tool that asks a single question: "In the past year, how often have you used the following?" with a checklist of potentially addictive substances. If indicated, additional screening is conducted specific to the substance or substances used to further explore unhealthy or at-risk use. Furthermore, certain populations may require additional screening regardless of their response; specifically, the NIDA quick screening tool has not been tested with pregnant women (Parran, 2014). The following Screening

TABLE 3-2: SUMMARY OF *DSM-5* SUBSTANCE USE DISORDER DIAGNOSTIC CRITERIA

Must meet at least two of the following over 12 months, resulting in a pattern of problematic behavior:

1. The substance is often taken in larger amounts or over a longer period than was intended.

2. There is a persistent desire or unsuccessful effort to cut down or control use of the substance.

3. A great deal of time is spent in activities necessary to obtain the substance, use the substance, or recover from its effects.

4. Craving, or a strong desire or urge to use the substance, occurs.

5. Recurrent use of the substance results in a failure to fulfill major role obligations at work, school, or home.

6. Use of the substance is continued despite having persistent or recurrent social or interpersonal problems caused or exacerbated by the effects of its use.

7. Important social, occupational, or recreational activities are given up or reduced because of use of the substance.

8. Recurrent use of the substance occurs in situations in which it is physically hazardous.

9. Use of the substance is continued despite knowledge of having a persistent or recurrent physical or psychological problem that is likely to have been caused or exacerbated by the substance.

10. Tolerance has developed, as defined by either a need for markedly increased amounts of the substance to achieve intoxication or desired effect or markedly diminished effect with continued use of the same amount of the substance.

11. Withdrawal occurs, as manifested by either the characteristic withdrawal syndrome for that substance (as specified in the *DSM-5* for each substance) or substance (or a closely related substance) is taken to relieve or avoid withdrawal symptoms.

Note. Adapted from National Institute on Drug Abuse. (2016b). *The science of drug abuse and addiction.* Retrieved from https://www.drug abuse.gov/publications/media-guide/science-drug-abuse-addiction-basics

Instruments section provides more detail on specific tools that can be used in practice.

Screening instruments can be self-report tools or interviews. Regardless of the method used, results are discussed with the individual being screened. Unfortunately, no instruments have been found to be equally valid for all patients regardless of their gender, age, or culture. However, these factors should be kept in mind when selecting a screening instrument to ensure the results accurately reflect use in a specified population.

If individuals have a negative screen, the occasion is used as an opportunity to focus on prevention of substance misuse, particularly with at-risk populations, such as adolescents. When individuals use such statements as "I don't drink," follow-up questions are useful to differentiate between abstinence as a lifelong state or because of previous misuse. If the latter, such individuals may be at risk for substance use; misuse is prone to relapse and is assessed as a chronic condition.

A positive screening is not a diagnosis, but it does require the clinician to provide a brief intervention and implement the SBI process. The five *As* is an effective framework developed for assessing and treating tobacco use in primary care settings. The five *As* is a tool that will also help clinicians identify and deliver appropriate intervention for risky substance use.

The five *As*:

1. Ask
2. Advise
3. Assess
4. Assist
5. Arrange

The first *A* is to (1) ask about substance use as described earlier in the screening process. The second *A* is to (2) advise. Clear, focused statements from a healthcare provider, tailored to the individual, are effective brief interventions that have been linked to behavior change (Fiore et al., 2008). Statements may include something like, "Your alcohol use is heavier than most and can be contributing to your abnormal test results. I recommend you consider abstaining from alcohol. I can help."

At this point, a referral can be made, or if the clinician feels competent in doing so, he or she can complete the five *As* process by (3) assessing readiness to change, (4) assisting with treatment, and (5) arranging for follow-up or referral. A shortened version of the five *As* – ask, advise, and refer – is also used in many healthcare settings.

Generally, patients identified as being at risk should be offered referral for a more comprehensive assessment and treatment. This referral for treatment is an additional component of SBI, referred to as SBIRT (screening, brief intervention, and referral for treatment). SBIRT has been endorsed by many professional organizations, including the American Academy of Pediatrics (AAP Committee on Substance Use and Prevention, 2016). When choosing the referral for further treatment, the clinician needs to consider the type of substance misused, the level of risk, and individual preference. Emergent referrals should be provided for patients who present an immediate risk to themselves or others.

Technology can greatly assist systematic implementation of SBIRT into treatment settings. Many electronic health records have screening prompts and tools. The Substance Abuse and Mental Health Services Administration (SAMHSA) has a website dedicated to SBIRT and evidence-based screening tools, including web-based forms.

Screening Instruments

A variety of tools exists for substance use and misuse screening. The most commonly used tools with good evidence to support their use are listed here. These tools vary in sensitivity and specificity and should be used to assess the defined substance in the target population. (See the Resources section at the end of this course for a list of the websites where these tools can be found.)

Alcohol

- Alcohol Use Disorders Identification Test (AUDIT) is a 10-item instrument designed as a brief healthcare interview administered by a clinician or as a self-report. The AUDIT has been validated cross-culturally.

- AUDIT-C is a modified three-question version of the AUDIT and provides feedback on alcohol use as compared with national norms.

- CAGE (which stands for the question topics of cut down, annoyed, guilty, eye opener) is a widely used four-item questionnaire, components of which have been incorporated into other instruments. A modified version, the CAGE Questions Adapted to Include

Drugs (CAGE-AID), is used to screen for alcohol and other substance misuse.

- CRAFFT (which stands for the question topics of car, relax, alone, forget, friends, trouble) is a six-item questionnaire designed to identify at-risk alcohol use in adolescents. It has been translated into multiple languages and can be either clinician-administered or self-administered.

- The National Institute on Alcohol Abuse and Alcoholism has an additional two-question initial screen with follow-up questions for use with youth ages 9 to 11, 11 to 14, and 14 to 18.

- For pregnant women and women of childbearing age, the TWEAK test (which stands for the question topics of tolerance, worried, eye opener, amnesia, cut down) and T-ACE (similar to the CAGE and standing for take [number of drinks], annoyed, cut down, eye opener) are recommended.

- Michigan Alcoholism Screening Test (MAST) is a 22-question self-test focusing specifically on alcohol use. There are other versions of this screening test: shortened (SMAST) and geriatric (MAST-G).

Other Drugs

- The Drug Abuse Screening Tool (DAST) has a 10-item version used to screen for substance misuse in older adolescents and adults.

- The Alcohol, Smoking, and Substance Involvement Screening Test (ASSIST) is a comprehensive assessment tool developed by clinicians for the World Health Organization (WHO).

Assessing Withdrawal

When a substance has been used, clinicians inquire if the individual has ever had withdrawal symptoms when not using the substance. For example, individuals may report hand trem-

ors when not consuming alcohol. Common withdrawal symptoms are listed in Table 3-3. It is important to distinguish reported withdrawal symptoms from other medical conditions. Not all misused substances have clear or easily identified withdrawal symptoms. (The presence or absence of withdrawal symptoms will be reviewed in the chapters associated with each category of substances.)

Withdrawal from alcohol can be assessed with the Addiction Research Foundation Clinical Institute Withdrawal Assessment for Alcohol-Revised (CIWA-AR). This tool evaluates orientation and the degree of withdrawal symptoms, such as nausea and vomiting; tremor; sweats; agitation; headache; and tactile, auditory, and visual disturbances or hallucinations. The tool takes about 5 minutes to administer. It is important to monitor for withdrawal because some symptoms (e.g., convulsions, withdrawal seizures) can be life-threatening.

The Clinical Opiate Withdrawal Scale (COWS) is used to assess opiate withdrawal symptoms and will be discussed in more detail in Chapter 10. (See the Resources section at the end of the course for the websites of these assessment tools.)

Treatment History

Prior experience with treatment can reveal valuable information regarding what has worked or not worked in the past. It can also provide information regarding the perceived benefit (or lack) of treatment modalities. Inquiries should include dates, duration, place, and form of substance misuse treatment, including medications used and efforts directed at self-treatment (e.g., "cold turkey" attempts). For each treatment episode, the clinician asks about the outcome – specifically, how long the individual was substance free, noting the longest substance-free period. This can be helpful when exploring what

TABLE 3-3: COMMON WITHDRAWAL SYMPTOMS FOR SELECTED DRUGS			
Alcohol	**Opioids**	**Cocaine**	**Benzodiazepines**
Hand tremors	Irritability	Irritability	Confusion
Grand mal seizures	Anxiety	Depression	Restlessness
Transient visual or auditory hallucinations or illusions	Nausea	Suicidal thoughts	Insomnia
	Vomiting	Anxiety	Anxiety
Sweating	Abdominal cramps		Hallucinations
Rapid heart rate	Diarrhea		Tingling extremities
Agitation	Chills		Muscle cramps
	Yawning		Blurred vision
	Runny nose		
	Watery eyes		
	Problems sleeping		
	Bone or muscle pain		

Note. Adapted from National Institute on Drug Abuse (2016a). *Commonly abused drugs charts.* Retrieved from https://www.drugabuse.gov/drugs-abuse/commonly-abused-drugs-charts

has worked or not worked for each individual and each mode of treatment. This then provides the clinician with an opportunity to engage the patient in tailoring the treatment process.

Consequences of Substance Use

It is critical to assess acute substance intoxication or toxicity, risk or presence of withdrawal symptoms, and coexisting disorders, including indications that the individual is a potential danger to others or himself or herself. If patients are at high risk for an emergent event, they should be promptly referred for crisis management in an emergency treatment setting.

Consequences of substance use may be grouped under medical, psychiatric, family/social, employment/support, and legal concerns affected by drug and alcohol use. The Addiction Severity Index (ASI) is a multidimensional 161-item structured interview on the areas potentially affected by substance use. It takes about 45 minutes to administer (see Resources section). The ASI also has a modified version (ASI-Lite, with 22 fewer questions), which can be administered in around 30 minutes.

Certain medical illnesses can be associated with substance use:

- Hepatitis
- Human immunodeficiency virus (HIV)
- Sexually transmitted infections
- Esophagitis
- Gastrointestinal bleeding
- Pancreatitis
- Gastritis
- Thrombophlebitis
- Cellulitis
- Cardiomyopathy
- Endocarditis
- Osteomyelitis
- Seizures

Documentation of past illnesses includes the date of onset. A current medical history includes the names and doses of medications prescribed, along with the frequency and amount actually used.

A psychiatric history includes active disorders and whether they preceded or were subsequent to initiation of substance use. This is critical to understanding if an underlying mental illness was a risk factor for substance misuse or if the substance use precipitated an acute psychiatric event. It is important to note any history of psychiatric care (inpatient and outpatient) and thoughts of or attempted suicide. If the patient gives permission to do so, corroborators, such as close family members and friends, can be very helpful in assessing substance use disorders in patients with psychiatric symptoms or mental illness.

A family history includes any history of substance use disorders in other family members, including first-degree and second-degree relatives. It also includes information on the patient's marital status; members of his or her household; the quality of his or her relationships with family members; and history of physical, emotional, or sexual abuse.

A social history includes education, housing, and exposure to other substance users and use in the household. An employment and legal history includes whether substance use has ever affected job performance and if the patient was ever arrested or incarcerated as a result of substance use.

Physical and Mental Status Evaluation

Physical signs suggestive of active substance use vary and depend on the following five factors:

1. Substance used: For example, stimulants can cause symptoms of increased heart rate and weight loss. Sedatives can cause lethargy and decreased levels of alertness. Certain stimulants, such as amphetamines and cocaine, can present with symptoms similar to alcohol intoxication (tachycardia, pupil dilation, and diaphoresis). There is no one defining symptom cluster associated with all substance types.

2. Route of administration: For injected substances, track or needle marks can be apparent. Local irritation can be found in those using a nasal route of administration.

3. Acute intoxication versus chronic use: As tolerance develops for many addictive substances, the signs of acute intoxication, such as slurred speech with alcohol, may become less or even unapparent for similar amounts of the substance used.

4. Individual characteristics: There may be variation in individual metabolism of substances, causing intoxication symptoms to appear with greater or lesser amounts of substance used. Individual expectations related to the effects of a particular substance may also affect the physical presentation. The presence or absence of altered liver or kidney function – often a sequelae of specific substance misuse, such as alcohol – can also affect the elimination time of substances and prolong or enhance intoxication.

5. Dose of the substance used and time since use: Substances have varying half-lives, causing a dose-related and time-related effect for symptom presentation. For example, for a substance with a short half-life and notable withdrawal symptoms, it is important to distinguish whether the presenting symptoms are related to intoxication or withdrawal.

In general, many substances commonly cause alterations in psychomotor functioning, perception, reasoning, and judgment during both acute and chronic intoxication and potentially during withdrawal (American Psychiatric Association, 2013).

A mental status evaluation is critical because cognitive function can affect an individual's ability to participate and engage in treatment. Furthermore, diagnoses can be made for other conditions that present similarly to substance use, such as dementia or neurologic disorders. The Mini-Mental State Examination (MMSE) is one widely used tool to screen for baseline cognitive impairment (Folstein, Folstein, & McHugh, 1975). It is a brief examination that measures orientation and recall, and tests ability to perform some additional functional skills.

If concerns are raised regarding cognitive ability, a neuropsychiatric assessment by a specialist is helpful. Use of many substances, most notably alcohol, can cause brain injury. Results of this evaluation can then be used to tailor treatment and rehabilitation, helping them to be more successful. For example, individuals with significant cognitive impairment are less likely to benefit from counseling or insight-oriented therapy as their main treatment component.

LABORATORY TESTING

Laboratory testing can help distinguish between substance-related and nonsubstance-related disorders. Because of the relatively short half-lives of most substances, a positive test result usually confirms recent substance use. This can make it challenging to differentiate between chronic use and intermittent or first-time use.

Laboratories should use certified testing procedures, such as those from the NIDA or the Department of Defense. What constitutes a positive test can vary from one laboratory to another (Warner & Lorch, 2014). It is important to know the cutoff for the specific substance tested. This can be affected by the concentration of the drug and how it remains over time. (Limits of drug detection times for urine are listed in Table 3-4.)

Newer testing techniques have made detection more reliable. But the caveat is that these results should always be interpreted in a clini-

cal context. Test results support a substance use diagnosis, but when used alone, they are inadequate to help make a diagnosis.

Steps for Drug Testing

Drug testing is often completed as a two-step process. The first step is the initial screen, followed by the confirmatory testing. Initial screening methodologies include an immunoassay, which yields a qualitative result reported as positive or negative based on a given range of detectable values, indicating the presence or absence of the drug, not the amount of the drug in the sample. Immunoassays include enzyme-linked immunosorbent assay or radioimmunoassay analysis. These tests depend on antibodies that react with either the drug or its metabolites and are quick and economical. Immunoassays are less sensitive than spectrometry confirmatory tests, generally yielding more false-positive results because of cross-reaction with similar chemical substances, such as cold and allergy medications and pain relievers. These assays are also commercially available for testing both urine and oral fluid.

Gas chromatography mass spectroscopy (GC/MS) is used as confirmatory testing and generally yields a negative finding if the immunoassay result is a false positive. GC/MS is highly sensitive and more expensive than immunoassay, but it can accurately distinguish between similar chemicals, correctly identifying both the presence and quantity of drugs detected.

Validating Urine Samples

Urine samples may be altered by adding, substituting, or otherwise changing the specimen to attain a negative, or "clean," test result. For example, urine may be diluted by adding water or overhydrating to reduce the concentration of a drug to less than its detectable limit. Although GC/MS is sensitive enough to detect the drug's presence, specimens that initially test

TABLE 3-4: DETECTION TIMES FOR COMMON DRUGS IN URINE TESTING*	
Drug	**Detection Time**
Amphetamines	1 to 3 days
Anabolic steroids – oral	Up to 3 weeks
Anabolic steroids – parenteral	Up to 1 year
Barbiturates – short acting	1 to 4 days
Barbiturates – long acting	1 to 3 weeks
Benzodiazepine	1 to 14 days
Cannabinoids	Single joint use: 1 to 3 days
	Heavy use: up to 30 days
Cocaine	1 to 3 days
Codeine	1 to 2 days
Cyclizine	1 to 2 days
Gamma hydroxybutyrate (GHB)	Up to 72 hours
Heroin or morphine	1 to 2 days
Ketamine	1 to 2 days
Lysergic acid diethylamide (LSD)	Up to 8 hours
Methadone	1 to 3 days
Methamphetamine	3 days
Methaqualone	1 to 7 days
Phencyclidine (PCP)	7 days
Propoxyphene	1 to 3 days
Rohypnol	1 to 3 days

*Detection times can vary and depend on the dose, route of administration, use pattern, laboratory testing methodology, and individual metabolism.

Note. Adapted from Warner, E., & Lorch, E. (2014). Laboratory diagnosis. In R. K. Reis (Ed.), *The ASAM principles of addiction medicine* (5th ed., pp. 332-343). Philadelphia, PA: Wolters Kluwer.

negative are not routinely subjected to GC/MS confirmatory testing. Therefore, it is important that urine samples be obtained under direct observation. To combat diluting, urine tested by laboratories is screened for additives and discarded if specific parameters, such as specific gravity, are not met. Administratively – depending on the purpose for testing, such as criminal justice – it is critical that a chain of sample-handling custody be verified. This is established when the sample is always within sight of a member of the drug-testing team until its arrival at the testing laboratory.

Specimens for Drug Testing

Urine testing is the most widely used and cost-effective method of detecting substance use. Other types of drug test specimens include blood, breath, hair, oral fluid or saliva, and sweat. Generally, blood testing is the most accurate method but also the most expensive and more invasive to obtain (Warner & Lorch, 2014).

Oral fluid or saliva, like urine, shows only recent substance use. Oral fluid is commonly used because direct observation is easier than it is for urine, and it is more difficult to tamper with the sample. But recent smoking can contaminate the results.

Hair testing can detect substance use further back in time – 6 months or longer. The longer the hair, the further back detection is possible; however, most laboratories use hair only within 3 to 5 cm from the scalp, limiting detection to 90 days. Variation can occur with the rate of hair growth, hair color (dark hair absorbs drugs more readily than lighter colored hair), and ethnicity (African American hair absorbs drugs more readily than other ethnic groups' hair). Hair testing is used especially for cocaine dependence. Compared with urine, hair is less sensitive for marijuana (Warner & Lorch, 2014).

Sweat tests can also be performed. Patches are placed on the skin for 10 to 14 days to detect substance use while the patch is in place. Cocaine, morphine, amphetamine, and ethanol have all been detected in sweat; however, there is substantial variability among individuals in how the drug concentrates in sweat. Although it is a useful approach when urine testing is not practical, there is marked biologic variability in individuals' rate of sweat production, leading to a greater variability of results and reliability of interpretation (Warner & Lorch, 2014).

Testing for Alcohol

Ethanol levels can be performed on blood, urine, saliva, or breath. Saliva and urine tests are least reliable. Breath testing is most convenient, and levels can be converted to approximate blood levels, which are most reliable. Alcohol testing is done in medical settings but is also important in certain legal proceedings (Warner & Lorch, 2014).

Blood alcohol concentration (BAC) reflects recent intake, measured in milligrams (mg) of alcohol per deciliter (dL) of blood and reported as a percentage. For example, 100 mg of alcohol in 1 dL of blood is reported as 0.10%. It then follows that two individuals with identical alcohol intake but different blood volumes (reflected in body weight) will have different BACs, with individuals having lower body weight testing at a higher BAC. This is part of the rationale for recommending lower safe drinking limits for women than for men (SAMHSA, 2012a).

Breath analysis is the most common method used to test for blood alcohol even though it is less accurate and not as reliable as blood testing. Breathalyzers estimate BAC, but cross-reactions may occur with acetone; patients who have diabetes mellitus in ketoacidosis may be confused with individuals who have ingested alcohol. Furthermore, breathalyzer results can be affected by the subject's breathing pattern or hematocrit level. Hyperventilation can produce falsely low readings, and low hematocrits can produce falsely high readings.

Other biomarkers, such as liver function testing, can reflect heaviness of alcohol use. Carbohydrate-deficient transferrin is a marker for chronic alcohol use. It is more accurate in men than in women. It is capable of detecting consecutive daily intake of 60 grams of alcohol over a period of 7 to 10 days. Gamma glutamyl transpeptidase (GGT) is a hepatic enzyme reflecting liver cell damage. It can be elevated with hyperthyroidism, anticonvulsant use, and nonalcoholic liver disease. Other laboratory tests supportive of alcohol abuse include increased mean corpuscular volume, increased mean corpuscular hemoglobin, hypercholesterolemia, and hyperglycemia (SAMHSA, 2012b). Although the latter tests are less sensitive than the GGT, such tests taken as a group should heighten the clinician's suspicions about alcohol abuse.

ASSESSING MOTIVATION FOR BEHAVIOR CHANGE

The stages of change, also known as the transtheoretical model of behavior change

(DiClemente, Schlundt, & Gemmell, 2004), is one model commonly applied to assessing and treating substance use. Appropriate interventions are planned based on assessment of the patient's current stage of change. The model consists of five stages that individuals progress through toward making a behavioral change:

1. Precontemplation: In precontemplation, the individual does not acknowledge that substance misuse is a problem and expresses no desire to change his or her pattern of use.

2. Contemplation: Contemplators begin to see substance use as a problem and are considering change, but not in the immediate future.

3. Preparation: Timing of action distinguishes the contemplation stage from the preparation stage. During contemplation, change is anticipated within the next 6 months; during preparation, it is expected within the coming month.

4. Action: The action stage is when the individual engages in treatment.

5. Maintenance/recovery: Maintenance or recovery is a time of relative stability. Efforts are dedicated to preventing relapse. This final stage involves the long-term outcome, which for many struggling with addiction involves potential recurrence of substance use.

(DiClemente et al., 2004)

The underlying rationale behind use of this model is to match the patient's level of readiness to change with the appropriate treatment modality. However, the process is not always linear, and regression or rapid progression between stages does occur.

Although stages can be useful ways to conceptually frame an assessment for tailoring interventions, the current understanding of addiction and the way it affects and alters the brain illustrates some potential limitations. Addiction is known to affect the go-stop systems in the prefrontal cortex of the brain. The go system relates to conscious decision making, planning, and goal-setting. Addictive substances can overactivate this system, leading to habitual craving and impulsive drug-seeking behaviors. Conversely, the stop system, which acts to check these impulses, becomes less activated in response to substance use (U.S. Department of Health and Human Services, 2016). Therefore, the decision-making capability of an addicted brain can be altered, making it challenging to engage patients in contemplative or preparatory activities.

An alternative and complementary method to enhance motivation to change is motivational interviewing (MI). MI is a patient-centered therapeutic approach that addresses ambivalence (Miller & Rose, 2009). The goal is to form a relationship with the patient through empathy, respect, and collaboration. This allows the patient to explore the discrepancies between his or her personal goals and substance-using behaviors. Working collaboratively with the patient also enhances a culturally sensitive approach to treatment.

Motivation can be fluid, so it is important to assess readiness regularly. This assessment should include measurements of confidence (self-efficacy), importance, and readiness. These can be assessed using a Likert scale, such as, "On a scale of 1 to 10, where 1 is not at all and 10 is extremely likely, how would you rank the importance of quitting (substance) at this time?" Additional questions can be framed that range from how confident the individual feels in being able to change to how ready he or she is to change at this time.

Principles of MI include the following techniques:

• Expressing empathy

• Developing discrepancies

• Rolling with resistance

• Supporting self-efficacy

- Evoking change talk
- Offering support

(Miller & Rose, 2009)

Key features of MI include replacing confrontation and giving out advice with active, reflective listening. Open-ended questions are used to explore ambivalence regarding substance-using behaviors and work toward affirming autonomy and positive-change talk.

DIAGNOSTIC SUMMARY

Data from the comprehensive assessment are used for the diagnostic summary that evaluates individuals' substance use problems in the context of their unique life situations. By the end of the assessment, there should be sufficient data to make a formal substance use disorder diagnosis and formulate a treatment plan. Two organizations have established diagnostic criteria for substance misuse. The American Psychiatric Association developed the *DSM,* now in its fifth edition, which is considered the national standard in the United States. The parallel system, the *International Classification of Disease,* now in its 10th revision *(ICD-10),* is used by the WHO (1992).

According to the *DSM-5,* the umbrella term substance-related disorders is subdivided between substance-induced disorders and substance use disorders. Substance-induced disorders are those that directly result from the pharmacologic effects of the drug, such as in withdrawal or intoxication. Other mental disorders can also be directly precipitated by drug effects.

Substance use disorders arise from the pattern of or consequences from substance use. Severity of the individual's problems is further described as mild, moderate, or severe, according to the number of symptoms met for the diagnosis. In general, mild is the presence of

two or three symptoms listed in the criteria, moderate by four or five symptoms, and severe by six or more symptoms. Severity can change over time to increase or decrease, so it should be reassessed periodically. Because these criteria are based on the individual's behavior or functional impairment resulting from the individual's substance use, these criteria apply to any drug (see Table 3-2).

Substance use can precipitate, reduce, aggravate, mimic, or obscure psychiatric symptoms, complicating the diagnostic process for either the substance use disorder or a mental illness. When substance use precipitates another psychiatric condition, the mental health symptoms are classified as a substance-induced disorder in the *DSM-5.* Populations with increased cooccurring disorder prevalence compared to the general U.S. population include people who are homeless, criminal justice offenders, and those with a history of infectious disease, such as hepatitis C or HIV/AIDS. It is critical that patients with a substance use disorder be screened for a psychiatric disorder because treating only one can negatively affect both disorders. Generally speaking, if the patient has abstained from substance use for at least 30 days, any remaining mental health symptoms should no longer be attributed to substance use (SAMSHA, 2009). It is critical that patients with a substance use disorder be also screened for a psychiatric disorder because treating only one can negatively impact both disorders. A time line of the person's life may also help in diagnosis with the primary diagnosis developing first (Ziedonis et al., 2014).

Similarities and differences exist between the *DSM* classifications of substance-related disorders and those found in the *ICD-10* codes. Similarities include specific listings and codes for specific substances and the many similar criteria used for diagnosis. Differences relate to the categorization and labeling of symptom clusters. *ICD-10* codes describe a specific condition but do not provide the specific criteria found in the *DSM-5*.

PATIENT CONFIDENTIALITY

Eliciting honest answers from patients with substance use disorders can be challenging. All questions should be asked in a nonjudgmental manner. Clinicians should clearly explain why the questions are important and the potential consequences that may occur if information given is inaccurate. Before beginning the interview, all individuals are informed about federal laws and regulations concerning confidentiality.

Federal law provides stringent requirements for disclosing patient information related to substance use. The goal of the regulations in Confidentiality of Alcohol and Drug Abuse Patient Records, 42 C.F.R. part 2, is to encourage people "to enter treatment without fear of stigmatization or discrimination as a result of information disclosure without the patient's express permission" (Center for Substance Abuse Treatment, 2013, p. 69). This law applies to facilities that provide substance use assessment and treatment as their primary mission. Ordinarily, federal regulations would not apply to general medical care facilities unless the clinician's primary function as part of providing care in that facility is substance use treatment and assessment, and if the facility receives federal assistance.

State laws may have additional requirements that vary among states. Some states have stricter confidentiality laws; however, all states must adhere to federal requirements as a minimum standard. All clinicians should be explicitly aware of whether they must comply with federal regulations and what additional, if any, state requirements apply. Awareness of existing regulations to protect patient information, along with communicating a genuine desire to help, should help convince individuals that truthful answers are in their best interest.

Confidentiality in assessing substance use can be a special concern when working with children and adolescents. For elementary and middle school age children, it is appropriate to involve a trusted adult. For older adolescents, this may be less clear and vary based on state law related to age of emancipation.

CASE STUDY 3-1

Gary is a 42-year-old male patient who works as a manager at a local grocery chain. He has come to the primary care clinic for help with persistent "heartburn" that he reports is no longer responding to OTC medications. He explains that his job has been really stressful lately, and he has been smoking over a pack of cigarettes a day to help him stay awake and alert during the day. He also reports needing to drink a bit more alcohol at night to help him "unwind" after a stressful day.

Gary appears slightly disheveled and fatigued, and his hands are trembling. He has a ruddy complexion and is tense, making little eye contact with the nurse. He says he just wants some medicine for his stomach and feels irritated that he has to answer so many questions. He tells the nurse this is why he hates coming to the clinic. He finds it hard to be away from work, but he has had to report to work late recently because he cannot sleep because of his stomach symptoms. He further explains that he has had a hard time keeping steady employment in the past, blaming "the bad economy." He states that he has been at his current job for 2 years and generally enjoys his work there.

His medical history is significant for hypertension for which he no longer takes medication because it "made me feel bad." He is divorced and lives alone, but he has contact with his grown children whom he is trying to help support while they are in college. He wants his kids to graduate college because he "barely finished" high school and it has limited his work choices in life. He explains that he feels financially stressed and has trouble making ends meet at times. He has found himself feeling increasingly isolated from social contacts because of his fatigue and limited finances. Other than his stomach symptoms, he feels like he is in "pretty good shape for his age." He states, "It's not like I'm going to go running races or anything like that at my age."

Upon physical examination, Gary's vital signs are heart rate 98 beats/min; blood pressure 165/98 mm Hg; and respiratory rate 18 breaths/min. Gary's weight is 265 pounds; his height is 5 feet, 11 inches. The nurse calculates Gary's body mass index to be 37. Gary's heart rhythm is regular with a normal point of maximal impulse noted. Gary's lungs are clear, but his respirations are mildly labored. His abdomen is obese with central adiposity and mildly diffuse tenderness in his upper abdomen with no guarding or rebound tenderness noted. Gary's bowel sounds are active in all quadrants. No masses are noted. He is alert and oriented, but the nurse detects a faint smell of beer on Gary's breath during the examination.

Questions

1. What is the nurse's initial approach in assessing Gary's symptoms and signs for a substance use disorder?

2. Which screening tool could the nurse use to assess Gary's alcohol use?

3. What is the nurse's response if Gary screens positive for alcohol use greater than the national norm?

4. Which medical conditions based on Gary's presentation and his report of increased alcohol intake at home does the nurse consider as higher risk for Gary?

5. What is the nurse's instruction to Gary regarding encouraging him to follow up about his stomach symptoms?

Answers

1. Start with open-ended questions and nonjudgmental responses. Expressing empathy will help Gary in understanding that the assessment questions are not meant to be probing but will help identify appropriate treatment for any problems that he may have. This type of an approach will assist in making Gary feel less defensive.

2. A brief screening tool, such as the three-question AUDIT-C, will help to reveal information about whether Gary's alcohol use exceeds established norms.

3. A positive alcohol screening result is an opportunity to engage in a brief intervention using motivational interviewing principles. Depending on Gary's responses, the nurse can begin to help Gary by assisting him with identifying discrepancies in his behavior. If he becomes aggravated and defensive after receiving feedback, she could roll with his resistance, offering to provide further information at a more convenient time and encouraging follow-up.

4. With positive alcohol screening, in addition to Gary's smoking history and current symptoms, the nurse considers that Gary may need further evaluation for gastrointestinal pathology, including gastritis, peptic ulcer, and liver disease. Additionally, Gary's blood pressure is high and requires reassessment and possible medical follow-up. It is also important to assess Gary for withdrawal symptoms and discuss management of these symptoms if they are noted.

5. The nurse explains to Gary that to help him with his stomach symptoms, she will need to arrange for more comprehensive assessment and treatment of his symptoms. Using a five *A*s behavioral counseling approach, the nurse arranges follow-up with Gary, which is a key element of maintaining a therapeutic relationship. If he agrees to laboratory tests to assess possible medical conditions associated with his alcohol and tobacco use, Gary's follow-up could be based on reviewing these results, which may feel less threatening to him. Relating his current symptoms to both alcohol and tobacco use may provide an opportunity to promote behavior change before a first follow-up visit with Gary.

SUMMARY

Assessment for substance use disorders requires a sensitive and organized approach. All individuals can benefit from screening, and it is important to use a nonjudgmental approach. SBIRT is an effective framework used to screen, briefly intervene, and refer for more intensive evaluation and treatment when appropriate. It is critically important for accuracy in screening that the appropriate instrument be used and that appropriate follow-up evaluation be undertaken. After an initial positive screen, a comprehensive assessment includes a detailed history, a physical, and a laboratory evaluation. Laboratory testing for substance use provides useful confirmation that can corroborate information provided in the assessment interview, but it is also subject to the limitations discussed.

Theoretical frameworks, such as the stages of change, can assist clinicians in determining how ready the patient is to change his or her behavior. Also important, MI interventions can foster the development of effective therapeutic

relationships needed to best assess and treat addiction. Tailoring interactions and therapeutic techniques based on these models is useful in establishing patient-centered relationships and guiding the therapeutic process.

As part of a comprehensive assessment for substance use disorders, it is important to determine other possible causes for unusual behavior in addition to substance misuse. Additional considerations are also needed for such populations as adolescents, women, older adults, and patients with comorbid conditions, such as mental illness.

EXAM QUESTIONS

CHAPTER 3
Questions 12–17

Note: Choose the one option that BEST answers each question.

12. A goal of a comprehensive substance use assessment is to

    a. measure the patient's blood alcohol concentration.

    b. perform a genitourinary examination.

    c. make a preliminary diagnosis.

    d. assess the patient's readiness to change.

13. Which screening instrument was developed specifically to assist clinicians in assessing risky alcohol use in adolescents?

    a. CAGE

    b. MAST

    c. CRAFFT

    d. AUDIT-C

14. Which statement about laboratory testing for substance use is correct?

    a. Test results can be used as the sole source of information for diagnosing a substance use disorder.

    b. Marijuana (cannabis) can be detected in the urine for up to 30 days after use.

    c. Results of drug tests are interpreted using universal standardized measures.

    d. Blood test results cannot differentiate between a chronic user and a first-time user.

15. Individuals in the precontemplation stage of change characteristically

    a. believe that they have a serious substance use problem.

    b. express tentative readiness to participate in a drug treatment program.

    c. express the belief that they do not have a drug problem.

    d. state, "It's time for me to do something about my problem."

16. A principle of motivational interviewing is

    a. providing brief advice.

    b. expressing empathy.

    c. reviewing health risks.

    d. arranging for follow-up.

17. According to *DSM-5,* substance use that precipitates a psychiatric condition is classified as a

    a. substance-induced disorder.

    b. mixed disorder.

    c. substance use disorder.

    d. mental disorder.

REFERENCES

American Academy of Pediatrics Committee on Substance Use and Prevention. (2016). Substance use screening, brief intervention, and referral to treatment. *Pediatrics, 138*(1), e20161210.

American Psychiatric Association. (2013). *Diagnostic and statistical manual of mental disorders* (5th ed.). Washington, DC: Author.

Center for Substance Abuse Treatment. (2013). *Enhancing motivation for change in substance abuse treatment.* (Treatment improvement protocol [TIP] Series, No. 35. HHS Publication No. [SMA] 13-4212 [update]). Rockville, MD: Substance Abuse and Mental Health Services Administration.

DiClemente, C. C., Schlundt, D., & Gemmell, L. (2004). Readiness and stages of change in addiction treatment. *American Journal of Addiction, 13*(2), 103-119.

Fiore, M. C., Jaén, C. R., Baker, T. B., Bailey, W.C., Benowitz, N., Curry, S. J., ... Wewers, M. E. (2008). *Treating tobacco use and dependence: 2008 Update.* Rockville, MD: U.S. Department of Health and Human Services.

Folstein, M. F., Folstein, S. E., & McHugh, P. R. (1975). Mini-mental state. A practical method for grading the cognitive state of patients for the clinician. *Journal of Psychiatric Research, 12*(3), 189-198.

Miller, W. R., & Rose, G. S. (2009). Toward a theory of motivational interviewing. *American Psychologist, 64*(6), 527-537.

National Institute on Drug Abuse. (2016a). *Commonly abused drugs charts.* Retrieved from https://www.drugabuse.gov/drugs-abuse/commonly-abused-drugs-charts

National Institute on Drug Abuse. (2016b). *The science of drug abuse and addiction.* Retrieved from https://www.drugabuse.gov/publications/media-guide/science-drug-abuse-addiction-basics

Parran, T. V. (2014). Assessment. In R. K. Reis (Ed.), *The ASAM principles of addiction medicine* (5th ed., pp. 344-352). Philadelphia, PA: Wolters Kluwer.

Substance Abuse and Mental Health Services Administration. (2009). *Treatment improvement protocol (TIP) series, No. 51.* Rockville, MD: Author.

Substance Abuse and Mental Health Services Administration. (2012a). *Results from the 2011 National Survey on Drug Use and Health: Summary of national findings* (NSDUH Series H-44, HHS Publication No. [SMA] 12-4713). Rockville, MD: Author.

Substance Abuse and Mental Health Services Administration. (2012b). *The role of biomarkers in the treatment of alcohol use disorders: 2012 Revision* (Advisory, Volume 11, Issue 2). Rockville, MD: Author.

U.S. Department of Health and Human Services, Office of the Surgeon General. (2016). *Facing addiction in America: The surgeon general's report on alcohol, drugs, and health.* Washington, DC: Author.

Van Ryzin, M. J., Fosco, G. M., & Dishion, T. J. (2012). Family and peer predictors of substance use from early adolescence to early adulthood: An 11-year prospective analysis. *Addictive Behaviors, 37*(12), 1314–1324.

Warner, E., & Lorch, E. (2014). Laboratory diagnosis. In R. K. Reis (Ed.), *The ASAM principles of addiction medicine* (5th ed., pp. 332-343). Philadelphia, PA: Wolters Kluwer.

World Health Organization. (1992). *International classification of diseases and related health problems* (10th revision). Geneva: Author.

Zgierska, A., & Fleming, M. F. (2014). Screening and brief intervention. In R. K. Reis (Ed.), *The ASAM principles of addiction medicine* (5th ed., pp. 295-331). Philadelphia, PA: Wolters Kluwer.

Ziedonis, D.M., Fan, X., Bizamcer, A.N., Wyatt, S.A., Tonelli, M.E. & Selson, D.A. (2014). Co-occuring addiction and psychotic disorders. In R. K. Reis (Ed.), *The ASAM principles of addiction medicine* (5th ed., pp. 1346-1364). Philadelphia, PA: Wolters Kluwer.

CHAPTER 4

TREATMENT OF
SUBSTANCE USE DISORDERS

LEARNING OUTCOME

After completing this chapter, the learner will be able to discuss the best therapy approaches and treatment settings for patients with substance use disorders.

CHAPTER OBJECTIVES

After completing this chapter, the learner will be able to:

1. Review the history of treating patients with substance use disorders.

2. Describe the principles of evidence-based practice for the treatment of substance use disorders.

3. Identify common medications used in the treatment of substance use disorders.

4. Summarize the current behavioral therapy approaches in the treatment of substance use disorders.

INTRODUCTION

Substance use disorders are medical illnesses characterized by evidence of impaired control, social impairment, risky use, and pharmacological criteria. Substance use disorders are classified as mild, moderate, or severe to indicate the level of severity, which is determined by the number of criteria outlined in the 5th edi-

tion of the *Diagnostic and Statistical Manual of Mental Disorders* met by a patient (American Psychiatric Association [APA], 2013). Substance use disorders develop when the "recurrent use of alcohol and/or drugs causes clinically and functionally significant impairment, such as health problems, disability, and failure to meet major responsibilities at work, school, or home" (Substance Abuse and Mental Health Services Administration [SAMHSA], 2015). According to the 2014 National Survey on Drug Use and Health (NSDUH), approximately 22.5 million people aged 12 years or older needed treatment for substance use or dependence (SAMHSA, 2015). Unfortunately, only 4.1 million received treatment (about 5.9% of those needing it). Of the estimated 4.1 million people who received treatment, 2.6 million received treatment at a specialty facility. The most common substances misused were alcohol (15.7 million people), illicit drugs (7.7 million people; see Figure 4-1), and cannabis (4.0 million people).

Treatment of substance use disorders is defined as "a service or set of services that may include medication, counseling, and other supportive services designed to enable an individual to reduce or eliminate alcohol and/or other drug use; address associated physical or mental health problems; and restore the patient to maximum functional ability" (U.S. Department of Health and Human Services [HHS], 2016, p. 4-3).

FIGURE 4-1: ILLICIT DRUG USE

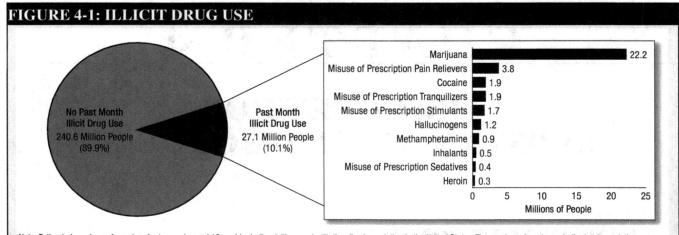

Note: Estimated numbers of people refer to people aged 12 or older in the civilian, noninstitutionalized population in the United States. The numbers do not sum to the total population of the United States because the population for NSDUH does not include people aged 11 years old or younger, people with no fixed household address (e.g., homeless or transient people not in shelters), active-duty military personnel, and residents of institutional group quarters, such as correctional facilities, nursing homes, mental institutions, and long-term care hospitals.

Note: The estimated numbers of current users of different illicit drugs are not mutually exclusive because people could have used more than one type of illicit drug in the past month.

NSDUH = National Survey on Drug Use and Health.

Note. From Center for Behavioral Health Statistics and Quality. (2016). *Key substance use and mental health indicators in the United States: Results from the 2015 National Survey on Drug Use and Health.* (HHS Publication No. [SMA] 16-4984, NSDUH Series H-51). Retrieved from https://www.samhsa.gov/data/sites/default/files/NSDUH-FFR1-2015/NSDUH-FFR1-2015/NSDUH-FFR1-2015.pdf

The treatment setting and approach to the treatment of substance use disorders are shifting from specialty care to primary care practices, especially for patients with disorders falling in the severity level of mild to moderate. Why this change in treatment setting? Research shows that intervening at the earliest possible opportunity before the condition becomes problematic is the most effective way to help someone with a substance use problem (National Institute on Drug Abuse [NIDA], 2014). Screening, brief intervention, and referral to treatment (SBIRT) is an evidenced-based approach to screen for and raise awareness of substance use. The goals of SBIRT intervention are to identify risky drinking and provide early intervention based on level of risk. These interventions are brief and patient centered. The healthcare provider uses concepts of motivational interviewing (MI) to (1) foster the patient's motivation to change, (2) evoke change talk from the patient, and (3) explore and resolve ambivalence discrepancy (Miller & Rollnick, 2013).

The length of treatment also plays a critical role in patient outcomes. Overall, good outcomes are observed, particularly after 90 days of treatment. However, research has shown that beneficial outcomes are closely related to both treatment duration and setting – the longer the duration of treatment in the appropriate setting, the better the outcome. Settings vary and include inpatient, outpatient, residential, community, and office settings. Other related critical factors include patient engagement and participation in treatment (NIDA, 2014). There are three basic approaches to the treatment of substance use disorders: pharmacotherapy, behavioral treatment, and a combination of the two approaches.

HISTORICAL ASPECTS OF TREATMENT

In the 1800s, it was common to make medicines from opium (such as laudanum and paregoric), and in 1832, morphine was extracted from crude opium. Morphine was followed by codeine and the introduction of commercial heroin in 1898. Consumption rapidly escalated until federal laws limited importation of opium, resulting in vast problems with opium smuggling. In 1912, the Hague Treaty, an international agreement to encourage nations to develop stringent laws restricting opioid consumption to medical purposes only, was instituted. In response, formal drug treatment emerged, with clinics operated by police or health departments designed to maintain addicts on morphine. Two years later, the Harrison Act made nonmedical opiate use illegal, representing the beginning of a federal role in addressing substance misuse. With opiate use solely under the control of medical care, it was observed that morphine-addicted patients could be maintained on heroin in a manner permitting them to function in society. However, in 1919, it became illegal to prescribe opioid maintenance when addiction was the patient's sole problem (Musto, 2005).

In the same year, an experiment by the New York City Health Department used heroin to recruit persons addicted to morphine into a 6-week inpatient detoxification and rehabilitation program. This experiment ended after about 1 year when it was observed that even after detoxification was complete, addicts usually relapsed to heroin use, and all clinics were closed by 1925. With the subsequent incarceration of addicts, federal prisons quickly filled, necessitating the building of two opioid hospitals operated by the U.S. Public Health Service to treat addicts (Musto, 2005).

Treatment focusing on abstinence appeared first among organized religion, followed by the proliferation of self-help groups after World War II, permitting individuals using substances to remain in their communities rather than relocating to asylums. Group support was given through structured meetings based on stepwise activities to encourage recovery. Membership in such groups required that individuals publicly identify themselves as an alcoholic or addict and declare their dependence on a "higher power." Alcoholics Anonymous (AA), established in 1935, is the prototype of this approach (Musto, 2005).

In 1937, the Research Council on Problems of Alcohol brought prominent scientists into the study of alcohol-related problems, and in 1939, the book *Alcoholics Anonymous* was published. In 1944, Marty Mann founded the National Committee for Education on Alcoholism, which is now called the National Council on Alcoholism and Drug Dependence. In the 1950s, the National Institute of Mental Health established a special division on alcoholism; the American Medical Association created a special committee to solve the growing problem of alcoholism; AA membership surpassed 90,000; a halfway house movement was founded by the Association of Halfway House Alcoholism Programs of North America; the New York City Medical Society on Alcoholism, today known as the American Society of Addiction Medicine (ASAM), was established; and the Veteran's Health Administration began developing alcoholism treatment units. In the 1960s, alcohol educational programs were developed, the book *The Disease Concept of Alcoholism* was published, and the American Public Health Association adopted an official statement identifying alcoholism as a treatable illness. Federal funding for addiction counseling began, and methadone was introduced in the treatment of narcotic addiction. Insurance companies also began to reimburse for treatment, the National Center for the Prevention and Control of Alcoholism was created within the National Institute of Mental Health, and the Cooperative Commission on the Study of Alcoholism released its report *Alcohol Problems: A Report to the Nation.* In the 1970s, Congress passed the Comprehensive Alcohol Abuse and Alcoholism Prevention,

Treatment, and Rehabilitation Act, which established the National Institute on Alcohol Abuse and Alcoholism (NIAA). The *American Journal of Psychiatry* and *Annals of Internal Medicine* published "Criteria for the Diagnosis of Alcoholism." The Employee Assistance Professional Association was established, along with standards by the Joint Commission on Accreditation of Hospitals for alcoholism treatment programs. The U.S. Food and Drug Administration approved the use of methadone for treating heroin addiction. Fetal alcohol syndrome was described in children born to mothers who used alcohol during pregnancy. In the 1980s, Mothers Against Drunk Driving was formed, Cocaine Anonymous was founded, the National Minimum Drinking Age Act required all states to make the purchase or public possession of alcoholic beverages illegal for anyone under the age of 21, and the American Academy of Psychiatrists in Alcoholism and Addictions was founded. An executive order mandating a Drug-Free Federal Workplace program was also implemented. In the 1990s, Internet-based programs and online recovery support groups and services grew (White, 1998).

Today, emerging technologies are changing how health care is delivered and how treatments are provided. Telehealth and telemedicine are two promising technologies that are changing how assessment and treatment are delivered to patients with substance use disorders. There is hope that now, with the rapid expansion of the Internet and effective strategies and approaches, substance use disorders will be reduced or eliminated.

PRINCIPLES OF EFFECTIVE TREATMENT

The National Institute on Drug Abuse (NIDA) has detailed 13 key principles of effective treatment programs for adults and adolescents with substance use disorders. These principles represent common methods of intervention for patients with substance use disorders and apply regardless of the treatment setting or type of substance use disorder (HHS, 2016; NIDA, 2012, 2014; see Table 4-1).

In addition, *Facing Addiction in America: The Surgeon General's Report on Alcohol, Drugs, and Health* (HHS, 2016) was created in response to the many social and health problems resulting from alcohol and drug misuse in the United States. This report describes a comprehensive approach to addressing substance use problems in the United States. The following subsections describe components of this approach.

Continuum of Care

The continuum of care is an "integrated system of care that guides and tracks a person over time" (HHS, 2016, p. 4-3). It refers to promoting optimum health; addressing individual patient and environmental risk factors; screening for and determining substance use problems early; intervening through medication, counseling, and other supportive services; and providing recovery support.

The American Society of Addiction Medicine (ASAM, 2013) recommends that five broad levels of care be constantly assessed to determine the appropriate level of treatment for each patient. Within a level, the patient may move up or down to receive the necessary intensity of services based on need without increasing the broad level of care. The five broad levels of care are as follows:

- Early interventions
- Outpatient services
- Intensive outpatient/partial hospitalization services
- Residential/inpatient services
- Medically managed, intensive inpatient services

TABLE 4-1: PRINCIPLES OF EFFECTIVE TREATMENT OF SUBSTANCE USE DISORDERS	
1.	Substance use disorders are complex but treatable disorders that affect brain function and behavior.
2.	No single treatment is appropriate for everyone.
3.	Treatment needs to be readily available.
4.	Effective treatment attends to multiple needs of the patient, not just his or her substance misuse.
5.	Remaining in treatment for an adequate period of time is critical.
6.	Behavioral therapies – including individual, family, or group counseling – are the most commonly used forms of treatment for substance use disorders.
7.	Medications are an important element of treatment for many patients, especially when combined with counseling and other behavioral therapies.
8.	A patient's treatment and services plan must be assessed continually and modified as necessary to ensure that it meets his or her changing needs.
9.	Many patients with a substance use disorder also have mental disorders.
10.	Medically assisted detoxification is only the first stage of treatment and by itself does little to change long-term substance misuse.
11.	Treatment does not need to be voluntary to be effective.
12.	Substance use during treatment must be monitored continuously because lapses during treatment do occur.
13.	Treatment programs should test patients for the presence of HIV/AIDS, hepatitis B and C, tuberculosis, and other infectious diseases and should provide targeted risk-reduction counseling, linking patients to prevention and treatment of infection services if necessary.

Note. Adapted from National Institute on Drug Abuse. (2012). *Principles of drug addiction treatment: A research-based guide* (NIH Publication No. 12-4180). Rockville, MD: National Institutes of Health, U.S. Department of Health and Human Services. Retrieved from https://www.drugabuse.gov/publications/principlesdrug-addiction-treatment-research-basedguide-third-edition

The goals of treatment for substance use disorders are similar to those for other chronic illnesses: reduce the major symptoms of the illness; improve overall health, including social functioning; and empower patients through education and counseling to monitor their condition to prevent relapse (ASAM, 2013).

ASAM (2013) developed criteria to determine the needed level of care for the treatment of patients with addiction. Healthcare providers use the criteria to determine placement, continued stay, and transfer or discharge of patients. Six assessment dimensions assist in obtaining a holistic biopsychosocial assessment of a patient with a substance use disorder. The six dimensions are as follows:

• Dimension 1: Acute Intoxication and/or Withdrawal Potential

• Dimension 2: Biomedical Conditions and Complications

• Dimension 3: Emotional, Behavioral, or Cognitive Conditions and Complications

• Dimension 4: Readiness to Change

• Dimension 5: Relapse, Continued Use, or Continued Problem Potential

• Dimension 6: Recovery/Living Environment

(ASAM, n.d.)

Early Intervention

Early intervention services are usually delivered in settings such as school clinics, primary care offices, and outpatient mental health clinics. The patients who benefit most from these services fall in the substance use severity level of mild to moderate. The goals of early intervention are to reduce risks by providing strategies in quitting or reducing unhealthy substance use (SAMHSA, 2016b).

SBIRT, mentioned earlier in the chapter, is an example of an early intervention that research has shown to be effective in reducing or eliminating substance use. Screening using validated tools is the first step of the SBIRT process; such tools include the Alcohol Use Disorder Identification Test (AUDIT), which screens for alcohol use in adults, and the Car, Relax, Alone, Forget, Friends, Trouble (CRAFFT) tool, which screens for substance use in adolescents (SAMHSA, 2016b). Ideally, healthcare providers should screen all patients presenting in primary care, urgent care, psychiatric care, and emergency department settings for substance use; Table 4-2 lists screening tools for use in these settings (NIDA, 2015).

The second step in SBIRT is to provide feedback to patients regarding their level of use relative to safe limits (SAMHSA, 2016b). Brief intervention focuses on increasing insight and awareness regarding substance use and motivation toward behavioral change (see Table 4-3). Motivational interviewing (MI) is a technique or counseling style that research has shown to be effective in reducing ambivalence during brief interventions. MI is a patient-centered approach that assists the patient in discovering his or her desire to change and addressing any ambivalence to change. The counselor works with the patient to assist in making a plan to change. A brief intervention may be all that is needed if patients appear to have only mild substance use problems and if the goal is to prevent more severe problems. Brief interventions can be incorporated into nonspecialist settings such as primary care. These settings may be the most suitable site for patients with mild to moderate substance problems because specialist settings normally are designed for patients

with moderate to severe problems. Spontaneous remission of problematic substance use is not uncommon, and a short intervention may be all that is required. Furthermore, treatment in a primary care or similar setting is less likely to be socially stigmatizing compared with drug treatment settings, and it may also be the ideal location to integrate drug treatment with the treatment of other comorbid health problems.

The last step in the SBIRT process is to refer patients who need more specialized care for their substance use disorder. It is critical that the healthcare provider incorporates strategies to motivate patients to accept the referral and to navigate barriers to the treatment of substance use disorders (HHS, 2016).

Research on the SBIRT approach has shown it to be effective – more so for alcohol use than illicit drug use, for which fewer investigations have been conducted (U.S. Preventive Services Task Force, 2016). Specifically, brief interventions have been shown to be effective in reducing alcohol consumption up to 50% and are just as effective for women and patients from diverse cultures (Gebara, Bhona, Ronzani, Lourenço, & Noto, 2013). However, even though there is a gap in evidence in using brief interventions with adolescents, promising studies support the use of SBIRT in this population (Mitchell, Gryczynski, O'Grady, & Schwartz, 2013; Yuma-Guerrero et al., 2012). For many patients, a brief intervention serves as a good transition to specialist care if more comprehensive assessment and treatment are needed. Other patients whose screening results indicate the high-risk range may need inpatient treatment.

Evidence-Based Medications

Regardless of the substance use disorder, the healthcare provider is expected to offer individualized, evidence-based treatment. The National Registry of Evidence-Based Programs and

TABLE 4-2: SUBSTANCE USE SCREENING TOOLS

Screening Tool	Substance Type		Patient Age		How Tool Is Administered	
	Alcohol	Drugs	Adults	Adolescents	Self-Administered	Clinician-Administered
Prescreen						
NIDA Drug Use Screening Tool: Quick Screen	X	X	X	See APA Adapted NIDA-Modified (NM ASSIST) tools	See APA Adapted NM ASSIST tools	X
CRAFFT (Part A)	X	X		X	X	X
AUDIT-C	X		X		X	X
Opioid Risk Tool		X	X		X	
Full screens						
NIDA Drug Use Screening Tool	X	X	X			X
AUDIT	X		X			X
CAGE-AID	X	X	X			X
CAGE	X		X			X
DAST-10		X	X		X	X
CRAFFT	X	X		X	X	X
DAST-20: Adolescent version		X		X	X	X

NIDA = National Institute on Drug Abuse; APA = American Psychiatric Association; ASSIST = Alcohol, Smoking, and Substance Involvement Screening Test; CRAFFT = Car, Relax, Alone, Forget, Friends, Trouble; AUDIT = Alcohol Use Disorder Identification Test; CAGE-AID = Cut Down, Annoyed, Guilty, Eye Opener, Adapted to Include Drugs; CAGE = Cut Down, Annoyed, Guilty, Eye Opener; DAST-10 = Drug Abuse Screen Test (10-item version); DAST-20 = Drug Abuse Screen Test (20-item version).

Note. From National Institute on Drug Abuse. (2015). *Chart of evidence-based screening tools for adults and adolescents.* Retrieved from https://www.drugabuse.gov/nidamed-medical-health-professionals/tool-resources-your-practice/screening-assessment-drug-testing-resources/chart-evidence-based-screening-tools-adults

TABLE 4-3: COMPONENTS OF BRIEF INTERVENTION

Raise the subject	Ask permission to screen.
Provide feedback	Identify and inform regarding level of risk.
Enhance motivation	Ask, "On a scale of 1 to 10, how ready are you to cut back?"; also ask about patient confidence level and motivation to change.
Negotiate a plan	Encourage a specific plan to reduce or abstain from substance use and/or seek treatment referral.

Note. Western Schools, 2017.

Practices, which can be found on the SAMHSA website, is available to guide the healthcare provider and patient with a substance use disorder about treatment options (SAMHSA, 2016a).

Five medications have been approved by the U.S. Food and Drug Administration (FDA) to treat alcohol and opioid use disorder: buprenorphine (with naloxone or alone), methadone, naltrexone, acamprosate, and disulfiram (see Table 4-4). The FDA-approved medications listed in Table 4-4 have shown safety and effectiveness in improving outcomes for patients with opioid and

continued on page 62

TABLE 4-4: PHARMACOTHERAPIES USED TO TREAT ALCOHOL AND OPIOID USE DISORDERS (1 OF 2)

Medication	Use	Dosage Form	DEA Schedule[a]	Application
Buprenorphine/naloxone	Opioid use disorder	Sublingual film: 2 mg/0.5 mg, 4 mg/1 mg, 8 mg/2 mg, 12 mg/3 mg Sublingual tablet: 1.4 mg/0.36 mg, 2 mg/0.5 mg, 2.9/0.71 mg, 5.7 mg/1.4 mg, 8 mg/2 mg, 8.6 mg/2.1 mg, 11.4 mg/2.9 mg Buccal film: 2.1 mg/0.3 mg, 4.2 mg/0.7 mg, 6.3 mg/1 mg	CIII	Used for detoxification or maintenance of abstinence for individuals aged 16 or older. Physicians who wish to prescribe buprenorphine must obtain a waiver from the Substance Abuse and Mental Health Services Administration (SAMHSA) and be issued an additional registration number by the DEA.
Buprenorphine hydrochloride	Opioid use disorder	Sublingual tablet: 2 mg, 4 mg, 8 mg, 12 mg Probuphine implants: 80 mg × 4 implants for a total of 320 mg	CIII	This formulation is indicated for treatment of opioid dependence and is preferred for induction. However, it is considered the preferred formulation for pregnant patients, patients with hepatic impairment, and patients with sensitivity to naloxone. It is also used for initiating treatment in patients transferring from methadone, in preference to products containing naloxone, because of the risk of precipitating withdrawal in these patients. It is for those already stable on a low to moderate dose of buprenorphine. The administration of the implant dosage form requires specific training, and the implant must be surgically inserted and removed.

TABLE 4-4: PHARMACOTHERAPIES USED TO TREAT ALCOHOL AND OPIOID USE DISORDERS (2 OF 2)

Methadone	Opioid use disorder	Tablet: 5 mg, 10 mg Tablet for suspension: 40 mg Oral concentrate: 10 mg/mL Oral solution: 5 mg/5 mL, 10 mg/5 mL Injection: 10 mg/mL	CII	Methadone used for the treatment of opioid addiction in detoxification or maintenance programs shall be dispensed only by Opioid Treatment Programs (OTPs) certified by SAMHSA and approved by the designated state authority. Under federal regulations, it can be used in patients under age 18 at the discretion of an OTP physician.
Naltrexone	Opioid use disorder, alcohol use disorder	Tablets: 25 mg, 50 mg, 100 mg Extended-release injectable suspension: 380 mg/vial	Not scheduled under the Controlled Substances Act	Provided by prescription; naltrexone blocks opioid receptors, reduces cravings, and diminishes the rewarding effects of alcohol and opioids. Extended-release injectable naltrexone is recommended to prevent relapse to opioids or alcohol. The prescriber need not be a physician but must be licensed and authorized to prescribe by the state.
Acamprosate	Alcohol use disorder	Delayed-release tablet: 333 mg	Not scheduled under the Controlled Substances Act	Provided by prescription; acamprosate is used in the maintenance of alcohol abstinence. The prescriber need not be a physician, but must be licensed and authorized to prescribe by the state.
Disulfiram	Alcohol use disorder	Tablet: 250 mg, 500 mg	Not scheduled under the Controlled Substances Act	When taken in combination with alcohol, disulfiram causes severe physical reactions, including nausea, flushing, and heart palpitations. The knowledge that such a reaction is likely if alcohol is consumed acts as a deterrent to drinking.

DEA = Drug Enforcement Agency; CIII = Class III drug (indicates that drug has a high potential for abuse but less than that of Class I or Class II drugs); CII= Class II drug (indicates that drug has a high potential for abuse).

aThe DEA Schedule is a mandatory registration of controlled substances resulting in a "closed system" for distribution of these substances.

Note. Adapted from U.S. Department of Health and Human Services, Office of the Surgeon General. (2016). *Facing addiction in America: The surgeon general's report on alcohol, drugs, and health.* Washington, DC: Author. Retrieved from https://addiction.surgeongeneral.gov/surgeon-generals-report.pdf

alcohol use disorders. Only trained healthcare providers should prescribe these medications because of the potential for misuse and overdose. There are no medications approved to treat marijuana, amphetamine, or cocaine use disorders. The following sections present an overview of evidence-based medications and medication-assisted treatment for substance use disorders.

Medication-Assisted Treatment for Opioid Use Disorder

Methadone is a widely used drug for stabilization and maintenance of patients with opioid dependence. It is a long-acting opioid agonist that substitutes for the shorter-acting heroin. It is a broadly supported approach that permits patients who are opioid dependent to participate normally in their daily lives. Methadone maintenance programs may be located within comprehensive drug treatment centers, primary care clinics, or social service agencies. Regardless of location, treatment programs that include methadone dispensing are meticulously regulated by the federal government and state governments. Opioid treatment programs must be certified by SAMHSA and registered with the U.S. Drug Enforcement Administration (DEA). Federal eligibility requires at least 1 year of opioid use and current evidence of opioid dependence. However, exceptions to eligibility criteria are made if the patient is pregnant or recently discharged from a controlled facility, such as prison.

Methadone maintenance consists of three phases:

1. Stabilization, wherein patients adjust to their methadone dose (doses of 20 to 30 mg daily, gradually increased to 80 mg or more per day until craving and opioid misuse are reduced)

2. Treatment planning, during which other problems affected by drug use are addressed, such as employment and physical health

3. Continued methadone at the maintenance dose, with few other services associated with the previous phase

During the first phase, it is important to have daily contact under observation and then taper to once weekly in the maintenance phase.

Buprenorphine is a partial opioid agonist – it binds to and activates opioid receptors but is less intense than full agonists. It has a lower risk of overdose and a lower potential for misuse, but if used with tranquilizers and/or alcohol, there is a greater potential for overdose and misuse. The Comprehensive Addiction and Recovery Act of 2016 expanded buprenorphine prescribing privileges to nurse practitioners and physician assistants (Fornili & Fogger, 2017). This increase in providers facilitates greater access to the treatment of substance misuse.

Naltrexone is a long-acting opioid antagonist that blocks the effects of opioids to extinguish the conditioned cues that encourage drug use. It can also reduce alcohol craving. It is nonaddicting and has few adverse effects. Naltrexone is not a controlled substance and can be prescribed or administered by any physician, nurse practitioner, or physician assistant with prescribing authority. Naltrexone has two formulations: oral and extended-release injectable. The extended-release injectable is administered monthly and can be used in patients with poor compliance with oral naltrexone (HHS, 2016).

Medication-Assisted Treatment for Alcohol Use Disorder

Disulfiram interferes with the normal metabolism of alcohol and is perhaps the oldest drug used for alcohol treatment. When alcohol consumption follows disulfiram administration, patients experience uncomfortable nausea, headaches, dizziness, flushing, and palpitations. Liver injury and liver failure may also occur.

Although it is rare today, disulfiram-alcohol reactions have resulted in death (HHS, 2016).

Naltrexone is an opioid antagonist but can also counteract some of the pleasurable aspects of drinking. It comes in two formulations, as mentioned earlier: oral and extended-release injectable (HHS, 2016).

Acamprosate was designed to reduce alcohol craving. It helps to normalize brain function by affecting the activity of the neurotransmitters gamma-aminobutyric acid and glutamate, helping to reduce the symptoms of craving that can lead to a relapse. When paired with behavioral interventions, acamprosate can be effective in reducing relapse (Jonas et al., 2014).

Behavioral Therapies

Behavioral therapies constitute the bulk of treatment for substance use disorders and include cognitive-behavioral therapy, motivational interventions, and contingency management. Although behavioral therapy is not typically initiated during the detoxification period, if this period is extended, behavioral therapy can and should be initiated. Behavioral therapies are an important complement to pharmacotherapy because the strategies learned assist the patient in adhering to the medication regime and preventing substance use relapse (Dugosh et al., 2016).

The following sections describe behavioral therapies that research has shown to be effective in addressing substance use disorders.

Cognitive-Behavioral Therapy

Cognitive-behavioral therapy (CBT) may be the most researched behavioral therapy intervention. CBT is based on social learning theory and emphasizes modification of the patient's thoughts and behaviors. Techniques employed by the healthcare provider assist the patient in modifying dysfunctional thoughts that cause maladap-

tive behavior patterns (NIDA, 2012). The goal is to encourage abstinence by helping patients to learn and master effective coping skills that, in turn, help them to believe they can resist relapsing to substance use. The focus is on an exploration of the positive and negative consequences of substance use. This approach is the foundation for relapse prevention, where patients are taught the skills needed to prevent a return to substance use after treatment. CBT usually involves 12 to 24 weekly individual sessions.

Contingency Management

Contingency management is an approach that emphasizes rewards for positive behavior versus punishment for negative behavior. The basic principle of this approach is to learn new behaviors and change old behaviors by using positive reinforcement. Abstinence is reinforced with vouchers that can be redeemed for various desirable services or cash. Patients are rewarded if they exhibit the desired behaviors, such as drug-free urine tests or participation in therapy activities. This approach has been effective, with high rates of abstinence (Higgins, Heil, & Sigmon, 2013). Abstinence has been shown to occur regardless of the cash value of the vouchers, implying that it is the reinforcement that is important, not the actual voucher.

The community reinforcement approach plus vouchers is an intensive approach that provides incentives and reinforcers to patients who follow the program. This program is delivered over 24 weeks and requires the patient to attend one to two counseling sessions each week. These sessions focus on improving relationships, reconstructing social activities, and establishing a safety network to support recovery. Research has shown an overall improvement in psychosocial functioning and increased abstinence with this approach (NIDA, 2012).

Motivational Enhancement Therapy

Motivational enhancement therapy (MET) uses MI techniques to assist patients in resolving ambivalence to change. MET works by helping patients to reflect on their current functioning by promoting empathy and increasing patient awareness of the discrepancy between their goals and their unhealthy behavior. This method helps to avoid confrontation and supports self-efficacy to encourage motivation to change (Burlew, Montgomery, Kosinski, & Forcehimes, 2013; NIDA, 2012). MET and CBT are often used in combination, and research has found the combination to be effective in promoting behavior change (NIDA, 2012).

The Matrix Model

The matrix model is a behavioral treatment that has various components of behavioral interventions and includes relapse prevention, family therapy, group therapy, drug education, and self-help. The sessions are delivered over 16 weeks. This model has shown effectiveness in reducing not only substance misuse but also associated risky behaviors (NIDA, 2012).

Twelve-Step Facilitation Therapy

Twelve-step facilitation therapy (TSF) is based on individual therapy delivered over 12 weeks and helps to prepare individuals to become engaged in a 12-step group such as AA or Narcotics Anonymous (NA). Twelve-step groups usually follow the same format and guidelines of "working through the steps." Three key ideas emphasized in these programs are as follows:

- Acceptance – Individuals realize that their substance use is out of their control and that abstinence is the best alternative.

- Surrender – Individuals give the problem and themselves to a higher power.

- Participation – Individuals take part in a proven pathway to recovery.

Evidence shows that TSF programs can be effective, especially in the areas of AA participation and developing a network of abstinent friends (Litt, Kadden, Kabela-Cormier, & Petry, 2009).

Family-Based Treatment

Family behavior therapy is an evidence-based therapeutic approach that not only addresses substance use but also family conflict. It is delivered over 20 sessions that focus on setting behavioral goals and providing family members with the skills needed to improve overall functioning (NIDA, 2012).

Behavioral couples therapy is based on a daily sobriety contract between the affected patient and his or her spouse. Research has shown that this approach is effective in sustaining abstinence and improving the couple's relationship; it can also reduce the social costs of substance use and the incidence of intimate partner violence (Winters, Fals-Stewart, O'Farrell, Birchler, & Kelley, 2002).

Strategies to Reduce Harm

Harm-reduction strategies have been developed to help people who are not yet ready to participate in treatment. The goal of a harm-reduction approach is to reduce the negative effects of substance use. Examples include needle-exchange programs to reduce the incidence of HIV, programs that substitute methadone for heroin to facilitate healthier social functioning, and drinking-control strategies (e.g., avoiding heavy-drinking activities or situations) to control alcohol intake. An example of a newer harm-reduction strategy is the use of naloxone to reverse the effects of a potential lethal opioid overdose. As mentioned earlier, naloxone is an opioid-antagonist medication that has been approved by the FDA to reverse opioid overdose and comes in injectable and nasal spray forms (Hawk, Vaca, & D'Onofrio, 2015).

Treatment Settings

Treatment may take place in inpatient, outpatient, or residential settings. Within each setting, any of the previously discussed therapies can be used.

Inpatient

Inpatient hospitalization is the most intensive treatment, with around-the-clock supervision and treatment by a interdisciplinary team. These patients may require withdrawal management and treatment of co-occurring medical conditions (Millette & Cort, 2013).

Alcohol withdrawal syndrome (AWS) can be difficult for the nurse to recognize and manage. AWS can range from mild to severe. Symptoms of withdrawal can appear within the first 6 to 24 hours after the last drink. Delirium tremens and alcohol withdrawal seizures can be fatal if not recognized early and treated.

The Clinical Institute Withdrawal Assessment for Alcohol-Revised (CIWA-AR) has been recognized as the gold standard for patients admitted to drug treatment facilities. There has been inconsistency in managing patients in the acute setting. The Glasgow Modified Alcohol Withdrawal Score (GMAWS) was developed to assist the nurse and provides a simplified score for assessing the level of AWS and the associated vitamin deficiency of thiamine (vitamin B1) in patients who chronically misuse alcohol. The scale includes dosing for oral diazepam and intravenous diazepam when indicated based on the patient's level of withdrawal. When administering diazepam, it is critical that the nurse monitor the patient closely for oversedation. Other oral benzodiazepine medications include lorazepam and chlordiazepoxide (recommended for outpatient treatment in the community; Benson, McPherson, & Reid, 2012).

Residential

Residential treatment involves a live-in facility with 24-hour supervision. These settings use a structured living environment as an integral part of patients' treatment plans. The primary advantage of these settings is that patients are away from their drug-related environments. The best known residential treatment model is the therapeutic community (TC). Typically, residents will stay between 6 to 12 months. In this model, residents learn how to resocialize using the program's entire community, including the other residents and staff members, as an active component of treatment. Treatment is highly structured, and the focus is on the patient's development of personal accountability and responsibility (NIDA, 2012).

Outpatient

Outpatient treatment can be more or less intensive and may include medications for detoxification or maintenance. Less intensive outpatient treatment uses various individual, group, or family counseling and therapeutic techniques, such as skills training, and educational support (including drug-free approaches). This is the least standardized treatment approach. Most of these programs involve seeing patients only once or twice weekly and use some combination of counseling strategies, social work, and 12-step or self-help meetings.

Intensive outpatient treatment, also known as partial hospitalization, typically involves a minimum of 9 hours of weekly attendance, usually in increments of 3 to 8 hours per day for 5 to 7 days per week, typically Monday through Friday. This setting is often recommended for patients in the early stages of treatment or those transitioning from residential or inpatient hospital settings.

Telehealth is an emerging outpatient technology that has changed how health care is being delivered. This is a growing field of health care. Interventions can be delivered by a variety of media, including smartphones, the Internet, videoconferencing, wireless communications, and streaming media (HSS, 2016). There are many advantages to technology-based interventions. They can improve access to the underserved, including those in rural areas, and therefore reach more people, and they may not require the patient to leave home to receive the services. Research on the effectiveness of this delivery method is now emerging, but at this time, telehealth techniques can only be considered as "promising." Table 4-5 lists examples of technology-assisted interventions.

Relapse Prevention and Recovery

Recovery Support Services

SAMHSA (2012) defines recovery as "a process of change through which individuals improve their health and wellness, live a self-directed life, and strive to reach their full potential." The four major dimensions that support a patient in recovery are one's health, home, purpose, and community. The guiding principles of recovery are that it

- emerges from hope;
- is patient-driven;
- occurs via many pathways;
- is holistic;
- is supported by peers and allies;
- is supported through relationship and social networks;
- is culturally based and influenced;
- is supported by addressing trauma;
- involves individual, family, and community strengths and responsibility; and
- is based on respect.

Recovery support services help to engage and support patients during treatment and provide ongoing support after treatment (HHS, 2016). These services are delivered by trained individuals such as case managers and recovery coaches, who also can be peers. These trained individuals assist the patient in navigating systems of care and assist with integrating the patient back into the community without substance use.

CASE STUDY 4-1

Kevin is a 21-year-old male college student who is living away from his family for the first time. He attends a major university that is known for student partying. He plays baseball as a club sport.

Kevin returns home during his school break and goes to see the family nurse practitioner for his annual physical examination. During

TABLE 4-5: EXAMPLES OF TECHNOLOGY-ASSISTED INTERVENTIONS

Intervention	Overview
Addiction–Comprehensive Health Enhancement Support System (A-CHESS)	Smartphone-based application offering monitoring, information, communication, and support services
HealthCall	60 days of automated telephone calls using interactive voice response (IVR)
CBT4CBT	For self-monitoring of alcohol use and other health-related behaviors; for use as an adjunct to motivational interviewing
Reduce Your Use	Self-guided, web-based treatment program for cannabis use disorder based on cognitive, motivational, and behavioral principles

Note. Adapted from U.S. Department of Health and Human Services, Office of the Surgeon General. (2016). *Facing addiction in America: The surgeon general's report on alcohol, drugs, and health.* Washington, DC: Author. Retrieved from https://addiction.surgeongeneral.gov/surgeon-generals-report.pdf

the visit, Kevin describes drinking alcohol two to three times a week with friends on Thursday through Saturday nights. He admits to drinking five to six drinks a night when out with friends. He describes occasionally having more than seven drinks in one night. He has experienced having a hangover that prevented him from making his 8 a.m. class on more than one occasion, and he feels guilty for missing his class. He has to ask friends for notes to make up for the lecture content and assignments that he has missed.

Kevin denies drinking in the mornings. However, when he gets really drunk, he cannot remember all of the things he did the night before. He does describe getting into one fight due to drinking alcohol during high school, but no similar events have occurred in the past year. No one at college has spoken to him or expressed concern about the amount of alcohol he is consuming. He states that all of his friends have the same drinking habits.

The nurse practitioner begins the SBIRT process with an alcohol screening. Kevin's score on the Alcohol Use Disorder Identification Test (AUDIT) tool is 12, placing him in the at-risk range. His past medical history is unremarkable. He has been healthy, but recently he has noticed that his blood pressure has been high when he has checked it at the local drug store. The nurse practitioner checks Kevin's vital signs today, and they are within normal limits, including his blood pressure. Kevin's social history is pertinent for parents who are divorced because his father "became violent" when he drank alcohol. Kevin admits that he does not want to become like his father and develop a drinking problem.

Questions

1. What is the nurse practitioner's first step in addressing Kevin's substance use?

2. What is the nurse practitioner's role in reviewing Kevin's substance use with him?

3. Which tools can the nurse practitioner utilize to assess Kevin's level of motivation, confidence, and readiness to change his alcohol use?

4. If Kevin becomes confrontational about his drinking, what is the nurse practitioner's best approach?

5. Following the brief intervention, what is the nurse practitioner's next step in the SBIRT process?

Answers

1. Begin the brief intervention process by raising the subject: Ask Kevin for his permission to discuss the AUDIT score with him.

2. Provide feedback. Explain to Kevin that the AUDIT score indicates that he is in the at-risk range. Explain the health risks associated with drinking, such as aggression, irrational behavior, memory loss, premature aging, frequent colds, cancer of the throat and mouth, weakening of the heart muscle, heart failure, anemia, liver damage, trembling hands and numbness in the fingers, ulcer, and inflammation of the pancreas.

3. The nurse practitioner could use a scale to assess motivation by asking the question, "On a scale of 0 to 10, how ready are you to cut back your usage?" The nurse should assess readiness, motivation, and confidence to make a change.

4. Roll with the resistance. Help Kevin to see a discrepancy between his stated goals and his current behavior. Explore with Kevin the things that he likes about drinking and the things that he does not like about drinking.

5. Schedule a follow-up appointment to monitor Kevin's progress with his stated goals. It is important to have a plan for follow-up. Identify supports that he has to follow through with his plan to reduce or stop drinking alcohol. If Kevin shows a lack of

progress in meeting his goals, the intensity of services may need to change to outpatient treatment.

SUMMARY

In 2015, only 5.9% of individuals in the United States needing treatment for substance use disorders received it. Of the 5.9%, more than 2.86 million received treatment at a specialty facility, with alcohol being the most common substance misused (SAMHSA, 2015). Treatment of substance use disorders comprises pharmacotherapy and behavioral therapy and should include continuing care after discharge from the formal treatment setting. Providing harm-reduction interventions to reduce the adverse effects of substances, such as the use of naloxone, reduces the risk of harm when the patient is not quite ready to begin to address his or her substance use disorder.

There are many settings, including primary care, where behavioral therapies can be delivered. Using evidence-based strategies will ensure better outcomes for the patient with a substance use problem. The best treatment outcomes most likely will involve a combination of drug therapy and psychosocial interventions. All treatment should be followed by continuing care and follow-up.

Research has identified effective strategies to treat patients with substance use disorders, but there remains a shortage of healthcare professionals to deliver the appropriate interventions. Including substance use education in healthcare training programs is the first step in addressing this workforce shortage. The use of technology to deliver interventions to patients in remote areas and provide services that reach a larger number of individuals with substance use disorders shows promise. Screening all patients will identify those at risk earlier, with the hope

that interventions will be utilized so that substance use problems will not progress further into becoming substance use disorders.

EXAM QUESTIONS

CHAPTER 4
Questions 18–23

Note: Choose the one option that BEST answers each question.

18. Technology-assisted interventions used for patients with substance use disorders are

    a. supported by large-scale research studies.

    b. promising treatment options.

    c. designed to reach a limited number of patients.

    d. inappropriate for patients with mild substance use problems.

19. Which patients are targeted for screening of substance use disorders in primary healthcare settings?

    a. All patients

    b. Only patients with a known problem of substance use

    c. Only at-risk patients

    d. Only patients the provider thinks are using substances

20. In the treatment of patients with an opioid use disorder, naltrexone

    a. does not decrease cravings for alcohol.

    b. is addictive.

    c. can be prescribed by a physician or nurse practitioner.

    d. is a controlled substance.

21. Disulfiram's mode of action is to

    a. interfere with the normal metabolism of alcohol.

    b. block the euphoric effects of opioids.

    c. reduce cannabis withdrawal symptoms.

    d. control the anxiety and agitation seen with cocaine dependence.

22. Behavioral therapy for patients with substance use problems is used appropriately

    a. if limited to a group of individuals.

    b. if more than one session is required.

    c. for a limited number of used drugs.

    d. in conjunction with pharmacological treatment.

23. The use of cognitive-behavioral therapy in treating substance use disorders

    a. is an intervention that has been highly researched.

    b. is not as effective as other therapies.

    c. cannot be combined with other treatment.

    d. involves long-term therapy of 12 months or greater to be effective.

REFERENCES

American Psychiatric Association. (2013). *Diagnostic and statistical manual of mental disorders* (5th ed.). Arlington, VA: Author.

American Society of Addiction Medicine. (n.d.). *What is the ASAM criteria?* Retrieved from http://www.asam.org/quality-practice/ guidelines-and-consensus-documents/the-asam-criteria/about

American Society of Addiction Medicine. (2013). *The ASAM criteria: Treatment criteria for addictive, substance-related, and co-occurring conditions.* North Bethesda, MD: Author. Retrieved from http://www. asam.org/quality-practice/guidelines-and-consensus-documents/the-asam-criteria/text

Benson, G., McPherson, A., & Reid, S. (2012). An alcohol withdrawal tool for use in hospitals. *Nursing Times, 108*(26), 15-17.

Burlew, A. K., Montgomery, L., Kosinski, A. S., & Forcehimes, A. A. (2013). Does treatment readiness enhance the response of African American substance users to motivational enhancement therapy? *Psychology of Addictive Behaviors, 27*(3), 744-753.

Center for Behavioral Health Statistics and Quality. (2016). *Key substance use and mental health indicators in the United States: Results from the 2015 National Survey on Drug Use and Health* (HHS Publication No. [SMA] 16-4984, NSDUH Series H-51). Retrieved from https://www.samhsa.gov/data/sites/ default/files/NSDUH-FFR1-2015/NSDUH-FFR1-2015/NSDUH-FFR1-2015.pdf

Dugosh, K., Abraham, A., Seymour, B., McLoyd, K., Chalk, M., & Fetinger, D. (2016). A systematic review on the use of psychosocial interventions in conjunction with medications for the treatment of opioid addiction. *Journal of Addiction Medicine, 10*(2), 93-103. doi:10.1097/ADM.0000000000000193

Fornili, K., & Fogger, S. (2017). Nurse practitioner prescriptive authority for buprenorphine: From DATA 2000 to CARA. *Journal of Addictions Nursing, 28*(1), 43-48.

Gebara, C. F. de P., Bhona, F. M. de C., Ronzani, T. M., Lourenço, L. M., & Noto, A. R. (2013). Brief intervention and decrease of alcohol consumption among women: A systematic review. *Substance Abuse Treatment, Prevention, and Policy, 8*, 31. doi:10.1186/1747-597X-8-31

Hawk, K. F., Vaca, F. E., & D'Onofrio, G. (2015). Reducing fatal opioid overdose: Prevention, treatment and harm reduction strategies. *Yale Journal of Biology and Medicine, 88*(3), 235-245.

Higgins, S. T., Heil, S. H., & Sigmon, S. C. (2013). Voucher-based contingency management in the treatment of substance use disorders. In G. J. Madden, W. V. Dube, T. D. Hackenberg, G. P. Hanley, & K. A. Lattal (Eds.), *APA handbook of behavior analysis. Vol. 2: Translating principles into practice* (pp. 481-500). Washington, DC: American Psychological Association.

Jonas, D. E., Amick, H. R., Feltner, C., Bobashev, G., Thomas, K., Wines, R., & Garbutt, J. C. (2014). Pharmacotherapy for adults with alcohol use disorders in outpatient settings: A systematic review and meta-analysis. *Journal of the American Medical Association, 311*(18), 1889-1900.

Litt, M. D., Kadden, R. M., Kabela-Cormier, E., & Petry, N. M. (2009). Changing network support for drinking: Network support project 2-year follow-up. *Journal of Consulting and Clinical Psychology, 77*(2), 229-242.

Miller, W., & Rollnick, S. (2013). *Motivational interviewing: Helping people change* (3rd ed.). New York, NY: Guilford Press.

Millette, S., & Cort, B. (2013). *Treatment for substance use disorders – The continuum of care.* National Partnership on Alcohol Misuse and Crime. Retrieved from http://www.alcoholandcrime.org/the-voice/issues/jun13/Continuum-of-Care-The-Voice-June2013.pdf

Mitchell, S. G., Gryczynski, J., O'Grady, K. E., & Schwartz, R. P. (2013). SBIRT for adolescent drug and alcohol use: Current status and future directions. *Journal of Substance Abuse Treatment, 44*(5), 463-472.

Musto, D. (2005). Historical perspectives. In J. H. Lowinson, P. Ruiz, R. B. Millman, & J. G. Langrod (Eds.), *Substance abuse: A comprehensive textbook* (4th ed., pp. 1-15). Philadelphia, PA: Lippincott Williams & Wilkins.

National Institute on Drug Abuse. (2012). *Principles of drug addiction treatment: A research-based guide* (NIH Publication No. 12-4180). Rockville, MD: National Institutes of Health, U.S. Department of Health and Human Services. Retrieved from https://www.drugabuse.gov/publications/principles-drug-addiction-treatment-research-based-guide-third-edition

National Institute on Drug Abuse. (2014). *Principles of adolescent use disorder treatment: A research-based guide* (NIH Publication No. 14-7953). Rockville, MD: National Institutes of Health, U.S. Department of Health and Human Services.

National Institute on Drug Abuse. (2015). *Chart of evidence-based screening tools for adults and adolescents.* Retrieved from https://www.drugabuse.gov/nidamed-medical-health professionals/tool-resources-your-practice/screening-assessment-drug-testing-resources/chart-evidence-based-screening-tools-adults

Substance Abuse and Mental Health Services Administration. (2012). *SAMHSA's working definition of recovery: 10 guiding principles of recovery.* Rockville, MD: Author.

Substance Abuse and Mental Health Services Administration. (2015). *Substance use disorders.* Retrieved from https://www.samhsa.gov/disorders/substance-use

Substance Abuse and Mental Health Services Administration. (2016a). *National registry of evidence-based programs and practices* (NREPP). Retrieved from https://www.samhsa.gov/nrepp

Substance Abuse and Mental Health Services Administration. (2016b). *Screening, brief intervention, and referral to treatment (SBIRT).* Retrieved from https://www.samhsa.gov/sbirt

U.S. Department of Health and Human Services, Office of the Surgeon General. (2016). *Facing addiction in America: The surgeon general's report on alcohol, drugs, and health.* Washington, DC: Author. Retrieved from https://addiction.surgeongeneral.gov/surgeon-generals-report.pdf

U.S. Preventive Services Task Force. (2016). *Final research plan: Unhealthy alcohol use in adolescents and adults, including pregnant women: Screening and behavioral counseling interventions.* Retrieved from https://www.uspreventiveservicestaskforce. org/Page/Document/final-research-plan/ unhealthy-alcohol-use-in-adolescents-and-adults-including-pregnant-women-screening-and-behavioral-counseling-interventions

White, W. (1998). *Slaying the dragon: The history of addiction treatment and recovery in America.* Bloomington, IL: Chestnut Health Systems.

Winters, J., Fals-Stewart, W., O'Farrell, T. J., Birchler, G. R., & Kelley, M. L. (2002). Behavioral couples therapy for female substance-abusing patients: Effects on substance use and relationship adjustment. *Journal of Consulting and Clinical Psychology, 70*(2), 344-355.

Yuma-Guerrero, P. J., Lawson K. A., Velasquez, M. M., von Sternberg, K., Maxson, T., & Garcia, N. (2012). Screening, brief intervention, and referral for alcohol use in adolescents: A systematic review. *Pediatrics, 130*(1), 115-122.

CHAPTER 5

TOBACCO USE DISORDERS

LEARNING OUTCOME

After completing this chapter, the learner will be able to describe evidence-based screening and treatment strategies for patients with tobacco use disorders.

CHAPTER OBJECTIVES

After completing this chapter, the learner will be able to:

1. Describe the epidemiology and etiology of tobacco use and tobacco use disorders.

2. Discuss the health effects of tobacco use and nicotine withdrawal.

3. Explain appropriate screening and treatment strategies for patients with tobacco use disorders.

4. Discuss tobacco use in special populations of patients.

INTRODUCTION

Cigarette smoking is the leading cause of preventable death and disability in the United States, and the human and financial costs are staggering. From 1965 to 2014, more than 20 million people died in the United States from tobacco-related illnesses (U.S. Department of Health and Human Services [HHS], 2014). For every such death, at least 30 people develop tobacco-related disease, resulting in more than

$150 billion in lost productivity and healthcare costs of $170 billion annually from direct use of tobacco and indirect exposure to tobacco smoke (Centers for Disease Control and Prevention [CDC], 2016c). If current trends in the United States continue, estimates suggest that 5.6 million youth under the age of 18 will die prematurely from tobacco-related causes (HHS, 2014).

For the past century, cigarettes have been very efficient nicotine-delivery devices. Tobacco products contain nicotine, a highly addictive substance, and up to 7,000 other chemicals, some of them known carcinogens (HHS, 2014). In recent years, the landscape of use has been changing with the development and marketing of tobacco products other than conventional cigarettes. Although conventional cigarettes remain the most commonly used form of tobacco, their usage has declined in recent years (CDC, 2016a). However, both exclusive and dual use (multiple products) of roll-your-own and smokeless tobacco, cigars, pipes, and electronic smoking devices have increased (Wang, Kenemer, Tynan, Singh, & King, 2016). Tobacco products in today's marketplace include

- combustible cigarettes, which can be conventional or roll-your-own;

- cigars (small, large, or cigarillos);

- pipes;

- bidis;

- hookahs;

- smokeless tobacco (chew, dip, snus, or snuff); and

- newer electronic smoking devices (electronic cigarettes, vapes, and heat-not-burn cigarettes).

The *Healthy People 2010* goal was to decrease the prevalence of cigarette smoking to less than 12% in the United States. This was not met and was therefore retained in *Healthy People 2020* (Jamal et al., 2016). Unfortunately, current data indicate that the target will once again not be met. In 2015, 15.1% of U.S. adults were current cigarette smokers, compared with 20.9% in 2005. Although this represents a decline, there is concern that persistent disparities in smoking rates among subgroups of the population have contributed to keeping prevalence rates above the expected target. For example, rates for persons with psychological distress remain alarmingly high at more than 40% (Jamal et al., 2016).

HISTORY

Tobacco *(Nicotiana tobacum)* was first used in the Americas by the pre-Columbians for religious ceremonies (Ravenholt, 1990). In the United States, the first successful crop was cultivated in Virginia in the early 17th century. Initially, the most common method of use was smokeless tobacco, specifically snuff and chewing tobacco. Smoking cigarettes is a relatively recent 20th-century phenomenon linked to industrialized production in the early 1900s and mass product distribution. Smoking rates rose quickly during the first half of the century until 1964, when Surgeon General Luther Terry released a startling report linking smoking to lung cancer (HHS, 2014; U.S. Department of Health, Education, and Welfare [HEW], 1964).

More recently, the skillful marketing and product-development techniques employed by the tobacco industry have colluded to maintain high rates of both tobacco use and youth initiation. In 1999, several states brought a lawsuit against the larger tobacco companies to recoup the costs of treating the health consequences of tobacco use (Jones & Silvestri, 2010). The industry settled out of court in what has been called the Master Settlement Agreement, which provided significant monetary compensation and public access to industry documents (see Truth Tobacco Industry Documents in the Resources section at the end of this course). The settlement monies were intended for use by the states to help fund tobacco control and treatment efforts.

EPIDEMIOLOGY

Prevalence

Cigarette smoking is one of the substances first tried by youth age 18 and younger (Miech, Johnston, O'Malley, Bachman, & Schulenberg, 2016), with at least 80% initiating use at or before the age of 18 (Benowitz, 2010). Cigarette smoking is the most common method of tobacco use, with less than 10% of adult and adolescents using cigars, pipes, and smokeless tobacco products; however, electronic cigarette use has increased significantly in recent years and in 2014 surpassed conventional cigarette use (CDC, 2016b; HHS, 2016). This trend started to reverse slightly in 2015. These data underscore the vulnerability of youth to nicotine addiction. Adolescents are particularly vulnerable to the effects of nicotine, the substance in tobacco that is highly addictive (Leventhal et al., 2015). Nicotine changes the brain levels of dopamine and other neurotransmitters, producing pleasure and mood alteration. The developing brain is particularly vulnerable to these effects (HHS, 2014).

Significant disparities exist in the prevalence rate of cigarette smoking in the United States, which are most pronounced between states. A plausible explanation is related to variation in state tobacco control policies (smoke-free laws, tobacco taxes, and access to treatment). Prevalence rates for any form of tobacco use in 2014 ranged from a low of 11.3% in Utah to 32.2% in West Virginia. Generally, tobacco use is highest among men and among Indian and Alaskan Natives. The lowest rates of smoking are among Asian and Hispanic populations (Nguyen, Marshall, Brown, & Neff, 2016). Significant variations in use by sex and ethnicity based on the type of tobacco used, along with cultural variations, are also noted.

Tobacco use prevalence also differs based on socioeconomic status, education, and other variables. A high prevalence of smoking is found among adults who have only a general educational development degree and those who live below the poverty level. Additional groups experiencing disproportionately high rates of tobacco use include veterans and active military; people who identify as lesbian, gay, bisexual, or transgender; those with disabilities; and people living with HIV or mental illness (CDC, 2016a).

Nicotine: An Addictive Chemical

Nicotine is the drug that causes tobacco to be addictive. It is a highly addictive substance that crosses the blood-brain barrier and causes a cascade of neurobiological effects resulting in a sense of well-being, reduced stress, and enhanced concentration. The drug is readily absorbed by the brain, spleen, and liver and primarily metabolized in the liver. The nicotine molecule is shaped like the neurotransmitter acetylcholine and rapidly binds to the acetylcholine receptors, which are involved in muscle movement, respiration, heart rate, learning, and memory. Most importantly, acetylcholine and its receptors also cause the release of other neurotransmitters and hormones, specifically dopamine. Dopamine affects the brain pathways

that control reward, pleasure, and motivation. Changes in dopamine levels, both stimulation from nicotine exposure and subsequent withdrawal effects, play a critical role in the development of chemical addiction (Benowitz, 2010).

Within seconds of cigarette inhalation, symptoms of pleasure and increased energy are experienced. This leads to a positive-reinforcement effect of the drug. Typically, a cigarette user will take 10 puffs during a period of 5 minutes in an attempt to continue the drug's pleasurable effects and/or alleviate withdrawal symptoms. This cycle will repeat throughout the day. A patient who smokes 20 cigarettes a day (1 pack) inhales around 200 hits of nicotine to the brain each day (National Institute on Drug Abuse [NIDA], 2016). However, there can be significant variation in the amount of nicotine delivered based on the individual's metabolism and how the tobacco product is used (Ahijevych, 1999). This variability is an important consideration in the dosing and effectiveness of nicotine-replacement products.

The initial feelings of pleasure and increased energy that occur after cigarette smoking are followed by the negative emotional and physical states associated with nicotine withdrawal. Withdrawal symptoms occur within hours of abstinence and can persist for weeks (Jackson, Muldoonc, De Biasib, & Damajc, 2015). The user will attempt to relieve these symptoms of irritability, restlessness, and reduced concentration by increasing nicotine ingestion. This is termed nicotine abstinence syndrome or, more commonly, nicotine withdrawal. Withdrawal has been shown to be mediated by a variety of factors, including type and topography of tobacco use, gender, age, and genetic factors (Jackson et al., 2015; Krebs et al., 2016).

HEALTH EFFECTS

Adverse Physical Effects

The use of tobacco products has been found to have harmful effects on nearly every organ system in the body. Five out of 10 tobacco users will die of an illness that can be prevented by quitting. Exposure to tobacco smoke accounts for more than 85% of lung cancer deaths and around one-third of heart disease deaths (HHS, 2014). Effects on health include lung and oral cavity cancers, including cancer of the mouth, pharynx, larynx, esophagus, stomach, pancreas, cervix, prostate, kidney, ureter, and bladder. Cigarette smoking markedly increases cardiovascular disease, specifically cerebral vascular accidents (strokes), myocardial infarctions, angina, vascular disease, and aneurysms. Smokeless tobacco use has also been found to increase cardiovascular disease risk (Piano et al., 2010). In addition, cigarette smoking results in increased rates of emphysema, bronchial disorders, gastric ulcers, osteoporosis, diabetes mellitus, and macular degeneration (HHS, 2014).

Fetal Effects

In pregnant women, carbon monoxide and nicotine interfere with the oxygen supply to the fetus. Nicotine crosses the placenta and is concentrated in the fetal blood, amniotic fluid, and breast milk. Nicotine levels in the fetus can be as much as 15% higher than maternal levels (HHS, 2014). As a result, cigarette smoking by pregnant women leads to higher rates of fetal death, decreased fetal growth, and low-birth-weight infants. Smoking during pregnancy is also associated with orofacial cleft defects, learning and behavioral problems, and atrial septal heart defects in children (HHS, 2014).

Secondhand Smoke Effects

Exposure to secondhand smoke can cause cardiovascular disease, lung cancer, respiratory disease, ear infections in children, asthma, and sudden infant death syndrome. The Environmental Protection Agency considers environmental tobacco smoke (ETS) a known human carcinogen in the Class A category, along with radon, benzene, and asbestos (Centers for Disease Control and Prevention [US]; National Center for Chronic Disease Prevention and Health Promotion [US]; Office on Smoking and Health [US], 2010). Studies suggest that non-smokers exposed to ETS at work were 30% more likely to develop lung cancer than nonexposed workers. The scientific evidence indicates that there is no risk-free level of exposure to second-hand smoke, and exposure to even small amounts can cause harm (Centers for Disease Control and Prevention [US]; National Center for Chronic Disease Prevention and Health Promotion [US]; Office on Smoking and Health [US], 2010).

TOBACCO USE DISORDER

*T*he *Diagnostic and Statistical Manual of Mental Disorders,* fifth edition *(DSM-5)* describes tobacco use disorder as a problematic pattern of tobacco use leading to significant impairment or distress (American Psychiatric Association [APA], 2013). Most tobacco users recognize the negative health effects of tobacco on their health. Yet quitting can be hard, and many have made multiple quit attempts and have either not succeeded in quitting or relapsed.

Similar to other substance use disorders, the diagnostic criteria for tobacco use disorder include (APA, 2013) the following:

- Tolerance

- Withdrawal

- Substance being used in larger amounts or over a longer period than intended

- Persistent desire or unsuccessful efforts to cut down

- Great deal of time spent in activities to obtain the substance

- Giving up or reducing important social, occupational, or recreational activities because of substance use

- Continued use despite knowledge of having persistent or recurrent health problems that are likely caused by the substance use

To be diagnosed with tobacco withdrawal, the tobacco user must meet four of the following seven criteria within 24 hours of decreased tobacco use or cessation (APA, 2013):

- Depressed mood

- Insomnia

- Irritability, frustration, or anger

- Anxiety

- Difficulty concentrating

- Restlessness

- Increased appetite

The most common tobacco withdrawal symptoms are irritability, impaired concentration, and craving for nicotine.

Nicotine dependence is also assessed using measures such as the Fagerström Test for Nicotine Dependence and the Heaviness of Smoking Index (Baker et al., 2007; Heatherton, Kozlowski, Frecker, & Fagerström, 1991). Evidence from these studies suggests that two elements, the number of cigarettes smoked per day (10 or greater) and the time to the first tobacco use (<30 minutes) of the day, are the best predictors of the level of nicotine dependence.

SCREENING AND TREATMENT

Seventy percent of all tobacco users have a desire to quit (Prochaska & Benowitz, 2016). It is widely acknowledged that tobacco use should be addressed as a chronic, relapse-prone disorder (Steinberg, Schmelzer, Lin, & Garcia, 2010). According to the HHS Clinical Practice Guideline *Treating Tobacco Use and Dependence* (Fiore et al., 2008), it is essential that clinicians and healthcare delivery systems provide consistent identification, documentation, and treatment of every tobacco user who is seen in a healthcare setting. However, implementation of these standardized guidelines remains inconsistent and frequently fails to capture the increasing numbers of tobacco users who do not primarily use conventional cigarettes (Kruger, Shaw, Kahende, & Frank, 2012). Figure 5-1 presents a helpful algorithm to guide the process of identifying and referring patients with a tobacco use disorder for treatment.

Tobacco Use and Readiness-to-Quit Screening

The use of brief, motivational interventions is an evidence-based approach to helping patients facilitate behavior change. Clinicians screen each patient for tobacco use during every healthcare encounter. Assessing the patient's willingness to quit can guide the type of assistance provided. Clinicians should assess all patients who use tobacco and have a desire to abstain using the brief smoking cessation five *A*s strategy: ask, advise, assess, assist, and arrange. Clinicians educate current users of tobacco in any form on the adverse physical effects and offer resources and treatment options to quit. Studies have demonstrated that clinical intervention can have a powerful effect and can prompt quit attempts (Fiore et al., 2008).

If the patient is willing to make a quit attempt, the clinician assists by offering appropriate tobacco use treatment. This includes developing a quit plan; providing practical counseling; and promoting total abstinence by reviewing past quit experiences, identifying triggers, and helping the patient identify and develop a social support network. Unless medically contraindicated,

FIGURE 5-1: ALGORITHM FOR TREATING TOBACCO USE

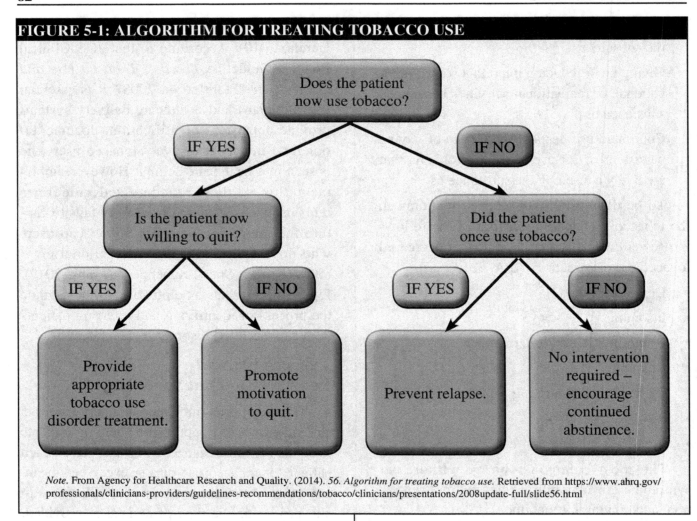

Note. From Agency for Healthcare Research and Quality. (2014). *56. Algorithm for treating tobacco use.* Retrieved from https://www.ahrq.gov/professionals/clinicians-providers/guidelines-recommendations/tobacco/clinicians/presentations/2008update-full/slide56.html

the clinician should discuss and recommend the use of pharmacological treatment. Nicotine-replacement medications can increase abstinence by targeting nicotine withdrawal symptoms. Lastly, the clinician should arrange for follow-up to monitor and support the patient's quit attempt. Table 5-1 describes the five *A*s in detail and suggests strategies for engaging the patient in the quit process.

In addition to the five *A*s, a three *A*s strategy, also referred to as the Ottawa Model, has been found to be effective in busy clinical settings (Papadakis et al., 2016). This method involves a more streamlined approach of ask, advise, and act. Although many clinicians and healthcare systems are consistent about screening for tobacco use and advising patients to quit, far fewer assess, fewer still assist with treatment, and very few arrange for

follow-up. In certain settings, implementing the three *A*s can effectively increase the delivery of evidence-based treatment.

If the patient is a current tobacco user who is unwilling to stop, the clinician should offer the patient a brief motivational intervention designed to encourage quit attempts. Motivational counseling focuses on the five *R*s: relevance, risks, rewards, roadblocks, and repetition (Fiore et al., 2008). Tobacco users may be unwilling to quit for a variety of reasons, such as misinformation, concern about nicotine withdrawal or lack of desired psychological effects, or reluctance because of prior unsuccessful quit attempts. Therefore, after asking about tobacco use, advising the smoker to quit, and assessing the willingness of the smoker to quit, it is important to provide the five *R*s of cessation motivation (see Table 5-2).

Clinicians should remind patients who have had previous unsuccessful attempts to quit smoking that it is common to experience repeated attempts to quit before being successful (Fiore et al., 2008). If the patient has a history of tobacco use but is currently abstinent, the clinician praises the accomplishment to reinforce tobacco avoidance in any form and continues to work with the patient to prevent relapse. Most relapses occur soon after the quit attempt; however, some people relapse months or even years after their quit date. Relapse prevention may include brief counseling interventions and pharmacotherapy. The key is to systematically identify tobacco use

TABLE 5-1: THE FIVE *A*s (1 OF 4)

Ask – *Systematically identify all tobacco users at every visit.*

Action	Strategies for Implementation
Implement an office-wide system that ensures that, for every patient at every clinic visit, tobacco use status is queried and documented. Repeated assessment is not necessary in the case of the adult who has never used tobacco or has not used tobacco for many years and for whom this information is clearly documented in the medical record.	Expand the vital signs to include tobacco use, or use an alternative universal identification system. Alternatives to expanding the vital signs are to place stickers indicating tobacco use status on all patient charts or to indicate tobacco use status using electronic medical records or computer reminder systems.

Vital Signs

Blood Pressure:_____

Pulse: _____ Weight: _____

Temperature: _____

Respiratory Rate: _____

Tobacco Use: (circle one) Current   Former   Never

Advise – *Strongly urge all tobacco users to quit.*

Action	Strategies for Implementation
In a clear, strong, and personalized manner, urge every tobacco user to quit.	Advice should be: • *Clear* – "It is important for you to quit smoking (or using chewing tobacco) now, and I can help you"; "Cutting down while you are ill is not enough"; "Occasional or light smoking is still dangerous." • *Strong* – "As your clinician, I need you to know that quitting smoking is the most important thing you can do to protect your health now and in the future. The clinic staff and I will help you." • *Personalized* – Link tobacco use to current health concerns, and/or its social and economic costs, and/or the impact of tobacco use on children and others in the household. "Continuing to smoke makes your asthma worse, and quitting may dramatically improve your health"; "Quitting smoking may reduce the number of ear infections your child has."

status and reinforce tobacco cessation each time the patient meets with the clinician.

Treatment

Pharmacotherapy

The use of medication is a critical component of tobacco cessation. The best treatment outcomes use both medication and counseling (Fiore et al., 2008). All tobacco users who are trying to quit should be offered pharmacotherapy as a treatment modality unless otherwise contraindicated. For those with medical comorbidities (e.g., acute coronary syndromes), pregnant and nursing women, adolescents, and light or intermittent tobacco users, medications are generally not indicated, and their use is considered off-label.

continued on page 86

TABLE 5-1: THE FIVE *A*s (2 OF 4)	
Assess – *Determine willingness to make a quit attempt.*	
Action	**Strategies for Implementation**
Assess every tobacco user's willingness to make a quit attempt at the time.	Assess the patient's willingness to quit: "Are you willing to give quitting a try?" • If the patient is willing to make a quit attempt at this time, provide assistance. • If the patient will participate in an intensive treatment, deliver such a treatment or refer to an intensive intervention. • If the patient clearly states that he or she is unwilling to make a quit attempt at this time, provide an intervention shown to increase future quit attempts. • If the patient is a member of a special population (e.g., adolescent, pregnant smoker, or racial or ethnic minority), consider providing additional information.
Assist – *Provide aids to quitting (e.g., counseling and medication).*	
Action	**Strategies for Implementation**
Help the tobacco user with a quit plan.	A patient's preparations for quitting should include the following: • Set a quit date – Ideally, the quit date should be within 2 weeks. • Tell family, friends, and coworkers about quitting, and request understanding and support. • Anticipate challenges to the planned quit attempt, particularly during the critical first few weeks. These include nicotine withdrawal symptoms. • Remove tobacco products from the environment before quitting, and avoid smoking in places where a lot of time is spent such as work, home, or car. Make home smoke-free.

TABLE 5-1: THE FIVE *As* (3 OF 4)	
Provide practical counseling (problem solving and skills training).	• *Abstinence* – Total abstinence is essential – not even a single puff after the quit date. • *Past quit experience* – Identify what helped and what hurt in previous quit attempts. Build on past success. • *Anticipate triggers or challenges in upcoming attempt* – Discuss challenges and triggers and how the patient will successfully overcome them (avoid triggers and alter routines). • *Alcohol* – Because alcohol can cause relapse, the patient should consider limiting and abstaining from alcohol while quitting. (Note that reducing alcohol intake could precipitate withdrawal in alcohol-dependent people.) • *Other smokers in the household* – Quitting is more difficult when there is another smoker in the household. Patients should encourage housemates to quit with them or to avoid smoking in their presence.
Provide intratreatment social support.	• Provide a supportive clinical environment while encouraging the patient in his or her quit attempt. "My office staff and I are available to assist you"; "I'm recommending treatment that can provide ongoing support."
Recommend the use of approved pharmacotherapy, except in special circumstances.	• Recommend the use of pharmacotherapies found to be effective. Explain how these medications increase smoking cessation success and reduce withdrawal symptoms. The first-line pharmacotherapy medications include bupropion, nicotine gum, nicotine inhaler, nicotine nasal spray, nicotine lozenge, nicotine patch, and varenicline. Second-line medications include clonidine and nortriptyline. There is insufficient evidence to recommend medications for pregnant women, smokeless tobacco users, light smokers, and adolescents (see Table 5-3).
Provide supplementary materials, including information on quit lines.	• *Sources* – Materials are available from federal agencies; nonprofit agencies; and local, state, or tribal health departments or quit lines and the national quit-line network (1-800-QUIT-NOW). • *Type* – Materials should be culturally, racially, educationally, and age appropriate for the patient. • *Location* – Materials should be readily available at every clinician's workstation.

TABLE 5-1: THE FIVE *A*s (4 OF 4)

Arrange – *Ensure follow-up contact.*

Action	Strategies for Implementation
Arrange for follow-up contact, either in person or via telephone.	• *Timing* – Follow-up contact should occur soon after the quit date, preferably during the first week. A second follow-up contact is recommended within the first month. Schedule further follow-up contacts as indicated. • *Actions during follow-up contact* – Identify problems already encountered, and anticipate challenges in the immediate future. Assess medication use and problems. Remind patients of quit-line support (1-800-QUIT-NOW). Address tobacco use at next clinical visit (treat tobacco use as a chronic disease.) For patients who are abstinent, congratulate them on their success. If tobacco use has occurred, review circumstances and elicit recommitment to total abstinence. Consider use of or a referral to more intensive treatment.

Note. From Fiore, M. C., Jaén, C. R., Baker, T. B., Bailey, W. C., Benowitz, N. L., Curry, S. J., … Leitzke, C. (2008). *Treating tobacco use and dependence: 2008 update.* Rockville, MD: U.S. Department of Health and Human Services.

TABLE 5-2: ENHANCING MOTIVATION TO QUIT TOBACCO – THE FIVE *R*s (1 OF 2)

Relevance – Encourage the patient to indicate why quitting is personally relevant, being as specific as possible. Motivational information has the greatest impact if it is relevant to a patient's disease status or risk, family or social situation (such as having children in the home), health concerns, age, gender, and other important patient characteristics (such as prior quitting experience or personal barriers to cessation).

Risks – The clinician should ask the patient to identify potential negative consequences of tobacco use. The clinician may suggest and highlight those that seem most relevant to the patient. The clinician should emphasize that smoking low-tar or low-nicotine cigarettes or using other forms of tobacco (such as smokeless tobacco, cigars, and pipes) will not eliminate these risks.

Examples of risks include the following:

• Acute: Shortness of breath, exacerbation of asthma, harm to pregnancy, impotence, infertility, and increased serum carbon monoxide

• Long-term: Heart attack and stroke, lung and other cancers (larynx, oral cavity, pharynx, esophagus, pancreas, bladder, cervix), chronic obstructive pulmonary diseases (chronic bronchitis and emphysema), long-term disability, and need for extended care

• Environmental: Increased risk of lung cancer and heart disease in spouses; higher rates of smoking in children of tobacco users; and increased risk for low birth weight, sudden infant death syndrome, asthma, middle ear disease, and respiratory infections in children of smokers

TABLE 5-2: ENHANCING MOTIVATION TO QUIT TOBACCO – THE FIVE *R*s (2 OF 2)

Rewards – The clinician should ask the patient to identify potential benefits of stopping tobacco use. The clinician may suggest and highlight those that seem most relevant to the patient.

Examples of rewards include the following:

- Improved health
- Setting a good example for children
- Improved sense of taste
- Healthier babies and children
- Improved sense of smell
- Not worrying about exposing others to smoke
- Saving money
- Improved physical health
- Improved self-esteem
- Performing better in physical activities
- Improved smell of home, car, clothing, and breath
- Reduced wrinkling and aging of skin and whiter teeth
- Not worrying about quitting

Roadblocks – The clinician should ask the patient to identify barriers or impediments to quitting and note elements of treatment (such as problem solving or pharmacotherapy) that could address barriers.

Typical barriers include the following:

- Withdrawal symptoms
- Lack of support
- Being around other tobacco users
- Fear of failure
- Depression
- Lack of knowledge of effective treatment options
- Weight gain
- Enjoyment of tobacco

Repetition – The motivational intervention should be repeated every time an unmotivated patient visits the clinical setting. Clinicians should tell tobacco users who have failed in previous quit attempts that most people make repeated quit attempts before they are successful.

Note. From Fiore, M. C., Jaén, C. R., Baker, T. B., Bailey, W. C., Benowitz, N. L., Curry, S. J., ... Leitzke, C. (2008). *Treating tobacco use and dependence: 2008 update.* Rockville, MD: U.S. Department of Health and Human Services.

There are seven first-line and two second-line pharmacotherapies for smoking cessation (Fiore et al., 2008). The first-line agents are as follows:

- Bupropion (Wellbutrin SR or Zyban)

- Varenicline (Chantix)

- Five types of nicotine-replacement therapy

  ◦ Nicotine gum (available over the counter)

  ◦ Nicotine lozenge (available over the counter)

  ◦ Nicotine patch (available over the counter)

  ◦ Nicotine inhaler and nasal spray (require a prescription)

Bupropion and varenicline require a prescription from a clinician. The agents in the previous list are all approved by the U.S. Food and Drug Administration (FDA) for the first-line treatment of tobacco use. The choice of pharmacotherapy is guided by individual patient factors and level of nicotine dependence. For example, nicotine-replacement dosing is based on the patient's current level of nicotine exposure. Table 5-3 provides a summary of the clinical guidelines for prescribing smoking cessation medication.

The second-line pharmacologic agents for the treatment of tobacco use are prescription clonidine and nortriptyline. *Treating Tobacco Use and Dependence* (Fiore et al., 2008) recommends that clinicians should consider these second-line agents for patients for whom first-line agents were not successful and for patients for whom first-line agents are contraindicated. Currently, these second-line agents are not FDA approved for treating tobacco use disorders and, therefore, are considered off-label.

A number of herbal and over-the-counter products, such as filters, herbal chew, and electronic cigarettes, claim efficacy for quitting tobacco, but they are not FDA approved, have not demonstrated effectiveness, and may be potentially harmful. If patients are using these products, it indicates an interest in quitting smoking. Clinicians must work with patients to help guide them in the use of evidence-based cessation methods that are most likely to promote successful outcomes without added harms.

Behavioral Counseling

There is a strong relationship between the intensity of tobacco use counseling and cessation outcomes. Counseling methods that involve person-to-person contact either individually, in groups, or via telephone (state quit line) or online are all evidence-based strategies, and effectiveness increases with greater frequency and duration of intervention. According to *Treating Tobacco Use and Dependence* (Fiore et al., 2008), research has found two types of counseling and behavioral therapies to be especially effective in nicotine-dependent patients who are attempting to quit: motivational interviewing and practical counseling. Motivational interviewing focuses on increasing the importance and salience of tobacco abstinence by facilitating the patient's self-identification of goals pertaining to smoking cessation. Practical counseling focuses on increasing confidence and self-efficacy for both cessation and maintenance of abstinence. Practical counseling involves problem-solving, skills training, and social support. Table 5-4 provides examples of these behavioral therapies.

Evidence suggests that even a brief intervention counseling session of 3 or fewer minutes results in a significant increase in long-term abstinence (Fiore et al., 2008). To enhance treatment success, more intensive intervention is appropriate for every tobacco user who has agreed to quit. Evidence has demonstrated that intensive interventions are more effective than brief interventions and should be used whenever possible. Table 5-5 lists the components of intensive interventions. Most health insurance plans and Medicare cover the cost of inten-

continued on page 90

TABLE 5-3: CLINICAL GUIDELINES FOR PRESCRIBING MEDICATION FOR TOBACCO USE DISORDERS (1 OF 2)	
Who should receive medication for tobacco use? Are there groups of smokers for whom medication has not been shown to be effective?	All smokers trying to quit should be offered medication, except when contraindicated or for specific populations for which there is insufficient evidence of effectiveness (i.e., pregnant women, smokeless tobacco users, light smokers, and adolescents).
What are the first-line medications recommended in this guideline update?	All seven of the medications approved by the U.S. Food and Drug Administration (FDA) for treating tobacco use are recommended: bupropion, nicotine gum, nicotine inhaler, nicotine lozenge, nicotine nasal spray, nicotine patch, and varenicline. The clinician should consider the first-line medications shown to be more effective than the nicotine patch alone. Unfortunately, there are no well-accepted algorithms to guide optimal selection among the first-line medications.
Are there contraindications, warnings, precautions, other concerns, and side effects regarding the first-line medications recommended in this guideline update?	All seven FDA-approved medications have specific contraindications, warnings, precautions, other concerns, and side effects. Refer to FDA package inserts for this complete information. (See following information regarding second-line medications.)
What other factors may influence medication selection?	Pragmatic factors also may influence selection, such as insurance coverage, out-of-pocket patient costs, likelihood of adherence, dentures when considering nicotine gum, or dermatitis when considering using the nicotine patch.
Is a patient's prior experience with a medication relevant?	Prior successful experience (sustained abstinence with the medication) suggests that the medication may be helpful to the patient in a subsequent quit attempt, especially if the patient found the medication to be tolerable and/or easy to use. However, it is difficult to draw firm conclusions from unsuccessful attempts with medication. Some evidence suggests that re-treating relapsed smokers with the same medication produces small or no benefit, whereas other evidence suggests that it may be of substantial benefit.
Which medications should a clinician use with a patient who is highly nicotine dependent?	The higher-dose preparations of nicotine gum, patch, and lozenge have been shown to be effective in highly dependent smokers. Also, there is evidence that combination nicotine-replacement therapy (NRT) may be particularly effective in suppressing tobacco withdrawal symptoms. Thus, it may be that NRT combinations are especially helpful for highly dependent smokers or those with a history of severe nicotine withdrawal.
Is gender a consideration in selecting a medication?	There is evidence that NRT can be effective with both sexes; however, evidence is mixed as to whether NRT is less effective in women than men. This may encourage the clinician to consider use of another type of medication with women, such as bupropion or varenicline.

TABLE 5-3: CLINICAL GUIDELINES FOR PRESCRIBING MEDICATION FOR TOBACCO USE DISORDERS (2 OF 2)

Are cessation medications appropriate for light smokers (i.e., <10 cigarettes/day)?	As noted previously, cessation medications have not been shown to be beneficial to light smokers. However, if NRT is used with light smokers, clinicians may consider reducing the dose of the medication. No adjustments are necessary when using bupropion or varenicline.
When should second-line agents be used for treating tobacco dependence?	Consider prescribing second-line agents (clonidine and nortriptyline) for patients unable to use first-line medications because of contraindications or for patients for whom the group of first-line medications has not been helpful. Assess patients for the specific contraindications, precautions, other concerns, and side effects of the second-line agents. Refer to FDA package inserts for this information. Use of clonidine or nortriptyline for smoking cessation is considered off-label use.
Which medications are considered for patients particularly concerned about weight gain?	Data show that bupropion and NRTs, in particular, 4 mg nicotine gum and 4 mg nicotine lozenge, delay – but do not prevent – weight gain.
Are there medications that should especially be considered for patients with a past history of depression?	Bupropion and nortriptyline (off-label) appear to be effective with this population, but NRT also appears to help individuals with a history of depression.
Should NRTs be avoided in patients with a history of cardiovascular disease?	No. The nicotine patch in particular has been demonstrated as safe for patients with cardiovascular disease. See FDA package inserts for more complete information.
May tobacco dependence medications be used long term (e.g., up to 6 months)?	Yes. This approach may be helpful with smokers who report persistent withdrawal symptoms during the course of medication treatment, relapse in the past after stopping medication, or a desire for long-term therapy. A minority of individuals who successfully quit smoking use ad libitum NRT medications (gum, nasal spray, inhaler) long term. The use of these medications for up to 6 months does not present a known health risk, and developing dependence on these medications is uncommon. Additionally, the FDA has approved the use of bupropion, varenicline, and some NRT medications for 6-month use.
Is medication adherence important?	Yes. Patients frequently do not use cessation medications as recommended (e.g., they do not use them at recommended doses or for recommended durations); this may reduce their effectiveness.
May medications ever be combined?	Yes. Among first-line medications, evidence exists that combining the nicotine patch long term (>14 weeks) with either nicotine gum or nicotine nasal spray, combining the nicotine patch with the nicotine inhaler, or combining the nicotine patch with bupropion increases long-term abstinence rates relative to placebo treatments. Combining varenicline with NRT agents has been associated with higher rates of side effects (e.g., nausea, headaches).

Note. From Fiore, M. C., Jaén, C. R., Baker, T. B., Bailey, W. C., Benowitz, N. L., Curry, S. J., ... Leitzke, C. (2008). *Treating tobacco use and dependence: 2008 update.* Rockville, MD: U.S. Department of Health and Human Services.

TABLE 5-4: ELEMENTS OF BEHAVIORAL COUNSELING AND THERAPIES

Common elements of practical counseling

Practical counseling (problem solving and skills training) treatment component	Examples
Recognize danger situations – Identify events, internal states, or activities that increase the risk of smoking or relapse.	• Negative affect and stress • Being around other smokers • Drinking alcohol • Experiencing urges • Smoking cues and cigarette availability
Develop coping skills – Identify and practice coping or problem-solving skills. Typically, these skills are intended to cope with situations of high temptation and opportunity.	• Learning to anticipate and avoid temptation • Learning cognitive strategies that will reduce negative moods • Accomplishing lifestyle changes that reduce stress, improve quality of life, and reduce exposure to smoking cues • Learning cognitive and behavioral activities to cope with smoking urges (such as distracting attention, changing routines)
Provide basic information – Provide basic information about smoking and successful quitting	• Any smoking (even a single puff) increases the likelihood of full relapse. • Withdrawal typically peaks within 1 to 2 weeks after quitting but may persist for months. • Withdrawal symptoms include negative mood, urges to smoke, and difficulty concentrating. • Smoking is addictive in nature.

Common elements of supportive behavioral strategies

Supportive treatment component	Examples
Encourage the patient in the quit attempt.	• Note that effective tobacco dependence treatments are now available. • Note that one-half of all people who have ever smoked have now quit. • Communicate belief in the patient's ability to quit.
Communicate caring and concern.	• Ask how the patient feels about quitting. • Directly express concern and willingness to help as needed. • Be open to the patient's expression of fears of quitting, difficulties experienced, and ambivalent feelings.
Encourage the patient to talk about the quitting process.	Ask about the following: • Reasons the patient wants to quit • Concerns or worries about quitting • Success the patient has achieved • Difficulties encountered while quitting

Note. From Fiore, M. C., Jaén, C. R., Baker, T. B., Bailey, W. C., Benowitz, N. L., Curry, S. J., ... Leitzke, C. (2008). *Treating tobacco use and dependence: 2008 update.* Rockville, MD: U.S. Department of Health and Human Services.

TABLE 5-5: STRATEGY COMPONENTS OF AN INTENSIVE INTERVENTION

Assessment	Readiness assessments should ensure that tobacco users are willing to make a quit attempt using an intensive treatment program. Additional assessments, such as determining level of nicotine dependence and barriers or facilitators to quitting, can provide information useful in counseling (e.g., stress level or dependence).
Program clinicians	Multiple types of clinicians are effective and should be used. One counseling strategy would be to have a medical or healthcare clinician deliver messages about health risks and benefits and prescribe pharmacotherapy, and then have nonmedical clinicians deliver additional psychosocial or behavioral interventions.
Program intensity	Because of evidence of a strong dose-response relationship, the intensity of the program should adhere to the following guidelines: • Session length – longer than 10 minutes • Number of sessions – four or more sessions • Total contact time – longer than 30 minutes
Program format	Either individual or group counseling may be used. Proactive telephone counseling also is effective. Use of adjuvant self-help material is optional. Follow-up assessment intervention procedures should be used.
Type of counseling and behavioral therapies	Counseling and behavioral therapies should involve practical counseling (problem solving or skills training).
Pharmacotherapy	Every smoker should be encouraged to use pharmacotherapies endorsed in the guidelines, except in the presence of special circumstances. The clinician should explain how these medications increase smoking cessation success and reduce withdrawal symptoms.
Population	Intensive intervention programs may be used with all tobacco users willing to participate in such efforts.

Note. From Fiore, M. C., Jaén, C. R., Baker, T. B., Bailey, W. C., Benowitz, N. L., Curry, S. J., ... Leitzke, C. (2008). *Treating tobacco use and dependence: 2008 update.* Rockville, MD: U.S. Department of Health and Human Services.

sive tobacco cessation counseling when conducted by providers eligible to bill for services. Individual, group, or proactive telephone counseling are viable options.

Many nicotine-dependent patients express a desire to explore alternative treatments for smoking cessation. Current clinical practice guidelines regarding alternative therapies for tobacco cessation include acupuncture, exercise, hypnosis, and biobehavioral feedback. The current evidence is inconclusive regarding the effectiveness of these treatments, with findings generally mixed or conflicting. Data regarding hypnosis and biobehavioral feedback were insufficient to determine the efficacy of these treatments, and the findings related to acupuncture and exercise were mixed (Fiore et al., 2008).

SPECIAL CONSIDERATIONS IN TOBACCO SCREENING AND TREATMENT

Types of Tobacco

Smokeless Tobacco

The two most common forms of smokeless tobacco in the United States are chewing tobacco and snuff (Nguyen et al., 2016). Chewing tobacco is generally a loose-leaf product but also comes in the forms of plug and twist. Snuff is finely ground tobacco that can be dry or moist or come in sachets, similar to tea bags. Generally, smokeless tobacco users place the product between the gum and cheek and suck on the tobacco, frequently spitting out the juices, but newer products, called snus, can be used without spitting. Smokeless tobacco contains 28 cancer-causing agents and exposes the user to high levels of nicotine, resulting in tobacco dependence.

A version of the Fagerström Test for Nicotine Dependence can be used with smokeless tobacco users to determine nicotine dependence (Fidler, Shahab, & West, 2010). Screening and treatment for smokeless tobacco users follow the same guidelines discussed earlier under tobacco use.

Electronic Cigarettes and Novel Tobacco Products

Electronic cigarettes and other novel tobacco products have been accessible and essentially unregulated for the past decade, with newer products in the tobacco industry pipeline, such as heat-not-burn technology. Clearly, combustible cigarettes have resulted in tremendous harm. The long-term effects from these newer products are currently "harm uncertain." Under a 2016 deeming regulation by the FDA, these products are being evaluated as potential reduced-exposure products (Zeller & Hatkusami, 2009). Although there is current debate regarding the use of these products, a few key considerations are warranted:

- Less harm does not equal no harm.

- Exposure to nicotine in any form puts youth at risk for dependence.

- There is no consistent evidence to support the use of these products for cessation.

- Vaporizing products emit small particulates that cause harmful effects to both the user and those exposed to the vapor.

Although it is important not to derail quit attempts in patients using these products, it is also important that healthcare providers promote access to evidence-based treatments.

Comorbid Substance Use and Mental Health Disorders

The prevalence of tobacco use in adults 18 years of age and older with mental illness and substance use disorders is markedly higher than in the general population. The prevalence of smoking in patients with other substance use disorders is extremely high, with estimates ranging above 70% (CDC, 2016a). Patients with comorbid chemical dependence and tobacco dependence have much higher rates of morbidity and mortality. Evidence demonstrates that abstinence from tobacco can enhance abstinence from other substances (Thurgood, McNeill, Clark-Carter, & Brose, 2016).

Concern regarding the use of cessation medications with potential neuropsychiatric adverse events has hindered the treatment of tobacco use disorder in patients with existing mental health disorders. A recently released large cessation trial evaluated the prevalence of these adverse events in patients with and without nicotine-replacement therapy (bupropion and varenicline) compared with placebo in patients with and without a psychiatric diagnosis. This study provides strong evidence regarding the safety and efficacy of cessation medications in patients with and without mental illness (Anthenelli et al., 2016).

Older Adult Smokers

All patients benefit from tobacco cessation, including patients older than age 70. Often, healthcare providers make the mistaken assumption that patients who continue to use tobacco into their 60s and 70s are not candidates for screening and treatment. Evidence supports the benefits of tobacco abstinence at older ages (Nash, Liao, Harris, & Freedman, 2016). Cessation of smoking and tobacco use in older adults can reduce their risk of death from coronary heart disease, chronic obstructive pulmonary disease, and lung cancer and decrease their risk of osteoporosis. Cessation interventions that have been effective in the general population have been proven to be as effective with older adults (Fiore et al., 2008).

CASE STUDY 5-1

*J*oey is a 36-year-old bisexual female who goes to the health clinic for respiratory symptoms and is seeing a nurse practitioner in the clinic for the first time. Joey says this is her third round of "bronchitis" this season. Joey states that she currently smokes and feels the menthol cigarettes seem to "open me up so I can breathe better."

Joey's medical history is significant for asthma in childhood ("but I grew out of it when I was 10"), chronic sinus problems, and depression without suicidal ideation. She states that she started smoking at age 16 years. She and her current partner, whom she lives with, both smoke.

Joey's current medications include an oral contraceptive, but she explains that she is going to stop using it "because I really don't need it right now, and besides, the doctor won't prescribe it for me anymore unless I quit smoking, and I don't want to do that right now." She also describes using inhalers of an unknown type for asthma symptoms on and off throughout the years.

Joey's family history is significant for her father having a heart attack at age 52 and her mother recently dying of lung cancer at age 64. She really misses her mom and is tearful when talking about her. She has five siblings, and all family members, except one brother, smoke. She

has an older sister who is having heart problems and is currently trying to quit smoking using varenicline, which is working pretty well for her.

When the nurse practitioner asks Joey about quitting smoking, she replies, "I'm way too stressed to even think about it now."

Joey explains that she recently lost her job and is feeling pressured financially. She has tried to quit smoking on her own in the past, but she found that she just felt irritated about everything. She states that she started to smoke again because it helps to calm her. She tried nicotine gum many years ago but did not like the taste. She notes that she used nicotine patches when she was in the hospital several years ago and that they worked pretty well, but she started smoking again after she was discharged.

Upon physical examination, Joey is afebrile with a heart rate and blood pressure that are within normal limits. She appears slightly anxious, as manifest through restlessness and tense muscles. Her respiratory rate is 20, and she coughs nonproductively. Joey's breath sounds are positive for wheezing.

Questions

1. What is the nurse practitioner's initial approach to discussing Joey's smoking habit?

2. What other information related to Joey's tobacco use does the nurse practitioner need to assess?

3. Which elements of motivational counseling are specifically relevant in employing the five *R*s strategy with Joey?

4. What is the nurse's action in encouraging Joey to follow up?

5. If Joey is agreeable to a smoking cessation trial at her follow-up visit, what is the nurse's action?

Answers

1. The nurse practitioner begins a discussion about Joey's smoking habit with open-ended questions and nonjudgmental responses. Expressing empathy about the recent loss of Joey's mother without focusing on her risk of getting lung cancer is another relationship-building approach.

2. The nurse practitioner asks about all forms of tobacco use with Joey because she may be using other forms, such as smokeless or electronic cigarettes. If time permits, the nurse provides for additional discussion of Joey's previous quit experiences.

3. Encouraging and supporting Joey's motivation to quit tobacco through the use of the five *R*s framework might include the following counseling techniques:

   • Relevance: Discuss how even a brief period of smoking abstinence could help her recovery and that help is available to manage her withdrawal symptoms in addition to treating her respiratory symptoms.

   • Risks: Although Joey feels that smoking may be helping her immediate symptoms, it is most likely contributing to her persistent bronchitis symptoms. In this situation, until the nurse establishes a relationship with Joey, it would be beneficial to focus on her most salient concerns.

   • Rewards: Explore benefits related not only to her physical health but also to being able to remain on oral contraceptives if this is an important future concern for her. Also, exploring the financial benefits of not smoking could be a very immediate reward.

   • Roadblocks: Being around others who smoke (e.g., her partner and most of her siblings) can certainly be a barrier. Discuss that she may get support from her sister who is trying to quit and potentially from engaging those around her in talking about quitting. Explore Joey's possible fear of failure resulting from her prior quit attempts.

   • Repetition: Revisit tobacco use at every follow-up visit with Joey using the five *R*s approach.

4. Schedule follow-up to ensure that Joey's recurring symptoms are resolving, and offer follow-up at any point that Joey may decide to take action in quitting smoking. An immediate follow-up visit may provide a window of opportunity to promote further discussion regarding tobacco cessation.

5. Review medication and counseling options with Joey, and encourage the use of both. Consider her prior experience (e.g., did not like gum, but patches worked well), and explore ways to manage triggers and enlist social support. Recommend a quit line or other counseling support, and set a follow-up visit.

SUMMARY

Tobacco use is the leading cause of preventable death and disability in the United States. Initiation of tobacco use most commonly occurs before age 18 and often results in nicotine dependence that continues throughout the patient's adult years. Nicotine is the drug in tobacco that causes addiction. It is a highly addictive substance that, when inhaled, quickly enters the brain. Although prevalence rates are declining for the general population, certain subgroups, such as persons with mental illness, continue to smoke at alarmingly high rates.

The clinical guideline *Treating Tobacco Use and Dependence* (Fiore et al., 2008) recommends that all adult and adolescent patients be screened for tobacco use; therefore, clinicians should ask all patients about their use of tobacco. If the patient is a current smoker or tobacco user, the clinician strongly advises the patient to quit and assesses the patient's willingness to quit. If the patient is willing to make a quit attempt, the clinician assists the patient by offering appropriate tobacco use treatment and arranging for follow-up. Treatment that includes the use of both behavioral counseling and medication, when indicated, is most effective.

If the patient is a current smoker who is not interested in quitting, the clinician is recommended to provide motivational interviewing and counseling that focus on why quitting is relevant, the health risks associated with continued use, the rewards associated with stopping, and the roadblocks to quitting, repeating this motivational intervention at every visit with the tobacco user. Patients who are currently abstinent from nicotine are offered counseling that reinforces their abstinence at every visit.

EXAM QUESTIONS

CHAPTER 5
Questions 24–28

Note: Choose the one option that BEST answers each question.

24. Nicotine has an onset of action in the brain that causes effects within

    a. 6 hours.
    b. 4 hours.
    c. 2 hours.
    d. seconds.

25. A common symptom of nicotine withdrawal is

    a. mood stabilization.
    b. irritability.
    c. weight loss.
    d. heartburn.

26. The best approach with a patient who wants to quit smoking is for the clinician to

    a. focus on the medical harm of smoking.
    b. encourage the patient to quit on his or her own.
    c. offer appropriate tobacco use disorder treatment.
    d. discourage the use of adjunct alternative therapies.

27. Mr. Smith has smoked 1 pack of cigarettes per day for 20 years and is currently unwilling to stop. His medical history is significant for high blood pressure. The clinician begins a brief intervention by stating, "Mr. Smith, I realize that you are not interested in stopping smoking today, but I am concerned that your smoking is increasing your blood pressure." This is an example of motivational counseling that focuses on personal

    a. repetition.
    b. rewards.
    c. roadblocks.
    d. relevance.

28. The prevalence of tobacco use is markedly increased in patients

    a. who are overweight.
    b. who attend college.
    c. with other substance use disorders.
    d. with a family history of heart disease.

REFERENCES

Agency for Healthcare Research and Quality. (2014). *56. Algorithm for treating tobacco use*. Retrieved from https://www.ahrq.gov/professionals/clinicians-providers/guide-lines-recommendations/tobacco/clinicians/presentations/2008update-full/slide56.html

Ahijevych, K. (1999). Nicotine metabolism variability and nicotine addiction. *Nicotine and Tobacco Research, 1,* S59-S62.

American Psychiatric Association. (2013). *Diagnostic and statistical manual of mental disorders* (5th ed.). Arlington, VA: Author.

Anthenelli, R. M., Benowitz, N. L., West, R., St. Aubin, L., McRae, T., Lawrence, D., ... Evins, A. E. (2016). Neuropsychiatric safety and efficacy of varenicline, bupropion, and nicotine patch in smokers with and without psychiatric disorders (EAGLES): A double-blind, randomised, placebo-controlled clinical trial. *Lancet, 387*(10037), 2507-2520.

Baker, T. B., Piper, M. E., McCarthy, D. E., Bolt, D. M., Smith, S. S., Kim, S., ... Transdisciplinary Tobacco Use Research Center (TTURC) Tobacco Dependence Phenotype Workgroup. (2007). Time to first cigarette in the morning as an index of ability to quit smoking: Implications for nicotine dependence. *Nicotine and Tobacco Research, 9*(Suppl. 4), 555-570.

Benowitz, N. L. (2010). Nicotine addiction. *New England Journal of Medicine, 362*(24), 2295-2303.

Centers for Disease Control and Prevention. (2016a). *Current cigarette smoking among U.S. adults aged 18 years and older*. Retrieved from https://www.cdc.gov/tobacco/campaign/tips/resources/data/cigarette-smoking-in-united-states.html

Centers for Disease Control and Prevention. (2016b). QuickStats: Cigarette smoking status among current adult e-cigarette users, by age group – National Health Interview Survey, United States, 2015. *Morbidity and Mortality Weekly Report, 65,* 1177.

Centers for Disease Control and Prevention. (2016c). *Smoking and tobacco use: Fast facts*. Retrieved from http://www.cdc.gov/tobacco/data_statistics/fact_sheets/fast_facts/index.htm#toll

Centers for Disease Control and Prevention (US); National Center for Chronic Disease Prevention and Health Promotion (US); Office on Smoking and Health (US). (2010). *How tobacco smoke causes disease: The biology and behavioral basis for smoking-attributable disease: A report of the surgeon general*. Atlanta, GA: Centers for Disease Control and Prevention (US).

Fidler, J. A., Shahab, L., & West, R. (2010). Strength of urges to smoke as a measure of severity of cigarette dependence: Comparison with the Fagerström Test for Nicotine Dependence and its components. *Addiction, 106,* 631-638. doi:10.1111/j.1360-0443.2010.03226.x

Fiore, M. C., Jaén, C. R., Baker, T. B., Bailey, W. C., Benowitz, N. L., Curry, S. J., ... Leitzke, C. (2008). *Treating tobacco use and dependence: 2008 update.* Rockville, MD: U.S. Department of Health and Human Services.

Heatherton, T. F., Kozlowski, L. T., Frecker, R. C., & Fagerström, K. O. (1991). The Fagerström Test for Nicotine Dependence: A revision of the Fagerström Tolerance Questionnaire. *British Journal of Addiction to Alcohol and Other Drugs, 86*(9), 1119-1127.

Jackson, K. J., Muldoonc, P. P., De Biasib, M., & Damajc, M. I. (2015). New mechanisms and perspectives in nicotine withdrawal. *Neuropharmacology, 96,* 223-234.

Jamal, A., King, B. A., Neff, L. J., Whitmill, J., Babb, S. D., & Graffunder, C. M. (2016). Current cigarette smoking among adults – United States, 2005-2015. *Morbidity and Mortality Weekly Report, 65,* 1205-1211.

Jones, W. J., & Silvestri, G. A. (2010). The Master Settlement Agreement and its impact on tobacco use 10 years later: Lessons for physicians about health policy making. *Chest, 137*(3), 692-700.

Krebs, N. M., Chen, A., Zhu, J., Sun, D., Liao, J., Stennett, A. L., & Muscat, J. E. (2016). Comparison of puff volume with cigarettes per day in predicting nicotine uptake among daily smokers. *American Journal of Epidemiology, 184*(1), 48-57.

Kruger, J., Shaw, L., Kahende, J., & Frank, E. (2012). Health care providers' advice to quit smoking, national health interview survey, 2000, 2005, and 2010. *Preventing Chronic Disease, 9,* E130.

Leventhal, A. M., Strong, D. R., Kirkpatrick, M. G., Unger, J. B., Sussman, S., Riggs, N. R., ... Audrain-McGovern, J. M. (2015). Association of electronic cigarette use with initiation of combustible tobacco product smoking in early adolescence. *Journal of the American Medical Association, 314*(7), 700-707.

Miech, R. A., Johnston, L. D., O'Malley, P. M., Bachman, J. G., & Schulenberg, J. E. (2016). *Monitoring the future national survey results on drug use, 1975-2015: Volume I, secondary school students.* Ann Arbor, MI: Institute for Social Research, University of Michigan. Retrieved from http://monitoring thefuture.org/pubs.html#monographs

Nash, S. H., Liao, L. M., Harris, T. B., & Freedman, N. D. (2016). Cigarette smoking and mortality in adults aged 70 years and older: Results from the NIH-AARP cohort. *American Journal of Preventive Medicine, 52*(3), 276-283. doi:10.1016/j.amepre.2016.09.036

National Institute on Drug Abuse. (2016). *Drug facts: Cigarettes and other tobacco products.* Retrieved from https://www.drugabuse.gov/publications/drugfacts/cigarettes-other-tobacco-products

Nguyen, K. H., Marshall, L., Brown, S., & Neff, L. (2016). State-specific prevalence of current cigarette smoking and smokeless tobacco use among adults – United States, 2014. *Morbidity and Mortality Weekly Report, 65,* 1045-1051.

Papadakis, S., Cole, A. G., Reid, R. D., Coja, M., Aitken, D., Mullen, K.-A., ... Pipe, A. L. (2016). Increasing rates of tobacco treatment delivery in primary care practice: Evaluation of the Ottawa Model for smoking cessation. *Annals of Family Medicine, 14*(3), 235-243.

Piano, M. R., Benowitz, N. L., Fitzgerald, G. A., Corbridge, S., Heath, J., Hahn, E., … Howard, G. (2010). Impact of smokeless tobacco products on cardiovascular disease: Implications for policy, prevention, and treatment: A policy statement from the American Heart Association. *Circulation, 122,* 1520-1544.

Prochaska, J. J., & Benowitz, N. L. (2016). The past, present, and future of nicotine addiction therapy. *Annual Review of Medicine, 67,* 467-486.

Ravenholt, R. (1990). Tobacco's global death march. *Population and Development Review, 16*(2), 213-240.

Steinberg, M. B., Schmelzer, A. C., Lin, P. N., & Garcia, G. (2010). Smoking as a chronic disease. *Current Cardiovascular Risk Reports, 4,* 413-420.

Thurgood, S. L., McNeill, A., Clark-Carter, D., & Brose, L. S. (2016). A systematic review of smoking cessation interventions for adults in substance abuse treatment or recovery. *Nicotine and Tobacco Research, 18*(5), 993-1001.

U.S. Department of Health and Human Services. (2014). *The health consequences of smoking: 50 years of progress. A report of the surgeon general.* Atlanta, GA: Author.

U.S. Department of Health and Human Services. (2016). *E-cigarette use among youth and young adults: A report of the surgeon general – Executive summary.* Atlanta, GA: Author.

U.S. Department of Health, Education, and Welfare. (1964). *Smoking and health: Report of the Advisory Committee to the Surgeon General of the Public Health Service* (PHS Publication No. 1103). Washington, DC: Author.

Wang, T. W., Kenemer, B., Tynan, M. A., Singh, T., & King, B. (2016). Consumption of combustible and smokeless tobacco – United States, 2000-2015. *Morbidity and Mortality Weekly Report, 65,* 1357-1363.

Zeller, M., & Hatkusami, D. (2009). The strategic dialogue on tobacco harm reduction: A vision and blueprint for action in the US. *Tobacco Control, 18,* 324-332.

CHAPTER 6

CAFFEINE

LEARNING OUTCOME

After completing this chapter, the learner will be able to describe the physiological effects, clinical signs and symptoms, and treatment interventions for patients with caffeine-related disorders.

CHAPTER OBJECTIVES

After completing this chapter, the learner will be able to:

1. Identify dietary sources and daily intakes of caffeine.

2. Describe the physiological effects associated with caffeine use.

3. Identify the common adverse effects and withdrawal symptoms associated with caffeine use.

4. Discuss the clinical interventions used to assist the patient in decreasing caffeine intake.

INTRODUCTION

Caffeine, a mild central nervous system stimulant, is the most commonly used mood-altering substance in the world. It occurs naturally as a plant alkaloid and is found in coffee, tea, the kola nut, and less commonly, the guarana and mate plants.

The use of caffeine as a mild stimulant has been well documented. Coffee was first dis-covered by Ethiopians, who would mix crushed dried coffee beans with fat that they rolled into balls for food. By the 14th century, Arabians had developed the process of roasting and grinding coffee beans. In addition, China has used tea for thousands of years.

Caffeine may also be produced synthetically, usually for soft drinks and medications. Caffeine may be found in multiple dietary sources and prescription and nonprescription drugs.

CAFFEINE CONSUMPTION

Eighty percent of the world's population consumes caffeine in some form. Research estimates that in North America, 80% to 90% of adults and children consume at least one caffeinated beverage every day (Mitchell, Knight, Hockenberry, Teplansky, & Hartman, 2014). Coffee is the most common source of caffeine for adults. The average daily intake of caffeine in the United States is about 200 mg per day among adults age 35 to 49 and 225 mg per day among adults age 50 to 64 years. Caffeinated soft drinks are the most common source of caffeine in children. Not surprisingly, 70% of all soft drinks contain caffeine; the consumption of soft drinks in children and adolescents has skyrocketed in the past few decades.

Consumption of energy drinks has also increased dramatically since their introduction to the market in 1997 (Sepkowitz, 2013).

Researchers estimate that Americans consumed about 6 billion energy drinks in 2010, compared to 2.3 billion in 2005. Sales of energy drinks are expected to reach $16 billion in 2017 (University of Maryland, 2014). Energy drinks are aggressively marketed to children, adolescents, and young adults. Regular energy drink consumption has been estimated at 31% of adolescents and 34% of college-age students (Centers for Disease Control and Prevention [CDC], 2015).

It is very difficult to estimate the exact amount of caffeine intake because the amount often depends on the serving size and method of preparation. Regular brewed coffee can contain about 95 mg of caffeine per 8 fluid ounces, whereas the caffeine content of espresso can range from 300 to 500 mg per 8 fluid ounces (Mitchell et al., 2014). The U.S. Food and Drug Administration (FDA) does not regulate the caffeine content in energy drinks, and manufacturers are not required to list caffeine content on ingredient lists of energy drinks in beverages classified as dietary supplements, because caffeine is a non-nutrient ingredient (Bailey, Salshana, Gahche, & Dwyer, 2014). However, an analysis by the FDA found that the caffeine content of energy drinks greatly exceeds that of soft drinks. For example, "Monster Energy" contained 160 mg caffeine per 16 fluid ounces and "Extreme Energy 5-Hour Shot" contained 220 mg of caffeine in 2 fluid ounces, compared to colas that contain 35-40 mg per 12 fluid ounces (University of Maryland, 2014). The Caffeine Awareness Alliance provides a website that is useful in estimating and calculating daily caffeine intake (see the Resources section at the end of this course).

An increasingly popular trend among adolescents and college students is mixing alcoholic beverages with energy drinks (CDC, 2015). Almost 60% of college-age students reported consuming alcohol mixed with energy drinks in the past month, either as cocktails, premixed caffeinated alcoholic beverages, or drinking alcohol and energy drinks separately during the same drinking episode (Howland & Rohsenow, 2012). Among college students, consumption of caffeinated beverages with alcohol is believed to offset the depressant and sedative effects of alcohol, reduce the subjective perception of intoxication, and reduce perceptions of headache, dry mouth, and weakness. Although subjective perceptions of intoxication are reduced, blood alcohol levels are not altered by caffeine, which increases the risk for continued alcohol consumption (Marczinski, Fillmore, Henges, Ramsey, & Young, 2013), resulting in dangerously high blood alcohol levels, risky behaviors, and injury (CDC, 2015).

BIOCHEMISTRY

Caffeine is a lipid-soluble molecule (similar to alcohol and nicotine) that acts as an inhibitor of adenosine receptors in the brain, which activates the release of excitatory neurotransmitters. The molecule quickly crosses the blood-brain barrier, with peak blood levels occurring within 30 to 120 minutes and a mean plasma half-life of 2.5 to 4.5 hours (Nehlig, 2016). It is this rapid absorption that results in the stimulant effect of caffeine on the central nervous system.

Caffeine is largely metabolized through the P450 liver enzyme system and results in three metabolites: paraxanthine, theophylline, and theobromine (Nehlig, 2016). Paraxanthine acts to increase lipolysis, elevating glycerol and free fatty acids; theobromine dilates blood vessels, increases urine volume, and contributes to the diuretic effect of caffeine; lastly, theophylline relaxes the smooth muscles of the bronchi. Tobacco increases the metabolism of caffeine, and several medications, such as cimetidine and hormonal contraceptives, decrease the rate of metabolism of caffeine.

PHYSIOLOGICAL EFFECTS

Caffeine consumption is considered safe and even beneficial in low to moderate doses (Addicott, 2014; Mitchell et al., 2014; Nehlig, 2016). Low doses of caffeine (50 to 200 mg) improve alertness, vigilance, sense of well-being, sociability, concentration, and mood (Addicott, 2014; Meredith, Juliano, Hughes, & Griffiths, 2013; Mitchell et al., 2014; Nehlig, 2016). Among daily caffeine users, these pleasant mood-altering effects may have more to do with the suppression of such low-grade withdrawal symptoms as fatigue and sleepiness than with the direct effect of caffeine.

Adverse Effects

The FDA states that daily intake of up to 400 mg of caffeine, the equivalent of about 4 cups of regular brewed coffee per day, is not associated with adverse health effects (Mitchell et al., 2014; Nehlig, 2016). However, intake of higher doses of caffeine, such as 400 to 800 mg in one sitting, can cause irritability, anxiety, nausea, restlessness, sleep disturbances, and headaches. These adverse effects are mitigated by an individual's tolerance and are usually short in duration. Patients with anxiety disorders are particularly vulnerable to the effects of caffeine, and many will self-limit their caffeine intake to decrease anxiety and panic symptoms. Other common adverse health effects include insomnia, gastroesophageal reflux disorder, mild increases in blood pressure, and urinary incontinence. Women who are pregnant or trying to become pregnant are counseled to decrease or abstain from caffeine intake.

Caffeine acts as a reinforcer. That is, individuals will continue to self-administer the drug if they consume it in dosages that increase its mood-altering effects. Tolerance, which describes the process of decreasing responsiveness to a drug after repeated exposures (American Psychiatric Association [APA], 2013), occurs as well.

Withdrawal Symptoms

Caffeine withdrawal is characterized by symptoms that occur with cessation of caffeine intake. Peak withdrawal occurs 1 to 2 days after cessation of caffeine consumption, but gradually resolve after a few days (Smith, 2013). The severity of withdrawal is usually reflective of the amount of daily consumption. Significant withdrawal symptoms occur with as little as 100 mg of caffeine per day – the equivalent of one cup of regular brewed coffee. The following are the most common withdrawal symptoms, in order of frequency (APA, 2013):

- Headache
- Marked fatigue
- Drowsiness
- Difficulty concentrating
- Work difficulty
- Irritability
- Dysphoric mood/depressed mood
- Flulike symptoms (e.g., nausea, vomiting, muscle pain/stiffness)

CAFFEINE-RELATED DISORDERS: DIAGNOSTIC CRITERIA

The *Diagnostic and Statistical Manual of Mental Disorders,* 5th edition (*DSM-5;* APA, 2013) lists these caffeine-related diagnoses: caffeine intoxication, caffeine withdrawal, other caffeine-induced disorders, and unspecific caffeine-related disorder not otherwise specified (Addicott, 2014). The World Health Organization (WHO), in its parallel system, the *International Classification of Disease,* 10th revision (*ICD-10;* 1992), recognizes caffeine dependence as a diagnosis. The *DSM-5* does not recognize the diagnosis of caffeine dependence but instead proposes that the diagnostic category of caffeine use disorder warrants further study and consideration for future versions of the *DSM.*

Caffeine intoxication or caffeine poisoning is a result of a significant ingestion of caffeine – at least 250 mg but more likely more than 500 mg. Common signs of caffeine intoxication include restlessness, nervousness (anxiety), excitement, insomnia, a flushed face, diuresis, gastrointestinal disturbance, twitching muscles, rambling thoughts and speech, tachycardia or cardiac arrhythmia, periods of inexhaustibility, and psychomotor agitation (Sadock, Sadock, & Ruiz, 2015). These symptoms cause impairment in functioning and are not caused by another medical condition (APA, 2013). The psychiatric co-morbidities typically associated with caffeine intoxication include depressive disorders, bipolar disorders, psychotic disorders, eating disorders, sleep disorders, and other substance-related disorders (APA, 2013). Caffeine-induced disorders include caffeine-induced anxiety disorder and caffeine-induced sleep disorder (APA, 2013). Caffeine-induced anxiety disorder is characterized by symptoms of anxiety that occur soon after ingestion of caffeine. Symptoms are similar to generalized anxiety disorder; patients will be overly talkative and irritable and report feeling "wired" with poor sleep (Sadock et al., 2015, p. 642). Caffeine-induced sleep disorder is characterized by difficulty with sleeping, including difficulty falling asleep, awakening in the middle of the night, and early morning awakening (Sadock et al., 2015). Unspecified caffeine use disorder is caffeine use that causes clinically significant distress or impairment in functioning, but does not meet full diagnostic criteria for caffeine-use disorders (APA, 2013).

NURSING ASSESSMENT AND CLINICAL INTERVENTIONS TO REDUCE CAFFEINE INTAKE

When obtaining a patient's history, it is important to elicit a thorough caffeine intake; this includes beverages, foods, and prescription and nonprescription drugs. Sensitivity to culture and ethnicity is also important in recognizing alternative methods of caffeine ingestion. Although it can be challenging to determine an accurate intake, if a patient is consuming more than 200 mg of caffeine per day, he or she should be carefully questioned about the presence of adverse physical symptoms and negative mood-altering symptoms and counseled to cut intake slowly.

In counseling a patient on caffeine reduction, it is important to identify the patient's goal clearly. Is the goal complete elimination of caffeine or a reduction in the amount of caffeine consumed? If the goal is reduction, what is the reduction goal in terms of milligrams? First, educate the patient on the dietary, pharmacological, and nonpharmacological sources of caffeine. Estimate with the patient his or her current daily caffeine intake. It is often helpful to have the patient keep a food diary for 1 to 2 weeks to determine accurate caffeine intake. Provide handouts and patient education materials with common sources of caffeine and the milligrams of caffeine associated with these sources. Encourage the patient to slowly decrease caffeine by 10% to 25% every few days until he or she reaches the identified goal. Suggesting noncaffeinated alternatives to replace the usual sources of caffeine is another helpful intervention.

Similar to strategies used for substance use reduction and abstinence, clinicians often employ motivational interviewing and the counseling relationship to help patients with caffeine use disorders. Motivational interviewing and counseling include expressing empathy, developing insights, and supporting self-efficacy. Nurses can assist by encouraging the patient to set specific goals and share these goals with a close friend or significant other who can offer support, identifying potential barriers to decreased caffeine intake, reframing withdrawal as a temporary process, and following up with the patient to monitor progress in meeting established goals.

Other substance use therapies for caffeine-related diagnoses are cognitive-behavioral therapy, group therapy, and 12-step self-help programs. Cognitive-behavioral therapy teaches coping skills and awareness of triggers and feelings preceding the use of caffeine. Group therapy is effective in helping group members to identify behaviors in each other that they may not be able to see in themselves. Members learn to express feelings and learn new coping skills in a therapeutic environment. A specific 12-step program for caffeine use has not yet been created, although this type of support group is useful for patients who misuse caffeine.

SUMMARY

Caffeine is a mild central nervous system stimulant. Moderate amounts of caffeine (20 to 200 mg) generally produce a pleasant, mood-altering feeling. Significant amounts of caffeine (more than 200 mg) may result in negative, mood-altering effects such as nervousness, increased anxiety, jitteriness, and upset stomach. Patients with anxiety disorders are particularly vulnerable to the effects of caffeine.

The most common symptoms of caffeine withdrawal are headache, fatigue, drowsiness, difficulty concentrating, difficulty working, irritability, depression, and flulike symptoms (APA, 2013). There are four caffeine-induced psychiatric disorders: caffeine intoxication, caffeine withdrawal, other caffeine-induced disorders, and unspecified caffeine-related disorders (APA, 2013). In obtaining a patient's history, it is important to elicit a thorough caffeine intake. In counseling a patient on caffeine reduction, it is important to identify the patient's goal clearly. Encourage the patient to slowly decrease caffeine by 10% to 25% every few days until he or she reaches the goal.

EXAM QUESTIONS

CHAPTER 6
Questions 29–32

Note: Choose the one option that BEST answers each question.

29. The average adult intake of caffeine in the United States is

    a. 160 to 180 mg per day.

    b. 200 to 225 mg per day.

    c. 280 to 325 mg per day.

    d. 320 to 350 mg per day.

30. Which type of effect does caffeine have on the central nervous system?

    a. A depressant effect

    b. A stimulant effect

    c. A modifier effect

    d. An antagonist effect

31. The most common symptom of caffeine withdrawal is

    a. drowsiness.

    b. irritability.

    c. headache.

    d. flulike symptoms.

32. When counseling patients on decreasing their caffeine intake, the practitioner recommends to reduce caffeine by 10% to 25% every

    a. day until the patient's goal is reached.

    b. other day until the patient's goal is reached.

    c. few days until the patient's goal is reached.

    d. week until the patient's goal is reached.

REFERENCES

Addicott, M. A. (2014). Caffeine use disorder: A review of the evidence and future implications. *Current Addictions Report, 1*(3), 186-192.

American Psychiatric Association. (2013). *Diagnostic and statistical manual of mental disorders* (5th ed.). Arlington, VA: Author.

Bailey, R. L., Saldanha, L. G., & Dwyer, J. T. (2014). Estimating caffeine intake from energy drinks and dietary supplements in the United States. *Nutrition Reviews, 72*(Supplement S1), 9-13.

Centers for Disease Control and Prevention. (2015). *Fact sheets: Caffeine and alcohol.* Retrieved from https://www.cdc.gov/alcohol/fact-sheets/caffeine-and-alcohol.htm

Howland, J., & Rohsenow, D. J. (2012). Risks of energy drinks mixed with alcohol. *Journal of the American Medical Association, 309*(3), 245-246.

Marczinski, C. A., Fillmore, M. T., Henges, A. L., Ramsey, M. A., & Young, C. R. (2013). Mixing an energy drink with an alcoholic beverage increases motivation for more alcohol in college students. *Alcohol Clinical and Experimental Research, 37*(2), 276-283.

Meredith, S. E., Juliano, L. M., Hughes, J. R., & Griffiths, R. R. (2013). Caffeine use disorder: A comprehensive review and research agenda. *Journal of Caffeine Research, 3*(3), 114-130.

Mitchell, D. C., Knight, C. A., Hockenberry, J., Teplansky, R., & Hartman, T. J. (2014). Beverage caffeine intake in the U.S. *Food and Chemical Toxicology, 63,* 136-142.

Nehlig, A. (2016). Effects of coffee/caffeine on brain health and disease: What should I tell my patients? *Practical Neurology, 16,* 89-95.

Pohler, H. (2010). Caffeine intoxication and addiction. *Journal for Nurse Practitioners, 6*(1), 49-52.

Sadock, B. J., Sadock V. A., & Ruiz, P (2015). *Kaplan & Sadock's synopsis of psychiatry, behavioral sciences/clinical psychiatry* (11th Ed.). Philadelphia: Wolters Kluwer.

Smith, A. P. (2013). Caffeine and caffeinated energy drinks. In P. M. Miller (Ed.). *Principles of addiction: Comprehensive addictive behaviors and disorders, 1,* 777-785. San Diego: Elsevier Press.

Smith, A. P. (2013). Caffeine and caffeinated energy drinks. In P. M. Miller (Ed.). *Principles of addiction: Comprehensive addictive behaviors and disorders, 1,* 777-785. San Diego: Elsevier Press.

University of Maryland, Francis King Cary School of Law, Legal Resource Center for Public Health Policy (2014). *Energy drinks fact sheet.* Retrieved from https://www.law.umaryland.edu/programs/publichealth/documents/LRC_Energy_Drinks_Fact_Sheet.pdf

World Health Organization. (1992). *The ICD-10 classification of mental and behavioural disorders: Clinical descriptions and diagnostic guidelines.* Geneva: World Health Organization.

CHAPTER 7

ALCOHOL

LEARNING OUTCOME

After completing this chapter, the learner will be able to describe the screening, diagnosis, and treatment of patients with alcohol use disorders.

CHAPTER OBJECTIVES

After completing this chapter, the learner will be able to:

1. Identify the prevalence of alcohol use disorders in the United States.

2. Discuss the potential health effects of alcohol use disorders in patients.

3. Explain the screening process for alcohol use disorders in patients.

4. Discuss behavioral therapy and medications for patients with alcohol use disorders.

INTRODUCTION

Alcohol is a widely used psychoactive substance in the United States (National Institute on Alcohol Abuse and Alcoholism [NIAAA], 2017). Alcohol is consumed at meals, for medicinal or religious purposes, in celebrating special occasions, and as a social facilitator. Moderate use of alcohol – no more than one (female) or two (male) drinks per day – appears to convey health benefits, whereas at-risk drinking behaviors (e.g., drinking too much on one occasion, drinking too often) and alcohol use disorder result in significant morbidity and mortality. More than half of individuals in the United States aged 12 or older report being current drinkers (Center for Behavioral Health Statistics and Quality [CBHSQ], 2016b). Identifying at-risk drinking, with or without dependence, is critical to help patients gain an understanding of the physical, social, and psychological risks associated with alcohol consumption.

EPIDEMIOLOGY AND PREVALENCE

The most common type of alcohol consumed in the United States is beer, followed by spirits and wine. Figure 7-1 shows the historical trend by beverage type. Among people in the United States aged 12 years and older, 51.7% report alcohol use (CBHSQ, 2016b). Current alcohol use is defined as consuming at least one drink or more in the past 30 days. This translates to an estimated 138.3 million people in the U.S. population currently using alcohol. Current alcohol use numbers have decreased from 2014 (NIAAA, 2015a). However, in spite of the slight downward trend, the United States continues to be 10% above the target goal for the overall level of per-capita consumption of alcohol established by the *Healthy People 2020* national objectives to maintain the optimum health of individuals (Office of Disease Prevention and Health Promotion, 2016).

FIGURE 7-1: U.S. PER-CAPITA ALCOHOL (ETHANOL) CONSUMPTION BY BEVERAGE TYPE, 1977-2013

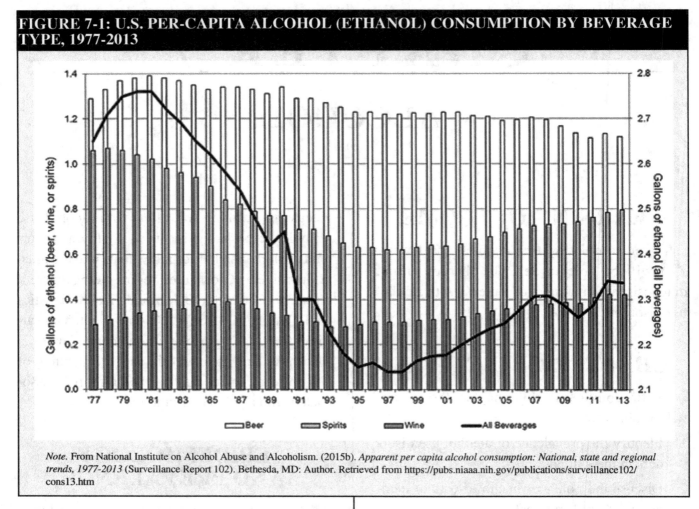

Note. From National Institute on Alcohol Abuse and Alcoholism. (2015b). *Apparent per capita alcohol consumption: National, state and regional trends, 1977-2013* (Surveillance Report 102). Bethesda, MD: Author. Retrieved from https://pubs.niaaa.nih.gov/publications/surveillance102/cons13.htm

The National Survey on Drug Use and Health (NSDUH) benchmarks alcohol consumption in the United States (CBHSQ, 2016a). Administered annually, the survey includes specific and detailed questions about the consumption of alcoholic beverages. A standard drink is defined as any drink that contains 14 grams of pure alcohol, such as a can or bottle of beer, a glass of wine or a wine cooler, a shot of liquor, or a mixed drink with liquor in it. Figure 7-2 shows standard drink equivalents as defined by the NIAAA (2016b).

In the 2015 NSDUH, consistent with federal definitions and other federal data collections, the CBHSQ changed the definition for the number of alcoholic drinks constituting binge drinking for women from five to four drinks on the same occasion on at least 1 day in the past 30

days (CBHSQ, 2016a). Nearly half of current alcohol users reported binge alcohol use. Binge drinking for males remained unchanged and is defined as drinking five or more drinks on the same occasion on at least 1 day in the past 30 days. Heavy alcohol use is defined as binge drinking on 5 or more days in the past 30 days based on the thresholds that were described previously for males and females. Any alcohol use, binge drinking, and heavy drinking are not mutually exclusive categories of use; heavy use is included in estimates of binge and current use, and binge use is included in estimates of current use (CBHSQ, 2016a; see Figure 7-3).

In 2015, approximately 66.7 million people aged 12 or older were binge alcohol users in the past 30 days. This equates to 1 in 4 people aged 12 or older (24.9%). Of those reporting binge

continued on page 114

FIGURE 7-2: STANDARD DRINK EQUIVALENTS

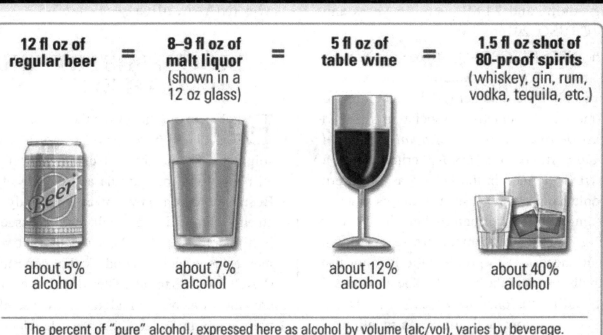

Note. From National Institute on Alcohol Abuse and Alcoholism. (2016b). *What is a standard drink?* Retrieved from https://www.niaaa.nih.gov/alcohol-health/overview-alcohol-consumption/what-standard-drink

FIGURE 7-3: PAST-MONTH BINGE USE AND HEAVY ALCOHOL USE AMONG PEOPLE AGE 12 OR OLDER, BY AGE GROUP, 2015

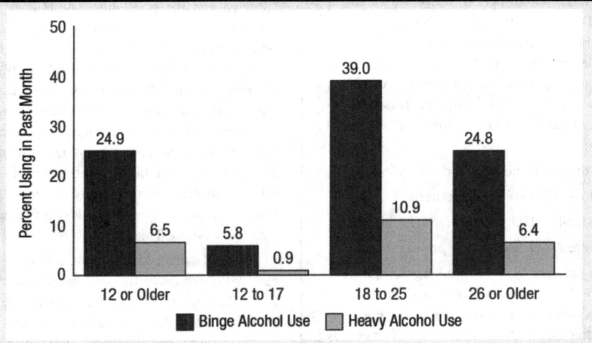

In 2015, the threshold for determining binge alcohol use for females changed from five or more drinks on an occasion to four or more drinks on an occasion.

Note. From National Institute on Alcohol Abuse and Alcoholism. (2016a). *Drinking levels defined.* Retrieved from https://www.niaaa.nih.gov/alcohol-health/overview-alcohol-consumption/moderate-binge-drinking

drinking, 5.8% were adolescents, 39% were young adults, and 24.8% were 26 years and older (CBHSQ, 2016a). 35

The NSDUH (CBHSQ, 2016a) report indicated that 15.7 million Americans met criteria for an alcohol use disorder (AUD) according to the American Psychiatric Association's (APA) *Diagnostic and Statistical Manual of Mental Disorders,* fifth edition *(DSM-5)* criteria (2013). An AUD is defined in the *DSM-5* as "a pattern of problematic alcohol use that causes distress and significant impairment. There is a strong craving and a persistent desire to cut down without success. The problematic alcohol use eventually impacts the patient's social, occupational, and recreational activities. An AUD can result in hazardous activities, continuation of alcohol use in spite of negative consequences (physical or psychological), and may result in tolerance and/or withdrawal" (APA, 2013, pp. 490-491). A patient meeting any 2 of the 11 *DSM-5* criteria for AUD (see Figure 7-4) during the same 12-month period receives a diagnosis of AUD. A severity scale for alcohol use has been added to better define the extent of alcohol use. The severity of an AUD – mild, moderate, or severe – is based on the number of *DSM-5* diagnostic criteria met. Using the *DSM-5* diagnostic criteria, an AUD diagnosis is classified as follows:

- No diagnosis: no criteria or one criterion

- Mild AUD: two or three criteria

- Moderate AUD: four or five criteria

- Severe AUD: six or more criteria

For women, low-risk drinking is defined as no more than three drinks on any single day and no more than seven drinks per week. For men, it is defined as no more than four drinks on any single day and no more than fourteen drinks per week. Low-risk drinking for healthy people over the age of 65 is defined as no more than one drink in a day and no more than seven drinks in a week (NIAAA, 2016a; see Figure 7-5).

BIOCHEMISTRY AND HEALTH EFFECTS

Ethyl alcohol (ethanol) is the substance found in alcoholic beverages. Ethanol is a water-soluble molecule that diffuses uniformly into all body water, both inside and outside of cells. Because women have lower lean body mass, ethanol elimination per unit of lean tissue mass is higher in women. This means that women may achieve higher blood alcohol concentration (BAC) levels than men after drinking equivalent amounts of alcohol. In addition, because of ethanol's solubility, it readily crosses the blood-brain barrier, profoundly affecting the central nervous system (CNS); it also crosses the placenta and thus affects fetal development, and it affects every organ in the body (Cederbaum, 2012).

Ethanol is primarily absorbed from the stomach and the small intestine (Cederbaum, 2012; Saunders et al., 2016). The age-old recommendation of "eat before you drink" is based on the fact that food in the stomach delays gastric emptying and the absorption of ethanol into the system. An empty stomach increases gastric emptying, and therefore absorption is increased. Thus, drinking on an empty stomach increases BAC levels. Other factors that appear to affect ethanol absorption include medications, illicit drugs, nicotine, and estrogen levels (Center for Substance Abuse Treatment, 2009).

Ethanol is considered to be a CNS depressant with both protective and harmful qualities. According to the World Health Organization (WHO, 2011), the link between alcohol consumption and consequences depends on the amount consumed, patterns of drinking, and toxic and beneficial biochemical effects. An example of beneficial biochemical effects in a moderate

FIGURE 7-4: *DSM-5* ALCOHOL USE DISORDER CRITERIA	
1	Had times when you ended up drinking more or longer than you intended?
2	More than once wanted to cut down or stop drinking, or tried to but couldn't?
3	Spent a lot of time drinking? Or being sick or getting over other aftereffects?
4	Wanted a drink so badly you couldn't think of anything else?
5	Found that drinking – or being sick from drinking – often interfered with taking care of your home or family? Or caused job troubles? Or school problems?
6	Continued to drink even though it was causing trouble with your family or friends?
7	Given up or cut back on activities that were important or interesting to you, or gave you pleasure, in order to drink?
8	More than once gotten into situations while or after drinking that increased your chances of getting hurt (such as driving, swimming, using machinery, walking in a dangerous area, or having unsafe sex)?
9	Continued to drink even though it was making you feel depressed or anxious or adding to another health problem? Or after having had a memory blackout?
10	Had to drink much more than you once did to get the effect you want? Or found that your usual number of drinks had much less effect than before?
11	Found that when the effects of alcohol were wearing off, you had withdrawal symptoms, such as trouble sleeping, shakiness, restlessness, nausea, sweating, a racing heart, or a seizure? Or sensed things that were not there?

The presence of two or more of these criteria during the same 12-month period indicates an alcohol use disorder (AUD).

Note. Adapted from American Psychiatric Association. (2013). *Diagnostic and statistical manual of mental disorders* (5th ed.). Arlington, VA: Author.

drinker would be the protection against blood clot formation and prevention of coronary artery disease. Moderate drinking also appears to confer benefits against diabetes, gallbladder disease, and ischemic stroke (due to blood clots) and improve lipid levels (Klatsky, 2015).

Harmful use of alcohol ranks among the top five risk factors for disease, disability, and death throughout the world (WHO, 2011). In 2012, 3.3 million deaths, or 5.9% of deaths globally, were attributed to alcohol (WHO, 2014). The harmful effects of alcohol in patients who drink heavily, misuse alcohol, or are alcohol dependent are profound and significant. Several recent studies have linked more than 30 disease conditions to the toxic effects of alcohol and have identified it as a contributing factor to many more (NIAAA, 2012; Rehm & Shield, 2013). Disease categories that have a direct or indirect link to alcohol include infectious disease, cancer (especially of the head, neck, and gastrointestinal tract), diabetes, neuropsychiatric disease, cardiovascular disease, digestive tract problems (e.g., gastritis), liver-pancreas-gallbladder disease (e.g., cirrhosis, pancreatitis, gallstones), and unintentional and intentional injury (NIAAA, 2012). Prenatal exposure to alcohol increases the risk for infant low birth weight, prematurity, intrauterine growth retardation, and spontaneous abortion. Fetal alcohol spectrum disorders, which include fetal alcohol syndrome, are the most common preventable causes of intellectual disabilities in the United States (Tan, Denny, Cheal, Sniezek, & Kanny, 2015).

The evidence is as yet unclear regarding the exact association between alcohol dependence and depressive disorders. It is often unclear whether the alcohol problem precedes the depression or the depression precedes the alcohol problem. However, the presence of comor-

FIGURE 7-5: INTERPRETATION OF THE AUDIT SCORE

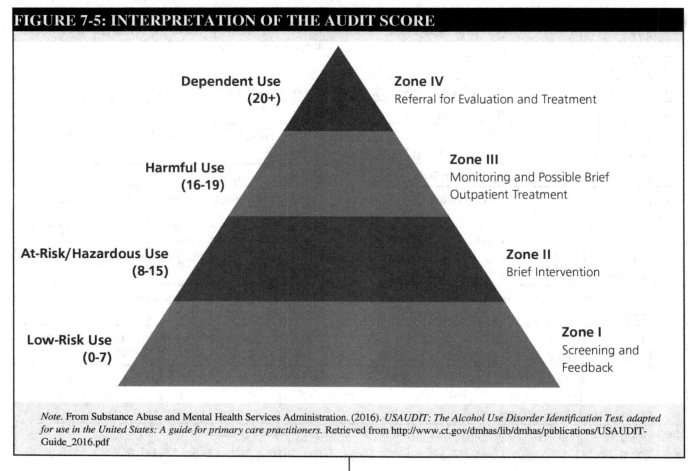

Dependent Use
(20+)

Zone IV
Referral for Evaluation and Treatment

Harmful Use
(16-19)

Zone III
Monitoring and Possible Brief
Outpatient Treatment

At-Risk/Hazardous Use
(8-15)

Zone II
Brief Intervention

Low-Risk Use
(0-7)

Zone I
Screening and
Feedback

Note. From Substance Abuse and Mental Health Services Administration. (2016). *USAUDIT: The Alcohol Use Disorder Identification Test, adapted for use in the United States: A guide for primary care practitioners.* Retrieved from http://www.ct.gov/dmhas/lib/dmhas/publications/USAUDIT-Guide_2016.pdf

bid depression must be considered in every patient who presents with an AUD (WHO, 2014) due to alcohol being a CNS depressant.

Alcohol use is a major contributing factor to accidents, injuries, and trauma (including motor vehicle accidents, head injuries, spinal cord injuries, burns, and drowning; WHO, 2014). Alcohol use is also associated with assault, homicide, and family violence. According to the National Council on Alcoholism and Drug Dependence (NCADD, 2015), alcohol use is reported to have been a factor in a majority of crimes. Nearly 50% of jail and prison inmates are clinically addicted, and 80% of offenders misuse drugs or alcohol. Alcohol is a factor in 40% of violent crimes (NCADD, 2015).

Whether an individual becomes addicted to alcohol is determined by one's genetic makeup and environment. Researchers have found that about half of one's risk for alcoholism is influ-

enced by genetics. The remaining risk is related to one's environment, including personal stressors, and family risk factors for developing an AUD (NIAAA, n.d.). Protective factors and societal factors also play a role in whether an individual becomes addicted to other misused substances, such as illicit drugs (American Society of Addiction Medicine [ASAM], 2011).

Women have increased vulnerability to alcohol due to their typically lower body weight, smaller liver capacity, and increased proportion of body fat, which are factors resulting in increased blood alcohol levels at a much more rapid rate than men (NIAAA, 2015a). Women with an AUD are at risk for liver disease, heart disease, and breast cancer, and prenatal alcohol exposure can cause learning and behavior problems in the developing fetus (NIAAA, 2015a).

An AUD not only affects the patient but also may have an impact on people other than the drinker. Family disruption, financial difficulties, and employment problems have been cited as common problems associated with problem drinking (NIAAA, 2012).

SCREENING

Screening for alcohol use and alcohol-related problems enables the clinician to identify people who are likely to have an alcohol problem. Screening is recommended to be conducted before or during a routine health history and physical examination, when prescribing a medication that interacts with alcohol, when treating patients in emergency departments or urgent care centers, and when caring for women who are pregnant or trying to conceive. Screening is also appropriate for patients who are likely to drink heavily, such as smokers, adolescents, and young adults; patients who have health problems that may be alcohol induced; and patients with a chronic illness that is not responding to treatment as expected (NIAAA, 2007).

The NIAAA (2007) recommends that alcohol screening follow these steps: ask about alcohol use, assess for an AUD, advise and assist the patient, and follow up with continued support. One study has shown that a positive response to the question, "On any single occasion during the past 3 months, have you had more than five drinks containing alcohol?" assists in identifying a patient who meets either the NIAAA criteria for at-risk drinking or the *DSM-5* criteria for alcohol use disorder (APA, 2013; NIAAA, 2007).

The NIAAA (2007) has recommended that the clinician begin to screen a patient for alcohol use by asking, "Do you sometimes drink beer, wine, or other alcoholic beverages?" If the patient answers "no," then the screening is complete. If the patient answers "yes," the clinician should ask, "How many times in the past year have you had five or more drinks in a day?" (for men) or "four or more drinks in a day?" (for women). If the patient responds that he or she drinks at these levels, the screening is considered positive, and the clinician should ask the patient, "On average, how many days per week do you have an alcoholic drink, and on a typical drinking day, how many drinks do you have?" From this information, the clinician should determine the weekly average of drinking by multiplying the number of days per week the patient drinks by how many drinks the patient consumes (see Figure 7-6).

Another method to screen for alcohol use is to use a standardized assessment tool. The Alcohol Use Disorders Identification Test (AUDIT) provides a reliable and valid baseline with which to assess alcohol use and may be completed by the patient before seeing a clinician. The AUDIT can be administered either as an oral interview or as a self-report questionnaire (see Table 7-1). This screen places the patient in an alcohol use category based on his or her identified level of risk. A negative prescreen is obtained when the patient

---

FIGURE 7-6: SCREENING FOR ALCOHOL USE

Step 1: Ask about alcohol use.

Step 2: Assess for alcohol use disorders.

Step 3: Advise and assist

- for at-risk drinking, and
- for alcohol use disorders.

Step 4: At follow-up, continue support

- for at-risk drinking, and
- for alcohol use disorders.

Note. From National Institute on Alcohol Abuse and Alcoholism. (2007). *Helping patients who drink too much: A clinician's guide* (updated 2005 ed., NIH Publication No. 07-3769). Retrieved from https://pubs.niaaa.nih.gov/publications/practitioner/CliniciansGuide2005/guide.pdf

scores between 0 and 7; no treatment is needed for patients in this category. For a score on the AUDIT between 8 and 15, the clinician would provide simple advice focused on the reduction of hazardous drinking. Scores between 16 and 19 indicate the need for brief counseling and continued monitoring, and scores of 20 or above clearly warrant further diagnostic evaluation for alcohol use disorder (see Figure 7-5). These are guidelines provided by the developers of the AUDIT and

TABLE 7-1: ALCOHOL USE DISORDERS IDENTIFICATION TEST (AUDIT)

Questions	SCORE				
	0	**1**	**2**	**3**	**4**
1. How often do you have a drink containing alcohol?	Never	Monthly or less	2 to 4 times per month	2 to 3 times per week	4 or more times per week
2. How many drinks containing alcohol do you have on a typical day when you are drinking?	1 or 2	3 or 4	5 or 6	7 to 9	10 or more
3. How often do you have six or more drinks on one occasion?	Never	Less than monthly	Monthly	Weekly	Daily or almost daily
4. How often during the past year have you found that you were not able to stop drinking once you had started?	Never	Less than monthly	Monthly	Weekly	Daily or almost daily
5. How often during the past year have you failed to do what was normally expected of you because of drinking?	Never	Less than monthly	Monthly	Weekly	Daily or almost daily
6. How often during the past year have you needed a first drink in the morning to get yourself going after a heavy drinking session?	Never	Less than monthly	Monthly	Weekly	Daily or almost daily
7. How often during the past year have you had a feeling of guilt or remorse after drinking?	Never	Less than monthly	Monthly	Weekly	Daily or almost daily
8. How often during the past year have you been unable to remember what happened the night before because of your drinking?	Never	Less than monthly	Monthly	Weekly	Daily or almost daily
9. Have you or someone else been injured because of your drinking?	No		Yes, but not in the past year		Yes, during the past year
10. Has a relative, friend, doctor, or other healthcare worker been concerned about your drinking or suggested you cut down?	No		Yes, but not in the past year		Yes, during the past year

Note. From Babor, T. F., Higgins-Biddle, J. C., Saunders, J. B., & Monteiro, M. G. (2001). *AUDIT: The Alcohol Use Disorders Identification Test. Guidelines for use in primary care* (2nd ed.). Geneva, Switzerland: World Health Organization. Retrieved from http://whqlibdoc.who.int/hq/2001/who_msd_msb_01.6a.pdf

should not replace clinical judgment by the clinician. The clinician should consider other factors such as family history and the patient's perceived honesty in responding to the AUDIT questions as well (Babor, Higgins-Biddle, Saunders, & Monteiro, 2001).

TREATMENT

Behavioral therapy options are available for the treatment of patients with an AUD. Behavioral counseling interventions recommended by the U.S. Preventive Services Task Force should be consistent with the five *As* approach:

1. Assess: Ask about/assess behavioral health risk(s) and factors affecting the choice of behavior-change goals/methods.

2. Advise: Give clear, specific, and personalized behavior-change advice, including information about personal health harms and benefits.

3. Agree: Collaboratively select appropriate treatment goals and methods based on the patient's interest and willingness to change the behavior.

4. Assist: Using behavior-change techniques (self-help and/or counseling), aid the patient in achieving agreed-upon goals by acquiring the skills, confidence, and social/environmental supports for behavior change, supplemented with adjunctive medical treatments when appropriate.

5. Arrange: Schedule follow-up contacts (in person or by telephone) to provide ongoing assistance/support and to adjust the treatment plan as needed, including referral to more intensive or specialized treatment.

(U.S. Preventive Services Task Force, n.d.)

An approach that has shown to be effective for patients with AUD is the Screening Brief Intervention and Referral for Treatment (SBIRT). During the screening stage, the clinician uses a tool such as the AUDIT to assess for risky alcohol behaviors. The SBIRT is most effective in addressing mild to moderate drinking disorders (Agerwala & McCance-Katz, 2012). The SBIRT also uses techniques of motivational interviewing (i.e., another behavioral approach) to motivate individuals to reduce or abstain from drinking. Brief interventions that are tailored to patients' specific concerns are preferred. The SBIRT process consists of the following steps:

- Raise the subject (ask permission to discuss the screen).

- Provide feedback (identify risk level, and explain the connection between substance use and the reason for the medical visit).

- Enhance motivation (use open-ended questions, affirmations, reflections, and summary).

- Negotiate a plan (encourage a specific plan or goal to reduce or abstain from alcohol; provide a referral, support autonomy, and make affirming statements).

Brief interventions are relatively simple counseling strategies that may occur one or more times. Research has shown that providing encouragement and educational information is effective in preventing or decreasing alcohol use. Clinical trials have demonstrated that brief interventions can decrease alcohol use significantly among those who drink more than the recommended limits but who are not alcohol dependent (NIAAA, 2007). Research studies have demonstrated a reduction in alcohol consumption and binge drinking of up to 33% in patients who were drinking at at-risk levels and received brief interventions. These reductions were significant and persisted over 3 years. Further, decreases in blood pressure readings, levels of gamma-glutamyl transferase (an enzyme found in the liver), psychosocial problems, hospital stays, and hospital readmissions for alcohol-related trauma were all significantly reduced. The evidence clearly supports the efficacy and sustainability of brief interventions. Every clinician can provide a brief intervention, and the data suggest that the more frequently the brief intervention is reinforced, the better the outcome. A physician's order or a definitive diagnosis is not required to address alcohol misuse; health behavior counseling decreases the morbidity and mortality of AUD, and clinicians should conduct brief interventions as needed (NIAAA, 2007).

If the patient is assessed to have an AUD based on the *DSM-5* criteria, the safest recommendation is for the patient to abstain from drinking. If a patient has an AUD and is willing to abstain from alcohol, it is important to provide additional resources. These resources may include (1) referral to an addiction specialist who can evaluate the severity of the patient's addiction, provide the resources needed in terms of inpatient or outpatient management, and determine whether the patient needs to be medically managed for withdrawal symptoms; (2) referral to a mutual-help group such as Alcoholics Anonymous (AA); and (3) a defined follow-up plan for the patient.

Research demonstrates that if the patient with an AUD is unwilling to abstain, repeated brief interventions result in significant decreases in the amount of alcohol consumed and in the cessation of alcohol consumption. For the patient with an AUD who is repeatedly hospitalized, or who seeks assistance and is in regular contact with a clinician, a 2-minute intervention should be done at each visit or hospitalization. The NIAAA (2007) recommends that the clinician take the following steps:

- Support efforts to cut down or abstain, with abstinence as the goal.

- Relate alcohol use to the patient's physical, emotional, and social problems.

- Address coexisting disorders.

- Consider additional resources, such as the following:
  ◦ An addiction specialist
  ◦ A mutual-help group
  ◦ Help from significant others
  ◦ Referral to a healthcare provider for medication management

Other Types of Behavioral Therapy

Several types of behavioral therapy are available to facilitate change and treat patients with an AUD, including cognitive-behavioral therapies (CBT), contingency management with a community reinforcement approach, motivational enhancement therapy (MET), 12-step interventions, mutual-help groups (e.g., AA), and family behavioral therapy; patients may also use a combination of these therapies.

CBT developed as a therapy to treat and prevent relapse of AUD. With CBT, patients learn to identify and correct problematic behaviors and to use the pyramid approach: how one thinks influences how one feels, which in turn influences how one acts.

Research has shown that contingency management can be an effective treatment by providing tangible rewards, such as vouchers for food items, movie passes, and other goods that promote a drug-free lifestyle, to promote positive behaviors such as abstinence (National Institute on Drug Abuse [NIDA], 2012).

Patients with an AUD can benefit from a type of outpatient therapy that involves an intensive, 24-week program consisting of a community reinforcement approach plus vouchers. The two goals of the approach are to eliminate positive reinforcers for drinking and enhance positive reinforcers for abstinence, which might include recreational, familial, social, and vocational reinforcers, as well as material incentives such as gift cards. The goal is to make a life without substance use more rewarding than a life with substance use. The treatment goals are for the patient who is drinking to learn new life skills and to reduce alcohol consumption (NIDA, 2012).

MET is a counseling approach that helps individuals resolve their ambivalence about engaging in treatment and stopping their alcohol use. MET is a brief, 2- to 4-hour session that combines assessment, feedback, and principles of motivational interviewing. MET is particularly effective for patients who are angry and resistant. Motivational interviewing principles are used to strengthen motivation and build a plan for change. Coping strategies for high-risk situations are suggested and discussed with the patient. In subsequent sessions, the therapist monitors the patient's change in alcohol use, reviews the cessation strategies being used, and continues to encourage commitment to change or sustained abstinence (NIDA, 2012).

Twelve-step facilitation therapy (e.g., AA) is an active-engagement strategy designed to increase the likelihood of a patient with an AUD becoming affiliated with and actively involved in 12-step self-help groups, thereby promoting abstinence. Three key ideas predominate in this therapy: (1) acceptance, which includes the realization that substance addiction is a chronic, progressive disease over which one has no control, that life has become unmanageable because of substance use, that willpower alone is insufficient to overcome the problem, and that abstinence is the only alternative; (2) surrender, which involves giving oneself over to a higher power, accepting the fellowship and support structure of other recovering addicted individuals, and following the recovery activities laid out by the 12-step program; and (3)

active involvement in 12-step meetings and related activities (NIDA, 2012).

With its combination of behavioral contracting and contingency management, family behavior therapy (FBT) can address issues that often co-occur with alcohol and other substance use problems, such as conduct disorders, child mistreatment, depression, family conflict, and unemployment, in addition to the substance use itself (NIDA, 2012).

Long-Term Treatment

The least restrictive environment provides the most efficient care and improved outcomes for the patient with an AUD. Unfortunately, 2.5 million patients participate in programs that are not appropriate for their needs. The ASAM has developed an expert consensus-based algorithm called CONTINUUM (a computer-based program) to determine the level of care that is recommended for patients based on their level of disease severity (ASAM, n.d.). Patient-treatment matching, which is recommended by the ASAM (2011), suggests that the clinician consider the following criteria when selecting an initial level of care:

- AUD severity level and likelihood of withdrawal syndrome
- Medical conditions and complications
- Emotional, behavioral, and cognitive conditions or complications
- Motivation to change
- Relapse or continued use potential
- Nature of the recovery environment

Clinicians should take the time to educate themselves about the available treatment programs in their community and to become familiar with the programs, staff, and facilities. Treatment facilities and programs may be found through the Substance Abuse and Mental Health Services Administration (SAMHSA, n.d.).

Behavioral change is difficult, and relapse is common. The first 12 months are particularly challenging, and relapse is most common during this time. AUD is a chronic disease similar to hypertension and diabetes, and recurrence of symptoms is common. Relapse rates for addiction are similar to those for other chronic diseases (NIDA, 2014). If relapse occurs, the patient is encouraged to recommit to abstinence. When a patient struggles to abstain, the NIAAA (2012) recommends that the clinician consider the following questions:

- Does the patient have a coexisting depression or anxiety disorder?

- What are the triggers for relapse?

- Is the patient a candidate for medication for alcohol dependence?

- Is the patient attending a mutual-help group or therapy?

- Is the patient receiving structured follow-up care?

Alcohol Withdrawal and Treatment

A patient with an AUD who suddenly stops drinking may experience alcohol withdrawal. As stated earlier, alcohol is a CNS depressant. The neurotransmitter gamma-aminobutyric acid (GABA) is influenced by the intake of alcohol. Normally, excitatory (glutamate) and inhibitory (GABA) neurotransmitters are in a state of homeostasis. Alcohol changes the GABA action, causing decreased CNS excitability. This in turn causes a decrease in the number of GABA receptors, requiring increasingly larger doses of ethanol to achieve the same euphoric effect. Chronic use of alcohol leads to an increased number of receptors and the production of more glutamate to maintain homeostasis. When the alcohol intake is stopped by the chronic user or by a hospitalization, the patient may experience increased CNS excitation, causing withdrawal symptoms. The severity of these withdrawal symptoms may range from feeling anxious and craving the substance to severe and generalized seizures (Kattimani & Bharadwaj, 2013).

Alcohol withdrawal symptoms usually begin within a few hours of abstinence and consist of mild to moderate tremors, irritability, sweating, elevated pulse and blood pressure, nausea, insomnia, and anxiety (Kattimani & Bharadwaj, 2013). Mild withdrawal is the most common form of withdrawal and can be managed successfully in the outpatient setting. A more severe syndrome, alcohol withdrawal delirium, occasionally follows. This generally begins between 24 to 72 hours after alcohol cessation and results in disorientation, poor short-term memory, altered sleep-wake cycle, hallucinations, delirium tremors, and/or seizures (Kattimani & Bharadwaj, 2013; Keys, 2011).

It is important to identify the patient who is at risk for alcohol withdrawal symptoms, particularly alcohol delirium. Patients who have higher levels of alcohol intake, who have had a longer duration of alcohol misuse, or who have developed alcohol withdrawal in the past are at increased risk of adverse withdrawal symptoms, and hospitalization should be considered. Patients who are older, have a history of delirium tremors or seizures or a comorbid acute illness, have elevated liver function tests, or who present with intense craving for alcohol are also considered to be at risk for withdrawal symptoms (Kattimani & Bharadwaj, 2013).

The Clinical Institute Withdrawal Assessment for Alcohol, revised (CIWA-Ar; Sullivan, Sykora, Schneiderman, Naranjo, & Sellers, 1989) is an instrument that rates 10 withdrawal features and has been found to identify the patient at risk for severe withdrawal symptoms. The higher the patient rates on the screening tool, the more severe in intensity the patient's withdrawal symptoms are likely to be (see Figure 7-7). A score on the CIWA-Ar from 0 to 9 indicates that the patient

continued on page 125

FIGURE 7-7: CIWA-Ar (1 OF 2)

Alcohol Withdrawal Assessment Scoring Guidelines (CIWA - Ar)

Nausea/Vomiting - Rate on scale 0 - 7

0 - None
1 - Mild nausea with no vomiting
2
3
4 - Intermittent nausea
5
6
7 - Constant nausea and frequent dry heaves and vomiting

Tremors - have patient extend arms & spread fingers. Rate on scale 0 - 7.
0 - No tremor
1 - Not visible, but can be felt fingertip to fingertip
2
3
4 - Moderate, with patient's arms extended
5
6
7 - severe, even w/ arms not extended

Anxiety - Rate on scale 0 - 7
0 - no anxiety, patient at ease
1 - mildly anxious
2
3
4 - moderately anxious or guarded, so anxiety is inferred
5
6
7 - equivalent to acute panic states seen in severe delirium or acute schizophrenic reactions.

Agitation - Rate on scale 0 - 7
0 - normal activity
1 - somewhat normal activity
2
3
4 - moderately fidgety and restless
5
6
7 - paces back and forth, or constantly thrashes about

Paroxysmal Sweats - Rate on Scale 0 - 7.
0 - no sweats
1- barely perceptible sweating, palms moist
2
3
4 - beads of sweat obvious on forehead
5
6
7 - drenching sweats

Orientation and clouding of sensorium - Ask, "What day is this? Where are you? Who am I?" Rate scale 0 - 4
0 - Oriented
1 – cannot do serial additions or is uncertain about date

2 - disoriented to date by no more than 2 calendar days

3 - disoriented to date by more than 2 calendar days
4 - Disoriented to place and / or person

Tactile disturbances - Ask, "Have you experienced any itching, pins & needles sensation, burning or numbness, or a feeling of bugs crawling on or under your skin?"
0 - none
1 - very mild itching, pins & needles, burning, or numbness
2 - mild itching, pins & needles, burning, or numbness
3 - moderate itching, pins & needles, burning, or numbness
4 - moderate hallucinations
5 - severe hallucinations
6 - extremely severe hallucinations
7 - continuous hallucinations

Auditory Disturbances - Ask, "Are you more aware of sounds around you? Are they harsh? Do they startle you? Do you hear anything that disturbs you or that you know isn't there?"
0 - not present
1 - Very mild harshness or ability to startle
2 - mild harshness or ability to startle
3 - moderate harshness or ability to startle
4 - moderate hallucinations
5 - severe hallucinations
6 - extremely severe hallucinations
7 - continuous hallucinations

Visual disturbances - Ask, "Does the light appear to be too bright? Is its color different than normal? Does it hurt your eyes? Are you seeing anything that disturbs you or that you know isn't there?"
0 - not present
1 - very mild sensitivity
2 - mild sensitivity
3 - moderate sensitivity
4 - moderate hallucinations
5 - severe hallucinations
6 - extremely severe hallucinations
7 - continuous hallucinations

Headache - Ask, "Does your head feel different than usual? Does it feel like there is a band around your head?" Do not rate dizziness or lightheadedness.

0 - not present
1 - very mild
2 - mild
3 - moderate
4 - moderately severe
5 - severe
6 - very severe
7 - extremely severe

Procedure:

1. Assess and rate each of the 10 criteria of the CIWA scale. Each criterion is rated on a scale from 0 to 7, except for "Orientation and clouding of sensorium" which is rated on scale 0 to 4. Add up the scores for all ten criteria. This is the total CIWA-Ar score for the patient at that time. Prophylactic medication should be started for any patient with a total CIWA-Ar score of 8 or greater (ie. start on withdrawal medication). If started on scheduled medication, additional PRN medication should be given for a total CIWA-Ar score of 15 or greater.
2. Document vitals and CIWA-Ar assessment on the Withdrawal Assessment Sheet. Document administration of PRN medications on the assessment sheet as well.
3. The CIWA-Ar scale is the most sensitive tool for assessment of the patient experiencing alcohol withdrawal. Nursing assessment is vitally important. Early intervention for CIWA-Ar score of 8 or greater provides the best means to prevent the progression of withdrawal.

FIGURE 7-7: CIWA-Ar (2 OF 2)

	Date											
Assessment Protocol a. Vitals, Assessment Now. b. If initial score ≥ 8 repeat q1h x 8 hrs, then if stable q2h x 8 hrs, then if stable q4h. c. If initial score < 8, assess q4h x 72 hrs. If score < 8 for 72 hrs, d/c assessment. If score ≥ 8 at any time, go to (b) above. d. If indicated, (see indications below) administer prn medications as ordered and record on MAR and below.	Time											
	Pulse											
	RR											
	O₂ sat											
	BP											

Assess and rate each of the following (CIWA-Ar Scale):   Refer to reverse for detailed instructions in use of the CIWA-Ar scale.

Nausea/vomiting (0 - 7)
0 - none; 1 - mild nausea ,no vomiting; 4 - intermittent nausea;
7 - constant nausea , frequent dry heaves & vomiting.

Tremors (0 - 7)
0 - no tremor; 1 - not visible but can be felt; 4 - moderate w/ arms
extended; 7 - severe, even w/ arms not extended.

Anxiety (0 - 7)
0 - none, at ease; 1 - mildly anxious; 4 - moderately anxious or
guarded; 7 - equivalent to acute panic state

Agitation (0 - 7)
0 - normal activity; 1 - somewhat normal activity; 4 - moderately
fidgety/restless; 7 - paces or constantly thrashes about

Paroxysmal Sweats (0 - 7)
0 - no sweats;   1 - barely perceptible sweating, palms moist;
4 - beads of sweat obvious on forehead;   7 - drenching sweat

Orientation (0 - 4)
0 - oriented; 1 - uncertain about date; 2 - disoriented to date by no
more than 2 days; 3 - disoriented to date by > 2 days;
4 - disoriented to place and / or person

Tactile Disturbances (0 - 7)
0 - none; 1 - very mild itch, P&N, ,numbness; 2-mild itch, P&N,
burning, numbness; 3 - moderate itch, P&N, burning ,numbness;
4 - moderate hallucinations; 5 - severe hallucinations;
6 – extremely severe hallucinations; 7 - continuous hallucinations

Auditory Disturbances (0 - 7)
0 - not present; 1 - very mild harshness/ ability to startle; 2 - mild
harshness, ability to startle; 3 - moderate harshness, ability to
startle; 4 - moderate hallucinations; 5 severe hallucinations;
6 - extremely severe hallucinations; 7 - continuous hallucinations

Visual Disturbances (0 - 7)
0 - not present;   1 - very mild sensitivity;   2 - mild sensitivity;
3 - moderate sensitivity;   4 - moderate hallucinations;   5 - severe
hallucinations;   6 - extremely severe hallucinations;   7 -
continuous hallucinations

Headache (0 - 7)
0 - not present; 1 - very mild; 2 - mild; 3 - moderate; 4 - moderately
severe; 5 - severe; 6 - very severe; 7 - extremely severe

Total CIWA-Ar score:

PRN Med: (circle one) Diazepam Lorazepam	**Dose given (mg):**											
	Route:											
Time of PRN medication administration:												
Assessment of response (CIWA-Ar score 30-60 minutes after medication administered)												
RN Initials												

Scale for Scoring:
Total Score =
  0 – 9: absent or minimal withdrawal
  10 – 19: mild to moderate withdrawal
  more than 20: severe withdrawal

Patient Identification (Addressograph)

Indications for PRN medication:
a. Total CIWA-AR score 8 or higher if ordered PRN only (Symptom-triggered method).
b. Total CIWA-Ar score 15 or higher if on Scheduled medication. (Scheduled + prn method)
Consider transfer to ICU for any of the following: Total score above 35, q1h assess. x more than 8hrs
required, more than 4 mg/hr lorazepam x 3hr **or** 20 mg/hr diazepam x 3hr required, or resp. distress.

Signature/ Title	Initials	Signature / Title	Initials

Alcohol Withdrawal Assessment Flowsheet (revised Nov 2003)

Note. From Sullivan, J. T., Sykora, K., Schneiderman, J., Naranjo, C. A., & Sellers, E. M. (1989). Assessment of alcohol withdrawal: The revised Clinical Institute Withdrawal Assessment for Alcohol scale (CIWA-Ar). *British Journal of Addiction, 84,* 1353-1357.

may experience only very mild withdrawal, 10 to 15 indicates mild withdrawal, 16 to 20 indicates moderate withdrawal, and 21 to 67 indicates severe withdrawal symptoms (UptoDate, 2017).

The healthcare provider assessing a patient for alcohol withdrawal must also consider other associated alcohol problems, including gastritis, gastrointestinal bleeding, liver disease, pancreatitis, electrolyte imbalances, folate and thiamine deficiency, and cardiomyopathy (Kattimani & Bharadwaj, 2013). Managing patients with severe withdrawal should include pharmacotherapy to reduce the risk of associated complications such as respiratory and cardiovascular symptoms. Timing from the last drink to the initiation of treatment is critical to reducing side effects from the withdrawal of alcohol.

Alcohol withdrawal has numerous complications. Minor symptoms include insomnia, tremors, mild anxiety, gastrointestinal upset, headaches, diaphoresis, and palpitations. These symptoms are present within 6 hours of the cessation of drinking and usually resolve with 24 to 48 hours. Usually, these symptoms are managed within an ambulatory setting.

Life-threatening signs and symptoms of alcohol withdrawal are delirium and seizures. Withdrawal seizures usually occur in patients with a long history of chronic alcohol use and occur in the fourth and fifth decades of life. These seizures are brief and occur over a shorter period of time. If these seizures are left untreated, they can progress to delirium tremens in some patients (UptoDate, 2017). Risk factors for delirium tremens include the following:

- A history of sustained drinking

- A history of previous delirium tremens

- Age greater than 30

- The presence of a concurrent illness

- Significant alcohol withdrawal in the presence of an elevated alcohol level

- More than 2 days from the last drink to the onset of withdrawal

Benzodiazepines are considered the medications of choice to treat withdrawal seizures because they improve symptoms and reduce the incidence of delirium tremens. They should be dosed using a validated assessment tool, such as the CIWA-Ar (UptoDate, 2017). All benzodiazepines appear to be equally effective; however, such long-acting agents as diazepam, chlordiazepoxide, and lorazepam are generally preferable to short-acting agents because of the decreased risk of rebound (Hoffman & Weinhouse, 2017). Benzodiazepines act on the GABA system and mimic the effects of alcohol. It takes several days for the neurotransmitters' equilibrium to be readjusted. As the patient's condition improves, the use of benzodiazepines can be tapered off (Keys, 2011).

Patients with moderate or severe alcohol withdrawal need close monitoring. Some patients may require care in an intensive care unit. Screening patients for substance use as part of the admission process may help to identify those patients who may be at risk for alcohol withdrawal and/or delirium. Medications that should not be used for alcohol withdrawal include ethanol, antipsychotics, and sustained anticonvulsant therapy. Antipsychotics lower the seizure threshold, and sustained anticonvulsant therapy is not indicated with isolated alcohol withdrawal seizures because they are usually self-limited (UpToDate, 2017).

CASE STUDY 7-1

*M*s. Jones is a 35-year-old female patient who has been married for 15 years and is the mother of two daughters, ages 5 and 7. Ms. Jones goes to the emergency department (ED) with a report of a severe headache, heartburn, and abdominal pain. She describes that she is often stressed because of the demands of her work and home life. She states, "I never seem to have enough time for myself. The evenings are the only time I have with my husband, and that is only for a few hours. I am constantly on the go to complete tasks at work or driving the girls to their activities, and then there is cleaning, washing clothes, and the list goes on." The nurse nods in agreement, acknowledging that all of her responsibilities can be overwhelming. The nurse further explores with Ms. Jones which activities she enjoys doing. Ms. Jones responds that she has difficulty remembering the last time that she did something that she enjoyed other than having a drink with her husband in the evening.

The clinician informs Ms. Jones that her exam findings were normal and that she is experiencing mild gastrointestinal reflux and a tension headache. The clinician proceeds in asking the patient the following questions:

Clinician: "Ms. Jones, do you sometimes drink alcohol, such as beer, wine, or spirits?"

Ms. Jones: "Yes, I do, but I'm not sure how that relates to why I'm here today."

Clinician: "Ms. Jones, the reason it is important is that it helps me get a better understanding of your health history. So, in the past year, has there been an occasion when you have had four or more drinks in one day?"

Ms. Jones: "Yes...generally just for special occasions like weddings and New Year's Eve, and then just sometimes during the week."

Clinician: "Ok, so on how many days per week do you have a drink?"

Ms. Jones: "Oh...maybe 1 to 2 days per week."

Clinician: "And on those days, how many drinks do you have?"

Ms. Jones: "Probably one or two glasses of wine."

Based on Ms. Jones's reported alcohol use, she is drinking at the maximum, 2 days a week with two glasses of wine, which is a total of four alcoholic beverages per week. The NIAAA considers this a moderate and safe drinking level for women. The clinician advises Ms. Jones of the risk of her drinking level. However, if Ms. Jones had responded differently, a follow-up plan including further discussion of strategies to address high-risk alcohol use may have been needed.

Questions

1. What is another way the clinician could have introduced the topic of drinking alcohol with Ms. Jones?

2. Although Ms. Jones's drinking falls within the low-risk category, which additional information could the ED staff have provided to her about drinking alcohol?

3. What is the purpose of the clinician using the AUDIT screen with Ms. Jones?

Answers

1. Rather than administering the AUDIT test immediately after reviewing Ms. Jones's diagnoses, the clinician could have first explained the purpose of using the AUDIT and described its routine use by clinicians in the ED. More detail about the tool's format and the length of time to administer the screen is other information the clinician could have shared. Then, the clinician should have asked Ms. Jones's permission to administer the AUDIT to her.

2. The ED staff can confirm that Ms. Jones understands the specific effects of alcohol on women. They can explain how women achieve higher BAC levels than men after drinking equivalent amounts of alcohol. They can also explain how drinking larger quanti-

ties of alcohol can lead to functional disturbances in the gastrointestinal tract, producing symptoms of gastritis or "heartburn." They can also describe how alcohol may produce effects on the neuropsychiatric system, leading to potential depressive disorders.

3. The AUDIT test is a validated screen for alcohol use disorders. It is not always obvious by appearance alone which patients are drinking alcohol regularly, especially for those falling in the at-risk to moderate range of drinking. Using the AUDIT to screen for substance use is becoming standardized care or evidence-based practice in most healthcare settings.

CASE STUDY 7-2

*M*s. Smith is a 36-year-old stay-at-home mother who presents to her primary care office for her annual physical examination. Ms. Smith completes the AUDIT screen prior to her seeing the clinician for her examination. Her score on the screen is 12. After her examination, the clinician engages in the following conversation with Ms. Smith regarding her AUDIT screen score.

Clinician: "I'd like to review your results from the AUDIT screen with you."

Ms. Smith: "Sure, but I only have a drink with my husband when the kids go to bed."

Clinician: "Ok, so how many days per week do you have a drink?"

Ms. Smith: "I probably drink 5 or 6 nights a week and no more than two or three glasses of wine."

Clinician: "Have you experienced any negative consequences over the last 6 to 12 months as a result of drinking alcohol?"

Ms. Smith: "Well, yes, it seems that sometimes my husband and I get into fights – not physical or anything – after we've been drink-

ing. It's hard on the kids because I think they can hear us. Sometimes after the fights, I have a hard time getting to sleep, and I don't get the kids to school on time the next day."

Clinician: "Have you ever experienced a period of time when your drinking interfered with your relationship with your kids or husband or some of your responsibilities?"

Ms. Smith: "You know, I'm a good mother, but I seem to have trouble managing the morning routine with the kids – getting them up, dressed, fed, and getting them to school – after one of those nights. I just seem to move more slowly sometimes after drinking the night before."

Clinician: "I see. So when you and your husband have been drinking and then fight, have you ever been frightened or concerned for your safety?"

Ms. Smith: "No, my husband is a good man; he would never hurt me or the kids."

Clinician: "Oh, that's good to know. So, have you ever wanted to stop or cut down on your drinking but tried and found that you couldn't?"

Ms. Smith: "No, not really."

Clinician: "Have you ever found that you have to drink much more than you once did to get the effect you want?"

Ms. Smith: "No, I'm sort of a cheap date – a few drinks are usually all I can handle."

Questions

1. Does Ms. Smith meet the *DSM-5* criteria for AUD?

2. What are the clinician's next steps in addressing Ms. Smith's current level of alcohol use?

3. What are other factors that would place Ms. Smith at risk for an AUD?

4. What is a possible follow-up plan for Ms. Smith?

Answers

1. Ms. Smith is drinking on 6 nights per week, maximum, with approximately three glasses of wine per night, which is a weekly total of 18 alcoholic beverages. Ms. Smith also reports having difficulty managing the normal morning routine for her children after nights when she drinks alcohol. Meeting two criteria for an AUD confirms that she is exhibiting symptoms of a mild AUD.

2. The clinician can explain his or her current concerns about Ms. Smith's drinking. For example, the clinician may state, "Ms. Smith, you are drinking more than is medically safe. Moderate drinking for women is one drink per day or no more than seven drinks per week. You are drinking 18 drinks per week, and I'm concerned that you are experiencing some symptoms related to your heavy drinking. Physically, your insomnia at night may be related to the amount of alcohol you are consuming. I'm also concerned about the arguments you are having at night and the difficulty you're having the morning after with your children. Alcohol lowers your inhibitions and is actually a depressant – it affects your behavior, perhaps including those nighttime arguments."

3. The clinician should also further assess Ms. Smith for an AUD. To determine this, the clinician can carefully assess whether Ms. Smith has experienced any significant negative consequences related to her drinking in the past 12 months. This includes consequences related to role failure, risk of bodily harm, run-ins with the law, and relationship trouble.

   The clinician must assess the extent and severity of Ms. Smith's alcohol-related symptoms and determine if Ms. Smith has any of the cardinal signs of AUD. Questions that assess alcohol dependence focus on the presence of three or more of these symptoms: tolerance, withdrawal, inability to stick to drinking limits, inability to stop or cut down, spending a lot of time drinking and less time on other matters, and drinking despite problems.

4. A possible follow-up plan for Ms. Smith includes first acknowledging that change is difficult. The clinician will ask a lot of open-ended questions to further assess Ms. Smith's intent to change and any obstacles to changing her drinking behavior. Next, the clinician can help Ms. Smith establish a goal to reduce or abstain from drinking alcohol. Resources such as referral to an addiction specialist or a mutual-help group may be warranted. The clinician also discusses steps to help support Ms. Smith's autonomy and makes affirming statements about her ability to reduce her at-risk drinking.

SUMMARY

Alcohol problems are common, and nurses and clinicians are in a unique position to identify patients with potential problems and intervene when appropriate. Every patient should be screened annually for alcohol use. Alcohol problems are related to the amount of alcohol consumed and the frequency of drinking. Patients who drink at moderate levels should be encouraged to abstain or drink alcohol within the recommended levels for their gender, age, and health condition. Patients who drink heavily or who are at risk for alcohol use disorders should be counseled to cut down on their alcohol consumption to moderate levels or abstain altogether.

Brief interventions are effective; reliable counseling techniques result in reduced alcohol consumption and binge drinking. Brief interventions should be factual and nonconfrontational. Clinicians should state their conclusions and recommendations clearly, focusing on moderate drinking limits and relating these to any concerns and medical findings related to the patient. Timely follow-up care should be arranged to reinforce these recommendations.

Patients who meet the criteria for an AUD are counseled to abstain. The clinician considers referring such patients for evaluation by an addiction specialist and recommending a mutual-help group.

EXAM QUESTIONS

CHAPTER 7
Questions 33–38

Note: Choose the one option that BEST answers each question.

33. The most common type of alcohol consumed in the United States is

    a. beer.

    b. wine.

    c. spirits.

    d. mixed drinks.

34. According to the National Survey on Drug Use and Health, binge drinking for women is defined as

    a. two drinks on the same occasion on at least 1 day in the past 30 days.

    b. three drinks on the same occasion on at least 1 day in the past 30 days.

    c. four drinks on the same occasion on at least 1 day in the past 30 days.

    d. five drinks on the same occasion on at least 1 day in the past 30 days.

35. The age group that is most associated with binge drinking is

    a. preadolescents aged 11 to 12.

    b. adolescents aged 12 to 17.

    c. young adults aged 18 to 25.

    d. adults aged 26 and older.

36. Further screening for alcohol use disorder is recommended for

    a. patients with musculoskeletal injuries or disorders.

    b. patients with chronic illness that is not improving with treatment.

    c. nonsmokers who are likely to drink occasionally.

    d. older adults in long-term care facilities.

37. Long-term treatment of alcohol use disorder generally includes

    a. benzodiazepine therapy.

    b. motivational enhancement therapy.

    c. negotiating a plan to reduce or abstain from alcohol.

    d. making a referral to community services.

38. The life-threatening signs and symptoms of alcohol withdrawal that are

    a. irritability and cravings.

    b. delirium and seizures.

    c. insomnia and mild tremors.

    d. sweating and anxiety.

REFERENCES

Agerwala, S. M., & McCance-Katz, E. F. (2012). Integrating Screening, Brief Intervention, and Referral to Treatment (SBIRT) into clinical practice settings: A brief review. *Journal of Psychoactive Drugs, 44*(4), 307-317.

American Psychiatric Association. (2013). *Diagnostic and statistical manual of mental disorders* (5th ed.). Arlington, VA: Author.

American Society of Addiction Medicine. (n.d.). *CONTINUUM*. Retrieved from https://www.asam.org/docs/default-source/membership/continuum(tm)-briefdescrip-tionbibliography-2016_01-27.pdf?sfvrsn=2

American Society of Addiction Medicine. (2011). *Public policy statement: Definition of addiction.* Retrieved from http://www.asam.org/docs/default-source/public-policy-statements/1definition_of_addiction_long_4-11.pdf?sfvrsn=2

Babor, T. F., Higgins-Biddle, J. C., Saunders, J. B., & Monteiro, M. G. (2001). *AUDIT: The Alcohol Use Disorders Identification Test. Guidelines for use in primary care* (2nd ed.). Geneva, Switzerland: World Health Organization. Retrieved from http://whqlibdoc.who.int/hq/2001/who_msd_msb_01.6a.pdf

Cederbaum, A. I. (2012). Alcohol metabolism. *Clinics in Liver Disease, 16*(4), 667-685. doi:10.1016/j.cld.2012.08.002

Center for Behavioral Health Statistics and Quality. (2016a). *Key substance use and mental health indicators in the United States: Results from the 2015 National Survey on Drug Use and Health* (HHS Publication No. [SMA] 16-4984, NSDUH Series H-51). Retrieved from https://www.samhsa.gov/data/sites/default/files/NSDUH-FFR1-2015/NSDUH-FFR1-2015/NSDUH-FFR1-2015.pdf

Center for Behavioral Health Statistics and Quality. (2016b). *Results from the 2015 National Survey on Drug Use and Health: Detailed tables, Table 2.41B.* Retrieved from https://www.samhsa.gov/data/sites/default/files/NSDUH-DetTabs-2015/NSDUH-DetTabs-2015/NSDUH-DetTabs-2015.htm#tab2-41b

Center for Substance Abuse Treatment. (2009). Physiological effects of alcohol, drugs, and tobacco on women. In *Substance abuse treatment: Addressing the specific needs of women* (Treatment Improvement Protocol [TIP] Series, No. 51, Chapter 3). Rockville, MD: Substance Abuse and Mental Health Services Administration. Retrieved from https://www.ncbi.nlm.nih.gov/books/NBK83244/

Hoffman, R., & Weinhouse, G. (2017). *Management of moderate and severe alcohol withdrawal syndromes.* Retrieved from https://www.uptodate.com/contents/management-of-moderate-and-severe-alcohol-withdrawal-syndromes

Kattimani, S., & Bharadwaj, B. (2013). Clinical management of alcohol withdrawal: A systematic review. *Industrial Psychiatry Journal, 22*(2), 100-108. doi:10.4103/0972-6748.132914

Keys, V. A. (2011). Alcohol withdrawal during hospitalization. *American Journal of Nursing, 111*(1), 40-44; quiz, 45-46. doi:10.1097/01. NAJ.0000393058.86439.9e

Klatsky, A. L. (2015). Alcohol and cardiovascular diseases: Where do we stand today? *Journal of Internal Medicine, 278*(3), 238-250. doi:10.1111/joim.12390

National Council on Alcoholism and Drug Dependence. (2015). *Alcohol, drugs and crime.* Retrieved from https://www.ncadd. org/about-addiction/addiction-update/alcohol-drugs-and-crime

National Institute on Alcohol Abuse and Alcoholism. (n.d.). *Genetics of alcohol use disorder.* Retrieved from https://www.niaaa. nih.gov/alcohol-health/overview-alcohol-consumption/alcohol-use-disorders/genetics-alcohol-use-disorders

National Institute on Alcohol Abuse and Alcoholism. (2007). *Helping patients who drink too much: A clinician's guide* (updated 2005 ed., NIH Publication No. 07-3769). Retrieved from https://pubs.niaaa.nih.gov/pub lications/practitioner/CliniciansGuide2005/ guide.pdf

National Institute on Alcohol Abuse and Alcoholism. (2012). *Alcohol's effects on immunity – Increasing the risks for infection and injury* (Alcohol Alert 89). Retrieved from https://pubs.niaaa.nih.gov/publications/ AA89/AA89.htm

National Institute on Alcohol Abuse and Alcoholism. (2015a). *Alcohol's effects on the body.* Retrieved from http://www.niaaa.nih. gov/alcohol-health/alcohols-effects-body

National Institute on Alcohol Abuse and Alcoholism. (2015b). *Apparent per capita alcohol consumption: National, state and regional trends, 1977-2013* (Surveillance Report 102). Retrieved from https://pubs. niaaa.nih.gov/publications/surveillance102/ cons13.htm

National Institute on Alcohol Abuse and Alcoholism. (2016a). *Drinking levels defined.* Retrieved from http://www.niaaa.nih.gov/ alcohol-health/overview-alcohol-consumption

National Institute on Alcohol Abuse and Alcoholism. (2016b). *What is a standard drink?* Retrieved from https://www.niaaa. nih.gov/alcohol-health/overview-alcohol-consumption/what-standard-drink

National Institute on Alcohol Abuse and Alcoholism. (2017). *Alcohol facts and statistics.* Retrieved from https://www.niaaa. nih.gov/alcohol-health/overview-alcohol-consumption/alcohol-facts-and-statistics

National Institute on Drug Abuse. (2012). *Principles of drug addiction treatment: A research-based guide* (3rd ed., NIH Publication No. 12-4180). Rockville, MD: National Institutes of Health, U.S. Department of Health and Human Services. Retrieved from https://www.drugabuse.gov/publications/ principles-drug-addiction-treatment-research-based-guide-third-edition

National Institute on Drug Abuse. (2014). *Drugs, brains, and behavior: The science of addiction.* Retrieved from https://www. drugabuse.gov/publications/drugs-brains-behavior-science-addiction

Office of Disease Prevention and Health Promotion. (2016). *Healthy people 2020.* Retrieved from http://www.healthypeople. gov/2020/

Rehm, J., & Shield, K. D. (2013). Global alcohol-attributable deaths from cancer, liver cirrhosis, and injury in 2010. *Alcohol Research, 35*(2), 174-183.

Saunders, J. B., Conigrave, K. M., Latt, N. C., Nutt, D. J., Ling, W., & Higuchi, S. (2016). *Addiction medicine* (2nd ed.). Oxford, UK: Oxford University Press.

Substance Abuse and Mental Health Services Administration. (n.d.). *SAMHSA treatment locator.* Retrieved from https://findtreatment.samhsa.gov/

Substance Abuse and Mental Health Services Administration. (2016). *USAUDIT: The Alcohol Use Disorder Identification Test, adapted for use in the United States: A guide for primary care practitioners.* Retrieved from http://www.ct.gov/dmhas/lib/dmhas/publications/USAUDIT-Guide_2016.pdf

Sullivan, J. T., Sykora, K., Schneiderman, J., Naranjo, C. A., & Sellers, E. M. (1989). Assessment of alcohol withdrawal: The revised Clinical Institute Withdrawal Assessment for Alcohol scale (CIWA-Ar). *British Journal of Addiction, 84,* 1353-1357.

Tan, C. H., Denny, C. H., Cheal, N. E., Sniezek, J. E., & Kanny, D. (2015). Alcohol use and binge drinking among women of child-bearing age – United States, 2011-2013. *Morbidity and Mortality Weekly Report, 64,* 1042-1046.

UptoDate. (2017). *Management of moderate and severe alcohol withdrawal syndrome.* Retrieved from https://www.uptodate.com/contents/managment-of-moderate-and-severe-alcohol-withdrawal-syndromes

U.S. Preventive Services Task Force. (n.d.). *The five As organizational construct for clinical counseling.* Retrieved from https://www.uspreventiveservicestaskforce.org/Page/Name/behavioral-counseling-interventions-an-evidence-based-approach#the-five-a39s-organizational-construct-for-clinical-counseling

World Health Organization. (2011). *The global status report on alcohol and health – 2011.* Geneva, Switzerland: Author. Retrieved from http://http://www.who.int/substance_abuse/publications/global_alcohol_report/msbgsruprofiles.pdf?ua=1

World Health Organization. (2014). *Global status report on alcohol and health – 2014.* Geneva, Switzerland: Author. Retrieved from http://www.who.int/substance_abuse/publications/global_alcohol_report/msb_gsr_2014_1.pdf?ua=1

CHAPTER 8

MARIJUANA/CANNABIS USE

LEARNING OUTCOME

After completing this chapter, the learner will be able to summarize the effects of using marijuana (cannabis), including any screening and treatment considerations for patients.

CHAPTER OBJECTIVES

After completing this chapter, the learner will be able to:

1. Identify the trends and patterns of marijuana use disorders among people in the United States.

2. List the biochemical actions of marijuana.

3. Describe marijuana's wide range of health effects.

4. Describe screening and treatment approaches for marijuana misuse.

5. Identify controversies surrounding the medical use of marijuana and legalization.

INTRODUCTION

Marijuana is a mind-altering drug composed of a dry, shredded mix of flowers, stems, seeds, and leaves from the hemp plant (*Cannabis sativa*). The term *cannabis* refers to marijuana and other formulations made from this plant (Welch & Malcolm, 2014). Table 8-1 lists various commercial and street names and other important facts about marijuana.

In 1965, the psychoactive ingredient in cannabis, delta-9-tetrahydrocannabinol (THC) was isolated (Welch & Malcolm, 2014). THC potency can vary and is determined by plant characteristics and product type. Marijuana is composed primarily of plant stems and leaves and typically has the lowest THC concentrations (0.5% to 5%) among all types of cannabis. Sinsemilla, a higher-grade marijuana from female plants cultivated to remain seedless, has concentrations ranging from 7% to 14%. Other hemp-derived drugs include hashish and hash oil. Hashish comes from dried resin and flowers, with THC concentrations of 2% to 8%. Hash oil contains THC extracted from hashish and has the highest potency, from 15% to 50% (Welch & Malcolm, 2014). In addition to cannabinoids from the marijuana plant, a range of synthetic cannabinoids ("spice" and related products) are widely available and unregulated by the U.S. Drug Enforcement Administration (DEA), which has made it challenging to determine use trends and clinical effects.

Most cannabis users smoke marijuana in hand-rolled cigarettes called joints, although some use pipes or water pipes called bongs. With legalization, food- and drink-based products are increasingly available. Hash oil, wax, or budder (which has a softer and more pliable texture) can be heated and aerosolized in electronic smoking or vaping devices. These, along with shatter, a solidified formulation, can have high concentrations of THC (National Institute

TABLE 8-1: COMMERCIAL AND STREET NAMES AND OTHER FACTS ABOUT MARIJUANA

Common Commercial Names	There are various brand names in states where the sale of marijuana is legal; for example, Marinol (dronabinol) contains THC that is synthetically derived and is a drug product approved by U.S. Food and Drug Administration (FDA).
Street Names	Marijuana: blunt, bud, dope, ganja, grass, green, herb, joint, Mary Jane, pot, reefer, sinsemilla, skunk, smoke, trees, weed Hashish: boom, gangster, hash, hemp, THC
Common Forms	Greenish-gray mixture of dried, shredded leaves, stems, seeds, and/or flowers (marijuana); resin (hashish); or sticky, black liquid (hash oil)
Common Administration Routes	Smoked or ingested (mixed in food or brewed as tea)
Drug Enforcement Administration (DEA) Schedule/Legal Status	Schedule I: illegal for both marijuana and THC, the active ingredient in marijuana, which is listed separately from marijuana Schedule III: FDA-approved drug product; legal by prescription only

Note. From U.S. Department of Health and Human Services, Office of the Surgeon General. (2016). *Facing addiction in America: The surgeon general's report on alcohol, drugs, and health.* Washington, DC: Author.

on Drug Abuse [NIDA], 2016a). Blunts, also popular, are cigars that have been opened so that the tobacco within can be mixed with or replaced by marijuana. Concerns have been raised that mixing tobacco and marijuana contributes to increased cannabis dependence in youth (Hindocha et al., 2015).

Cannabis use can be traced to ancient times and seems to have originated in Asian regions. Documentation of cannabis use for medicinal purposes dates to 2700 B.C., and it was listed in the *U.S. Pharmacopeia* until 1942. Recreational use became prevalent in the United States after Prohibition, and medicinal use ended shortly after when the Marijuana Tax Act was passed in 1937. In 1970, it was regulated by the U.S. Controlled Substance Act as a Schedule I (high potential for abuse and no accepted medical use) drug (Welch & Malcolm, 2014). The plant fibers (hemp) have been widely used for rope production.

EPIDEMIOLOGY OF MARIJUANA USE

Marijuana is the most commonly used illicit drug. According to the 2015 Center for Behavioral Health Statistics and Quality (CBHSQ) Report (Substance Abuse and Mental Health Services Administration [SAMHSA], 2015), 36.0 million people (13.5% of Americans) age 12 or older used marijuana in the prior year, and 117.9 million people (44.0%) reported use at some point during their lives. In the 2016 Monitoring the Future study, 15.5% of 8th graders, 31.1% of 10th graders, and 44.7% of 12th graders who participated in the survey reported using marijuana at least once in their lifetime (Miech, Johnston, O'Malley, Bachman, & Schulenberg, 2016). In this same study, 11.8% of 8th graders, 25.4% of 10th graders, and 34.9% of 12th graders reported using marijuana in the past year. Daily use was reported by 6% of 12th graders.

The overall trends of marijuana use show that annual marijuana use peaked among 12th-grade males at 51% in 1979. Since then, prevalence rates have fluctuated. A decline was noted for 13 years, evidenced by 22% of 12th graders reporting marijuana use in 1992. Beginning in 1993, a resurgence of use occurred among 8th, 10th, and 12th graders, with another peak in the late 1990s. Prevalence has leveled off in recent years (Johnston, O'Malley, Miech, Bachman, & Schulenberg, 2016). Data from 2016 indicate that this leveling off has persisted for 10th and 12th graders, along with a significant decline in daily (0.7%), past-month (5.4%), past-year (9.4%), and lifetime (12.8%) prevalence for 8th graders (NIDA, 2016b).

Marijuana use trends are of specific concern for those who use it regularly because they can experience an increased risk for dependence. In 2013, an estimated 8.1 million people had used marijuana in the previous month (Azofeifa et al., 2016). Among young adults ages 18 to 25, approximately 19.8% reported past-month marijuana use, compared with 6.5% of those 26 years and older (Johnston, O'Malley, Bachman, Schulenberg, & Miech, 2016). For those 12 years and older, a consistent trend toward daily use has occurred, and recent data show that this rate nearly doubled over a 10-year period, from 1.3% in 2004 to 2.5% in 2014 (Azofeifa et al., 2016).

In addition to being the most commonly used illicit drug, marijuana is the most consistently available illegal substance. Although it is still considered an illicit drug at the federal level, as of April 2017, the possession of small amounts of marijuana is legal in eight states (California, Maine, Massachusetts, Nevada, Colorado, Washington, Alaska, and Oregon) and the District of Columbia for medical and/or recreational use. In addition, 21 states (Alaska, California, Colorado, Connecticut, Delaware, Illinois, Maine, Maryland, Massachusetts, Minnesota, Mississippi, Missouri, Nebraska, Nevada, New York, North Carolina, Ohio, Oregon, Rhode Island, Vermont, and Washington) and the District of Columbia have decriminalized small amounts of marijuana, making possession of a small amount of the substance a civil or local infraction rather than a state crime (National Conference of State Legislators, 2017).

Paradoxically, in this climate of increased legalization, fewer youth from 12 to 17 years of age reported that marijuana was easily accessible, from 55% of youth in 2002 to 47.8% in 2014. However, among users of all age groups during this time frame, marijuana use for those reporting that they perceived no risk from marijuana more than doubled to nearly 20% for monthly use and 15.2% for use once or twice weekly (Azofeifa et al., 2016). In a climate of increased normalization of marijuana use, the perception of harm is fading. The long-term health outcomes and social consequences are currently unknown, however, because this is the beginning of the legalization and decriminalization era.

BIOCHEMISTRY

Although the marijuana plant synthesizes more than 500 chemicals, THC is the most psychoactive chemical. THC is one of over 100 cannabinoids found in the marijuana plant. Acute intoxication of THC produces a euphoric effect followed by a sense of relaxation, along with undesirable effects of anxiety, psychosis, dysphoria, apathy, and memory impairment (Martin-Santos et al., 2012). During the euphoric period, senses are heightened, and inhibitions are reduced. Reaction times are slowed, and sense of time may be distorted (U.S. Department of Health and Human Services [HHS], 2016).

The amount of THC determines the drug's potency. Over the past two decades, the average amount of THC found in marijuana available in the United States has more than doubled. A shift from traditional leaf or stem marijuana to increased sinsemilla with higher THC levels has been found, providing some explanation for this trend (ElSohly et al., 2016). The clinical consequences of using products with higher levels of THC can be increased potential for addiction and increased risk of intoxication.

Research is under way on endogenous cannabinoid molecules, THC, and other nonpsychoactive cannabinoids, such as cannabinol and cannabidiol, found in marijuana, which bind to cannabinoid receptors in the brain and throughout the body. The principle receptors are CB1 and CB2, with additional cannabinoid receptors still being identified (Welch & Malcolm, 2014). These pathways control an array of mental and physical processes in the brain and throughout the body, including memory and perception, fine motor coordination, pain sensations, immunity to disease, and reproduction. Research related to not just cannabinoids but also the pathways affected by them has led to several promising areas of clinical research. For example, dronabinol, a synthetically derived cannabinoid, is now approved for use in refractory emesis as a Schedule III medication.

THC attaches to cannabinoid receptors on nerve cells in the brain, leading to a disruption of the endogenous cannabinoids' normal function and increases in dopamine levels. This is the reward circuitry found with most misused substances (Welch & Malcolm, 2014). The regions of the brain in which cannabinoid receptors are abundant are the cerebellum (body movement), hippocampus (learning and memory), cerebral cortex (higher cognitive functions), nucleus accumbens (reward), and basal ganglia (movement control). This excessive neuronal activity of the overstimulated cannabinoid receptors produces the psychoactive effects, including psychosis, experienced by marijuana smokers. THC activates the reward system by stimulating the brain cells to release dopamine, causing the user

to feel euphoric or high; this is accomplished via the mesolimbic dopamine pathway, which is associated with positive symptoms (e.g., delusions, hallucinations) of psychosis. With time, the function of cannabinoid receptors may be altered, which, along with other changes in the brain, can lead to withdrawal symptoms and addiction (NIDA, 2016a).

When users smoke marijuana, the acute effects of THC begin rapidly and last for 1 to 3 hours. The psychological and cardiovascular effects occur within the first 5 to 10 minutes. Initially, the user may feel pleasant sensations, but this experience wanes, and feelings of sleepiness and depression then occur. Marijuana users may also feel increased anxiety, fear, distrust, or panic. Heavy use can impair working memory and the ability to recall events, and it may disrupt coordination and balance. The onset of these effects is determined by the route of administration. For example, if the user ingests cannabis in a food product, the onset is slower, around 30 to 60 minutes (NIDA, 2016a).

Controversy exists regarding addiction in the context of marijuana use. Tolerance and withdrawal symptoms are signs of addiction, and these have both been noted in marijuana users (Welch & Malcolm, 2014). Irritability, anxiety, and problems with sleep and appetite are symptoms of a withdrawal syndrome from marijuana (NIDA, 2016a). Up to 30% of marijuana users have been found to have problematic use (NIDA, 2016a), and the lifetime risk of dependence for regular users has been reported as 9% (Welch & Malcolm, 2014). The *Diagnostic and Statistical Manual of Mental Disorders,* fifth edition *(DSM-5)* identifies features of cannabis use disorder, in addition to intoxication, withdrawal, and other cannabis-induced disorders, such as delirium psychosis, anxiety, and sleep disorders (American Psychiatric Association [APA], 2013). Compulsive use can interfere with life activities, and chronic users can report a lack of control over use and continuing to use marijuana even when faced with adverse consequences. Females are more likely than males to develop dependence, and younger age of initiation is also a risk factor (Welch & Malcolm, 2014). One study found that among youth, compulsive, heavy users had an 8-point-lower IQ from the ages of 13 to 38, which did not return to normal (Meier et al., 2012). This did not occur in adults, providing evidence of the negative impact of marijuana use on the developing brain.

HEALTH EFFECTS

Marijuana use is associated with many health effects (NIDA, 2016a), including physical, psychological, and behavioral effects that can be divided into categories of acute, persistent, and long-term. Table 8-2 summarizes some of the key uses and potential health effects related to marijuana use.

Adverse Physical Effects

The danger of long-term respiratory problems from smoking marijuana, which is the most common way the product is used, is well confirmed. Smoking marijuana regularly may produce some of the same health problems as smoking cigarettes, including daily cough, phlegm production, chest illnesses, increased lung infections, and a greater tendency toward obstructed airways. There can be a burning and stinging of the mouth and throat with use. Marijuana smoke also contains carcinogenic hydrocarbons similar to tobacco smoke, but the evidence linking marijuana smoking to lung cancer is inconclusive (NIDA, 2016a). This may be a dose/exposure effect, but the evidence does not provide a clear explanation for this finding.

The short-term effects on brain functioning include problems with memory and learning, distorted perceptions, and difficulty in thinking and problem solving. THC alters the way in which information is processed by the hippocampus – the part of the brain responsible for memory formation. There is some evidence that cognitive impairments can last for days, weeks, or even longer depending on the amount of marijuana smoked. Youth have the highest risk for sustained impairment in working memory, reasoning, processing speed, and verbal comprehension (Meier et al., 2012). Marijuana also causes psychomotor disruption, resulting in altered coordination and reaction time. This is generally a timing- and dose-dependent effect (Welch & Malcolm, 2014).

There is additional evidence that marijuana affects the heart and the endocrine and immune systems (NIDA, 2016a; Welch & Malcolm, 2014). Marijuana increases the user's heart rate within 5 to 10 minutes of use and can cause orthostatic hypotension. This risk is greatest in people who are older, whose bodies are less able to compensate for these changes (NIDA, 2016a). Conversely, cannabinoids have also been found to have some potential antihypertensive action and are being considered for their therapeutic effects in certain heart conditions (Welch & Malcolm, 2014). Cannabinoids have an immunosuppressant effect and have been found to alter endocrine activity (specifically, pituitary hormones), but the clinical implications are complex and not completely understood (Zumbrun, Sido, Nagarkatti, & Nagarkatti, 2015).

Marijuana use can have a profound effect on the liver. It can slow liver metabolism and prolong the activity of certain drugs, such as barbiturates. Use can increase the risk of alcohol-induced steatosis and liver fibrosis and contribute to the progression of existing disease and should be avoided in people with these conditions (Welch & Malcolm, 2014).

TABLE 8-2: MARIJUANA USE	
Uses and Possible Health Effects	
Short-Term	Enhanced sensory perception and euphoria followed by drowsiness/relaxation; disinhibition, increased sociability; dry mouth; slowed reaction time; time distortion; impaired balance and coordination; increased heart rate and appetite; decreased blood pressure; problems with learning and memory; heightened imagination, hallucinations, and delusions; anxiety; panic attacks; psychosis
Long-Term	Mental health problems, chronic cough, frequent respiratory infections, increased risk for cancer, suppression of the immune system
Other Health-Related Issues	Breathing problems and increased risk of cancer of the head, neck, lungs, and respiratory tract *Youth:* Possible loss of IQ points when repeated use begins in adolescence *Pregnancy-related:* Babies born with problems with attention, memory, and problem solving
In Combination with Alcohol	Increased heart rate and blood pressure; further slowing of mental processing and reaction time
Withdrawal Symptoms	Irritability, trouble sleeping, decreased appetite, anxiety
Medical Uses	Marinol (dronabinol) is indicated for the treatment of anorexia associated with weight loss in patients with AIDS and the nausea and vomiting associated with cancer chemotherapy in patients who have failed to respond adequately to conventional antiemetic treatments.
Treatment Options	
Medications	There are no medications approved by the U.S. Food and Drug Administration (FDA) to treat marijuana addiction.
Behavioral Therapies	Behavioral treatments tested with adolescents Cognitive-behavioral therapy Contingency management and motivational incentives

Note. From U.S. Department of Health and Human Services, Office of the Surgeon General. (2016). *Facing addiction in America: The surgeon general's report on alcohol, drugs, and health.* Washington, DC: Author.

Marijuana use should be avoided in pregnancy because fetal effects of THC exposure have been noted, specifically, problems with attention, memory, and problem solving and behavior problems in exposed children (NIDA, 2016a). Research has also shown that marijuana use can induce galactorrhea and has as-yet poorly understood effects on reproductive function (Welch & Malcolm, 2014).

A paradoxical effect associated with heavy marijuana use called cannabinoid hyperemesis syndrome has also been extensively described in the literature. Generally, marijuana use has an associated antiemetic and appetite-stimulating effect. However, in some rare instances, a syndrome consisting of cyclic nausea and vomiting can occur with heavy use and generally resolves within 48 hours using supportive measures (Sun & Zimmerman, 2013). For unclear reasons, bathing in hot water alleviates the symptoms. There is concern that this condition may be misdiagnosed, which underscores the importance of screening for marijuana use (Sun & Zimmerman, 2013).

Beneficial Health Effects

As noted, marijuana use historically has been recognized for its beneficial effects on health. The current understanding of these effects presents a complex picture. Some of these effects are attributed to THC, but other cannabinoids, such as cannabidiol, which acts as an anticonvulsant, also play a role (Welch & Malcolm, 2014). There is increasing evidence for the clinical effectiveness of THC and cannabidiol in the management of chronic, intractable pain (Hill, 2015). Synthetic cannabinoids are used as antiemetics, and smoking marijuana has long been noted to stimulate appetite in people with AIDS, cancer, and cachexia. It is important to note, however, that the U.S. Food and Drug Administration (FDA) has not approved any medication that is smoked. Use can also lower intraocular pressure in treating glaucoma and moderating symptoms in neurologic conditions such as Parkinson's disease and multiple sclerosis.

Psychological Effects

The *DSM-5* (APA, 2013) and the *International Classification of Diseases* (*ICD-10*; World Health Organization [WHO], 2010) identify cannabis use disorders. Criteria to define cannabis use disorders follow the general criteria used for substance use disorders. These criteria include use of a substance in larger amounts and for a duration longer than expected, a persistent desire or unsuccessful efforts to reduce use, spending excessive amounts of time engaged in activities related to the use of the substance, an increase in cravings, disengagement from usual activities, using the substance with activities that can pose physical risk, and tolerance and withdrawal symptoms (APA, 2013). Withdrawal from cannabis was not recognized in the *DSM-4,* but research has produced sufficient evidence for its inclusion in the *DSM-5* (Hasin et al., 2013).

The *DSM-5* (APA, 2013) and the *ICD-10* (WHO, 2010) both include cannabis withdrawal and intoxication. Although historically there has been controversy about withdrawal symptoms, heavy use of cannabis results in what researchers often describe as cannabis withdrawal syndrome, which up to one-third of heavy users may experience (Wilkins, Danovitch, & Gorelick, 2014). Withdrawal symptoms include insomnia, anorexia, anxiety, irritability, depression, and tremor (Welch & Malcolm, 2014). As with tobacco use, when patients try to stop marijuana use, they often experience relapse. Cannabis intoxication is rare, is dose related, and can result in panic and paranoia. Symptoms associated with intoxication include pupil constriction, injected conjunctiva, headache, tremor, decreased coordination and urinary retention (Wilkins, Danovitch, & Gorelick, 2014). Both withdrawal and acute intoxication symptoms are self-limiting and can generally be managed with supportive measures.

The relationship between cannabis use disorders and psychiatric conditions, particularly schizophrenia, is also complex. Studies have detected increased levels of endocannabinoids in the cerebrospinal fluid of patients with schizophrenia, which led to several studies demonstrating that marijuana use is associated (not directly causal) with increased risk of developing the disease, worsening symptoms, and a poorer overall prognosis (Welch & Malcolm, 2014). This relationship between the cannabinoid system and psychosis has led to interest in the exploration of potential new treatments for schizophrenia and psychotic disorders (Iseger & Bossong, 2015).

Behavioral Effects

Most of the studies involving the behavioral effects of marijuana use have focused on motivation. Research has long noted that there is an association between decreased motivation, apathy, and chronic marijuana use. However, data that clearly link an amotivational syndrome with marijuana use have been challenging to parse out, and the nature of the relationship is still unclear. Animal and preclinical studies have demonstrated an association between decreased motivation toward reward-based learning and behaviors (Volkow et al., 2016). Yet because of other brain effects of marijuana, such as those on cognition, it is challenging for researchers to determine whether changes in motivation are causal, additive, or result from other cannabinoid effects. Youth who use marijuana have a higher risk of poor school performance and dropout compared with those who do not (Volkow, Baler, Compton, & Weiss, 2014).

Fetal Effects

Marijuana use among women who are pregnant and of childbearing age poses concerns. One concern is that fetal exposure to THC can alter brain development (NIDA, 2016a). Studies have suggested increased neural irritability and low birth weight in babies who were exposed to THC in utero, but these associations have been hard to clearly define (Gunn et al., 2016). THC passes to nursing infants through breastmilk, but the implications of this are not fully understood (NIDA, 2016a). A recent analysis (Brown et al., 2016) looked at trends in marijuana use over a 12-year period in women who were either pregnant or of childbearing age. They found a steady increase in marijuana use in these women, with an increase of 62% for past-month use by pregnant women. Prevalence rates overall were low in this group (3.85% in 2014); however, the growing trend is of concern in the context of increased normalization and legalization of marijuana use in the United States.

TREATMENT

Among marijuana users age 12 and older, 1.5% met the criteria for a diagnosis of cannabis use disorder in 2015 (HHS, 2016). Other research (NIDA, 2016a) found that those seeking treatment have generally tried to quit several times and have used marijuana for at least 10 years; severity of withdrawal symptoms and concurrent use of other substances also led users to seek treatment. Several other facilitators to seeking treatment have been identified (van der Pol et al., 2013). These include social support, heavy use with symptoms of dependency, external pressure, and favorable perception of and experiences with treatment.

Nurses and other healthcare providers should systematically assess patients' cannabis use through a clinical evaluation of the use, frequency, quantity of consumption, and complications from use. All adolescents should be asked about the use of drugs – including cigarettes, alcohol, and marijuana – at all routine health maintenance visits. Although there is no current evidence-based instrument specific to marijuana use, the drug is one of the substances included in the NIDA Quick Screening Tool and the WHO's Alcohol, Smoking, and Substance Involvement Screening Test (Zgierska & Fleming, 2014).

Since the 1980s, urine tests have been used to detect 11-nor-delta-9-tetrahydrocannabinol-9-carboxylic acid, a metabolite of THC. This is detectable in the urine from 5 to 30 days after use. The reason for this prolonged window is that THC is highly lipophilic and is stored in fat tissue. Other screening tests may include saliva, sweat patch, and hair tests, although there are limitations associated with these methods, and urine testing is most common (Warner & Lorch, 2014).

Many occupational settings require drug testing, and the cutoff point of 50 ng/ml for the THC metabolite is federally mandated (Warner

& Lorch, 2014). Confirmatory readings can be determined at a level of 15 ng/ml, and many factors can alter the detection time, including potency, method of administration, assay sensitivity, and chronicity of use (Warner & Lorch, 2014). Testing in schools was one of the recommended strategies of the Office of National Drug Control Policy (2002). The school recommendation assumed that drug testing can be a means of preventing and treating youth drug use. However, evidence suggests that if testing is done, it should not be a stand-alone approach but needs to be done in the context of other treatment and prevention measures. Although reasonable suspicion can be a prompt for testing, only students who participate in competitive extracurricular activities can legally be subject to random drug testing (NIDA, 2014).

In 1997, the U.S. government sponsored the Cannabis Youth Treatment (CYT) study, which resulted in innovative and effective treatment methodologies. Various approaches included the following:

- Motivational enhancement therapy (MET) plus cognitive-behavioral therapy (CBT). This consisted of two individual MET sessions and three group CBT sessions lasting 6 to 7 weeks. The MET component focused on assisting adolescents to resolve their ambivalence about whether they had a problem with cannabis or substances and increasing their motivation to stop using. The CBT component focused on teaching such skills as refusing offers of cannabis, establishing a social network in support of recovery, developing a plan for pleasant activities to replace cannabis activities, and coping with high-risk situations.

- A more in-depth MET+CBT treatment strategy consisting of 12 sessions. This was similar to the previously described strategy but with a longer time frame.

- A family support network. This approach used 12 sessions of MET+CBT with six parent education group meetings, four home visits, referral to a self-help group, and case management.

- Adolescent community reinforcement. This consisted of 10 individual sessions with adolescents, four sessions with caregivers, and limited case management.

- Multidimensional family therapy. This approach consisted of 12 to 15 sessions with adolescents and their family members and case management over 12 to 14 weeks.

(Dennis et al., 2004)

The effectiveness of these treatment modalities was studied in 600 cannabis users (predominately white males, age 15 to 16; Dennis et al., 2004). Overall, the CYT study found that all of these interventions resulted in significant pre- and post-treatment improvements during the 12 months for two main outcomes: days of abstinence and percent of adolescents in recovery.

CBT continues to be a mainstay of substance use treatment and is widely used in settings for people with co-occurring mental health disorders. This is generally a short-term approach to treatment (12 to 24 weeks) and is most beneficial when combined with other therapies (HHS, 2016). Some of these combined approaches include MET and contingency management, which uses tangible rewards to reinforce behavioral change. Currently, web-based treatments using these modalities show promise in reaching targeted groups and increasing access to treatment (HHS, 2016).

Although no medications are approved to treat marijuana dependence, research has found evidence of some efficacy for three medications: gabapentin, an anticonvulsant; N-acetylcysteine, a glutamate modulator; and buspirone, an anxiolytic (Wilkins, Hrymoc, & Gorelick, 2014).

Their mechanism of action is unclear, but evidence suggests that they result in decreased use in marijuana users with symptoms of dependency. Research is focused on blocking the cannabinoid receptors, which could potentially treat dependence and have implications for the use of cannabinoids in the treatment of other conditions (Wilkins, Hrymoc, & Gorelick,, 2014).

SPECIAL ISSUES

Special Populations

High-risk groups for the use of marijuana include youth and young adults, particularly women of childbearing age and those who are pregnant. In the 2015 National Survey on Drug Use and Health (Azofeifa et al., 2016), young adults ages 18 to 25 had the highest rates of use of illicit drugs. In this age group, over half (52.7%) reported ever using (one-time experimentation) marijuana, with 32.2% using in the prior year and 19.8% using in the previous month. This compares to lifetime use of 44%, past-year use of 13.5%, and past-month use of 8.3% for all people 12 and older. For youth ages 12 to 17, past-year use was 12.6%, and past-month use was 7%, with the highest past-year, past-month, and daily use rates found in 12th graders: 34.9%, 21.3%, and 6%, respectively (Miech et al., 2016). These statistics clearly indicate that youth and young adults are at particular risk. An analysis of 13,718 middle school and high school students found that the students' own and peer involvement with substances, delinquency, and school problems were the three risk factors that predicted marijuana use at all stages of marijuana involvement: initiation of experimental use, initiation of regular use, progression to regular use, failure to discontinue experimental use, and failure to discontinue regular use (van den Bree & Pickworth, 2005). Additional risk factors include less time spent with parents (Best, Gross, Manning, Gossop, &

Strang, 2005) and positive expectations of use (Chabrol et al., 2006).

The extent of marijuana use is evident in the findings from a former drug use monitoring system. The Drug Abuse Warning Network (DAWN) monitored the health impact of drugs and found that marijuana was mentioned in the medical record of more than 456,000 drug-related emergency department visits in the United States in 2011 (CBHSQ, 2013). Most of these patients were male (two-thirds), and 13% were between the ages of 12 and 17. There was a 21% increase in these findings over the study period from 2009 to 2011. The DAWN monitoring system was discontinued in 2011.

Considerable concern exists that substances commonly used by youth, such as marijuana, tobacco, and alcohol, can have a gateway effect – that is, can lead to the use and misuse of other illicit substances. Although the gateway theory has been debated for many years (Volkow et al., 2014), recent evidence has been building to support this effect (Hindocha et al., 2015; Secades-Villa, Garcia-Rodríguez, Jin, Wang, & Blanco, 2015). Secades-Villa et al. (2015) recently estimated that nearly 45% of people with lifetime cannabis use progress to the use of other illicit drug use at some point. This progression was particularly evident for people with mental health conditions. One explanation for this effect is related to the impact of marijuana and tobacco use on dopamine regulation in the developing brain, causing those who are younger and heavier users to rely on these substances in the activation of the brain reward cycle. A second explanation may be that these substances have a priming effect, causing a heightened response when exposed to certain substances (NIDA, 2016a).

Medicinal Use of Cannabis

The history of cannabis as a medicinal plant is extensive. The oldest known therapeutic description was given by an emperor in China who used it for beriberi, constipation, gout, malaria, and absentmindedness. It has also been used throughout the world, including the United States, for various ailments; the U.S. government outlawed its use in medical care in 1937. Because cannabis has been associated with appetite stimulation and pain relief in such illnesses as cancer and AIDS, there are increasing efforts to legalize cannabis (Welch & Malcolm, 2014). One review found high-quality evidence for the use of marijuana for chronic pain, neuropathic pain, and spasticity caused by multiple sclerosis, noting that this level of evidence does not exist for many other conditions (Hill, 2015). A recent meta-analysis of studies related to the medicinal use of cannabis concluded the following:

> There was moderate-quality evidence to support the use of cannabinoids for the treatment of chronic pain and spasticity. There was low-quality evidence suggesting that cannabinoids were associated with improvements in nausea and vomiting due to chemotherapy, weight gain in HIV infection, sleep disorders, and Tourette syndrome. Cannabinoids were associated with an increased risk of short-term AEs [adverse events]. (Whiting et al., 2015, p. 2456)

Several limitations pertain to developing sound evidence regarding the medical use of marijuana. Whiting et al. (2015) noted a lack of consistent use of standardized research design protocols in the studies examined. The scheduled status of marijuana (Schedule I) also makes it challenging to conduct research. Sociopolitical factors also come into play with the persistent controversies surrounding legalization.

Currently, there is a clinical trial under way regarding the use of a 99% liquid cannabidiol (nonpsychoactive) medication for the treatment of seizures in certain types of epilepsy affecting children who have not responded to other therapies (Kaur, Ambwani, & Singh, 2016). Although there have been anecdotal reports in the media regarding the use of marijuana to treat children's seizures, it is important to note that it is not marijuana smoke or THC that has demonstrated the potential therapeutic effect but a nonpsychoactive cannabinoid extracted from the plant. The current product being tested systematically in clinical trials has more potential to help while minimizing harm compared with Internet products claiming to be natural marijuana treatments, which clearly can pose harm (Sirven & Shafer, 2015).

Legalization Issues

Controversies related to legalizing marijuana remain pervasive, with more states legalizing marijuana for medicinal (and recreational) use. States and large industries, such as the tobacco industry, are positioned to gain significant financial benefits from legalization (Barry, Hiilamo, & Glantz, 2014).

Although THC and certain nonpsychoactive cannabinoids are recognized as ingredients that can be used to treat some medical problems, research has not yet proven marijuana as a smoked product to have benefits that outweigh harm for most conditions. There are currently many clinical trials under way to further study the potential uses of marijuana; in the meantime, it remains the conclusion of the DEA that marijuana smoke creates adverse events that do not outweigh the benefits (DEA, 2011). The DEA maintains that there are persistent concerns regarding efficacy and safety in the use of marijuana for medicinal purposes (DEA, 2011).

The U.S. government has maintained a strong stand against legalizing the medicinal use of marijuana in the United States. Under federal law, marijuana is regulated as a Schedule I controlled substance, and its use is prohibited. In 2005, the Supreme Court in *Gonzales v. Raich* declared that the U.S. government can ban possession of marijuana even in those states that have eliminated sanctions for its use in treating symptoms of illness (Rosenbaum, 2005). To date, the U.S. government has chosen not to interfere with state legalization despite having the legal right to do so.

As of January 2017, 28 states (Alaska, Arizona, Arkansas, California, Colorado, Connecticut, Delaware, Florida, Hawaii, Illinois, Maine, Maryland, Massachusetts, Michigan, Minnesota, Montana, Nevada, New Hampshire, New Jersey, New Mexico, New York, North Dakota, Ohio, Oregon, Pennsylvania, Rhode Island, Vermont, and Washington) and Washington, DC, maintained laws permitting marijuana use for medical purposes. Colorado, Alaska, Oregon, Washington, California, Maine, Massachusetts, and Nevada have all voted to legalize recreational use of marijuana (ProCon.org, 2016).

Until the U.S. Supreme Court rules directly on the constitutionality of state medical marijuana laws, a conflict remains between federal law that outlaws marijuana use and state laws that may permit its limited medical use. Generally, a physician's role is to certify the patient's confirmed diagnosis and state a recommendation for medicinal marijuana as a proposed treatment.

SUMMARY

Cannabis has an interesting history relating to recreational and medicinal use, and it is a drug with controversial underpinnings. The use of cannabis as a recreational drug continues to be a concern in U.S. society for several reasons: after several years of decline, marijuana use remains at a relatively steady rate among high school students, the potency of THC is increasing, and there has been a recent increase in the use of marijuana by women who are pregnant. These concerns are occurring in the context of increased legalization and normalization of marijuana use in society.

It is also important to consider the potential clinical benefits of cannabinoids. Although research is not conclusive, there is mounting evidence that certain cannabinoids are useful in the treatment of specific medical conditions, such as chronic pain. Healthcare providers must follow established processes of drug testing to ensure that the benefits of use in patients with these conditions clearly outweigh the potential harm.

Because marijuana is the most common illicit drug used among U.S. youth, with concerns regarding a gateway effect leading to the use of other illicit substances, it remains important to concentrate efforts on use prevention. Clearly, youth are most vulnerable to the long-term detrimental effects of regular marijuana use. It is important to continue to explore the longitudinal effects of both use patterns and health effects. Legalization will result in investigation of the consequences of increased access to cannabis and any unintended consequences, both good and bad, that universally accompany policy change.

Finally, it is challenging to communicate the scientific evidence regarding marijuana and use patterns. The knowledge base is continuing to evolve. Research on cannabinoids and cannabinoid receptors is promising for a variety of conditions, with the caveat of potential pitfalls. It is vitally important that as trusted practitioners, nurses remain committed to using evidence-based practice in their care of patients.

EXAM QUESTIONS

CHAPTER 8
Questions 39–45

Note: Choose the one option that BEST answers each question.

39. Marijuana is the most commonly used illicit drug and the most

    a. consistently banned substance with adverse drug effects.

    b. potent drug available.

    c. commonly abused drug by athletes.

    d. consistently available drug.

40. The intoxication effect of cannabis is a result of

    a. overstimulation of the cannabinoid receptors in the brain.

    b. stimulation of primarily one area of the brain.

    c. the need for an increased dose of marijuana.

    d. the lack of marijuana brain receptors.

41. Which of the following is a true statement about the health effects of marijuana use?

    a. Smoking marijuana regularly may produce some of the same health problems as smoking cigarettes.

    b. Behavioral effects related to job performance resulting from marijuana use are rare.

    c. Coordination, balance, and reaction time are improved with marijuana use.

    d. The heart rate of a person smoking marijuana decreases within the first 5 to 10 minutes.

42. Which of the following is a true statement regarding the treatment of patients with a marijuana use disorder?

    a. There is limited evidence that any type of treatment is effective over a short- or long-term period of follow-up.

    b. Comparable benefits have been found for adolescents in cognitive-behavioral groups and individual treatment, including motivational enhancement therapy.

    c. There is no evidence that any type of medication should be developed to treat marijuana dependence.

    d. Rewards are an ineffective treatment approach in promoting abstinence from marijuana use.

43. A risk factor that predicts marijuana use at all stages of marijuana involvement is

    a. being a 12th-grade student.

    b. having older siblings.

    c. having problems at home.

    d. having problems in school.

44. Research supports the use of evidence-based treatment practices involving marijuana for which health condition?

    a. Heart failure

    b. Liver disease

    c. Chronic pain

    d. Epilepsy

continued on next page

45. The Drug Enforcement Administration's current position on the medical use of marijuana is that

   a. marijuana smoke creates adverse events that do not outweigh the drug's benefits.

   b. its use should be regulated exclusively by state law.

   c. scientific evidence supports the positive health effects of marijuana use outweighing the adverse effects.

   d. there is no cause for further study of the medicinal value of marijuana.

REFERENCES

American Psychiatric Association. (2013). *Diagnostic and statistical manual of mental disorders* (5th ed.). Arlington, VA: Author.

Azofeifa, A., Mattson, M. E., Schauer, G., McAfee, T., Grant, A., & Lyerla, R. (2016). National estimates of marijuana use and related indicators – National Survey on Drug Use and Health, United States, 2002-2014. *Morbidity and Mortality Weekly Report Surveillance Summary, 65*(SS-11), 1-25.

Barry, R. A., Hiilamo, H., & Glantz, S. A. (2014). Waiting for the opportune moment: The tobacco industry and marijuana legalization. *Milbank Quarterly, 92*(2), 207-242.

Best, D., Gross, S., Manning, V., Gossop, M., & Strang, J. (2005). Cannabis use in adolescents: The impact of risk and protective factors and social functioning. *Drug and Alcohol Review, 24*(6), 483-488.

Brown, Q. L., Sarvet, A. L., Shmulewitz, D., Martins, S. S., Wall, M. M., & Hasin, D. S. (2016). Trends in marijuana use among pregnant and nonpregnant reproductive-aged women, 2002-2014. *Journal of the American Medical Association, 317*(2), 207-209.

Center for Behavioral Health Statistics and Quality. (2013). *Drug abuse warning network: 2011: Selected tables of national estimates of drug-related emergency department visits.* Rockville, MD: Substance Abuse and Mental Health Services Administration.

Chabrol, H., Chauchard, E., Mabila, J., Mantoulan, R., Adele, A., & Rousseau, A. (2006). Contributions of social influences and expectations of use to cannabis use in high-school students. *Addictive Behaviors, 31*(11), 2116-2119.

Dennis, M., Godley, S. H., Diamond, G., Tims, F. M., Babor, T., Donaldson, J., & Funk, R. (2004). The Cannabis Youth Treatment (CYT) study: Main findings from two randomized trials. *Journal of Substance Abuse Treatment, 27*(3), 195-196.

Drug Enforcement Administration. (2011). *The DEA position on marijuana.* Retrieved from http://www.justice.gov/dea/docs/marijuana_position_2011.pdf

ElSohly, M. A., Mehmedic, Z., Foster, S., Gon, D., Chandra, S., & Church, J. C. (2016). Changes in cannabis potency over the last 2 decades (1995-2014): Analysis of current data in the United States. *Biological Psychiatry, 79*(7), 613-619.

Gunn, J. K. L., Rosales, C. B., Center, K. E., Nuñez, A., Gibson, S. J., Christ, C., & Ehiri, J. E. (2016). Prenatal exposure to cannabis and maternal and child health outcomes: A systematic review and meta-analysis. *BMJ Open, 6*(4), e009986. doi:10.1136/bmjopen-2015-009986

Hasin, D. S., O'Brien, C. P., Auriacombe, M., Borges, G., Bucholz, K., Budney, A., ... Grant, B. F. (2013). *DSM-5* criteria for substance use disorders: Recommendations and rationale. *American Journal of Psychiatry, 170*(8), 834-851.

Hill, K. P. (2015). Medical marijuana for treatment of chronic pain and other medical and psychiatric problems: A clinical review. *Journal of the American Medical Association, 313*(24), 2474-2483.

Hindocha, C., Shaban, N. D. C., Freeman, T. P., Das, R. K., Gale, G., Schafer, G., ... Curran, H. V. (2015). Associations between cigarette smoking and cannabis dependence: A longitudinal study of young cannabis users in the United Kingdom. *Drug and Alcohol Dependence, 148,* 165-171.

Iseger, T. A., & Bossong, M. G. (2015). A systematic review of the antipsychotic properties of cannabidiol in humans. *Schizophrenia Research, 162*(1-3), 153-161.

Johnston, L. D., O'Malley, P. M., Bachman, J. G., Schulenberg, J. E., & Miech, R. A. (2016). *Monitoring the Future national survey results on drug use, 1975-2015: Volume II, college students and adults ages 19-55.* Ann Arbor, MI: Institute for Social Research, University of Michigan.

Johnston, L. D., O'Malley, P. M., Miech, R. A., Bachman, J. G., & Schulenberg, J. E. (2016). *Monitoring the Future national survey results on drug use, 1975-2015: Overview, key findings on adolescent drug use.* Ann Arbor, MI: Institute for Social Research, University of Michigan.

Kaur, R., Ambwani, S. R., & Singh, S. (2016). Endocannabinoid system: A multi-facet therapeutic target. *Current Clinical Pharmacology, 11*(2), 110-117.

Martín-Santos, R., Crippa, J. A., Batalla, A., Bhattacharyya, S., Atakan, Z., Borgwardt, S., ... McGuire, P. K. (2012). Acute effects of a single, oral dose of d9-tetrahydrocannabinol (THC) and cannabidiol (CBD) administration in healthy volunteers. *Current Pharmaceutical Design, 18,* 4966-4979.

Meier, M. H., Caspi, A., Ambler, A., Harrington, H., Houts, R., Keefe, R. S., & Moffitt, T. E. (2012). Persistent cannabis users show neuropsychological decline from childhood to midlife. *Proceedings of the National Academy of Sciences of the United States of America, 109*(40), E2657-E2664.

Miech, R. A., Johnston, L. D., O'Malley, P. M., Bachman, J. G., & Schulenberg, J. E. (2016). *Monitoring the Future national survey results on drug use, 1975-2015: Volume I, secondary school students.* Ann Arbor, MI: Institute for Social Research, University of Michigan.

National Conference of State Legislatures. (2017). *Marijuana overview: Legislation.* Retrieved from http://www.ncsl.org/research/civil-and-criminal-justice/marijuana-overview.aspx

National Institute on Drug Abuse. (2014). *Frequently asked questions about drug testing in schools.* Retrieved from https://www.drugabuse.gov/related-topics/drug-testing/faq-drug-testing-in-schools

National Institute on Drug Abuse. (2016a). *Marijuana.* Retrieved from https://www.drugabuse.gov/drugs-abuse/marijuana

National Institute on Drug Abuse. (2016b). *Monitoring the Future study: Trends in prevalence of various drugs.* Retrieved from https://www.drugabuse.gov/trends-statistics/monitoring-future/monitoring-future-study-trends-in-prevalence-various-drugs

Office of National Drug Control Policy. (2002). *What you need to know about drug testing in schools.* Retrieved from http://www.ncjrs.gov/ondcppubs/publications/pdf/drug_testing.pdf

ProCon.org. (2016). *28 legal medical marijuana states and DC.* Retrieved from http://medicalmarijuana.procon.org/view.resource.php?resourceID=000881

Rosenbaum, S. (2005). *Gonzales v. Raich*: Implications for public health policy. *Public Health Reports, 120*(6), 680-682.

Secades-Villa, R., Garcia-Rodríguez, O., Jin, C., J., Wang, S., & Blanco, C. (2015). Probability and predictors of the cannabis gateway effect: A national study. *International Journal on Drug Policy, 26*(2), 135-142.

Sirven, J. I., & Shafer, P. O. (2015). *Medical marijuana and epilepsy*. Retrieved from http://www.epilepsy.com/learn/treating-seizures-and-epilepsy/other-treatment-approaches/medical-marijuana-and-epilepsy

Substance Abuse and Mental Health Services Administration. (2015). *The Center for Behavioral Health Statistics and Quality (CBHSQ) report*. Rockville, MD: Author.

Sun, S., & Zimmermann, A. E. (2013). Cannabinoid hyperemesis syndrome. *Hospital Pharmacy, 48*(8), 650-655.

U.S. Department of Health and Human Services, Office of the Surgeon General. (2016). *Facing addiction in America: The surgeon general's report on alcohol, drugs, and health*. Washington, DC: Author.

van den Bree, M. B., & Pickworth, W. B. (2005). Risk factors predicting changes in marijuana involvement in teenagers. *Archives of General Psychiatry, 62*(3), 311-319.

van der Pol, P., Liebregts, N., de Graaf, R., Korf, D. J., van den Brink, W., & van Laar, M. (2013). Facilitators and barriers in treatment seeking for cannabis dependence. *Drug and Alcohol Dependence, 133*(2), 776-780.

Volkow, N. D., Baler, R. D., Compton, W. M., & Weiss, S. R. (2014). Adverse health effects of marijuana use. *New England Journal of Medicine, 370*, 2219-2227.

Volkow, N. D., Swanson, J. M., Eden Evins, A., DeLisi, L. E., Meier, M. H., Gonzalez, R., & Baler, R. (2016). Effects of cannabis use on human behavior, including cognition, motivation, and psychosis: A review. *JAMA Psychiatry, 73*(3), 292-297.

Warner, E., & Lorch, E. (2014). Laboratory diagnosis. In R. K. Reis (Ed.), *The ASAM principles of addiction medicine* (5th ed., pp. 332-343). Philadelphia, PA: Wolters Kluwer.

Welch, S. P., & Malcolm, R. (2014). The pharmacology of marijuana. In R. K. Reis (Ed.), *The ASAM principles of addiction medicine* (5th ed., pp. 217-234). Philadelphia, PA: Wolters Kluwer.

Whiting, P. F., Wolff, R. F., Deshpande, S., Di Nisio, M., Duffy, S., Hernandez, A. V., & Kleijnen, J. (2015). Cannabinoids for medical use: A systematic review and meta-analysis. *Journal of the American Medical Association, 313*(24), 2456-2473.

Wilkins, J. N., Danovitch, I., & Gorelick, D. A. (2014). Management of stimulant, hallucinogen, marijuana, phencyclidine, and club drug intoxication and withdrawal. In R. K. Reis (Ed.), *The ASAM principles of addiction medicine* (5th ed., pp. 692-694). Philadelphia, PA: Wolters Kluwer.

Wilkins, J. N., Hrymoc, M., & Gorelick, D. A. (2014). Pharmacologic interventions for other drug and multiple drug addictions. In R. K. Reis (Ed.), *The ASAM principles of addiction medicine* (5th ed., pp. 823-824). Philadelphia, PA: Wolters Kluwer.

World Health Organization. (2010). *International statistical classification of diseases and related health problems* (10th rev.). Geneva, Switzerland: Author.

Zgierska, A., & Fleming, F. M. (2014). Screening and brief intervention. In R. K. Reis (Ed.), *The ASAM principles of addiction medicine* (5th ed., pp. 297-331). Philadelphia, PA: Wolters Kluwer.

Zumbrun, E. E., Sido, J. M., Nagarkatti, P. S., & Nagarkatti, M. (2015). Epigenetic regulation of immunological alterations following prenatal exposure to marijuana cannabinoids and its long-term consequences in offspring. *Journal of Neuroimmune Pharmacology, 10*(2), 245-254.

CHAPTER 9

STIMULANTS

LEARNING OUTCOME

After completing this chapter, the learner will be able to describe stimulant use disorder, including its diagnostic criteria, effects on the body, and current treatment approaches.

CHAPTER OBJECTIVES

After completing this chapter, the learner will be able to:

1. Identify the prevalence of stimulant use for methylphenidate, amphetamines, methamphetamine, and cocaine.

2. Compare the routes of administration, mechanism, and biochemistry of stimulants, including methylphenidate, amphetamines, methamphetamine, and cocaine.

3. Describe the various effects of stimulants on the body.

4. Identify common psychological and physical symptoms of stimulant use disorder.

5. Explain current assessment and treatment approaches for stimulant use disorder.

INTRODUCTION

The class of drugs known as stimulants is commonly used because of the increased energy individuals experience beyond what would normally be expected. Stimulants may be taken to improve attention and focus, control impulses, facilitate weight loss, or boost sexual performance. Mild stimulants include nicotine and caffeine, whereas stronger ones include methylphenidate, amphetamines, and cocaine. At relatively low doses, use may be equated with perceptions of being more alert, intelligent, energetic, or stronger. At higher doses, euphoria is experienced, followed or accompanied by toxic effects (National Institute on Drug Abuse [NIDA], 2014).

Stimulants are prescribed to treat medical disorders such as attention-deficit hyperactivity disorder (ADHD) and sometimes depression. Current evidence indicates that when used as intended under medical supervision, stimulants used to treat ADHD do not typically trigger substance use disorders (Heal, Smith, Gosden, & Nutt, 2013). When taken in doses and via routes other than those prescribed, prescription stimulants can increase brain dopamine in a rapid and highly amplified manner (similar to other misused drugs, such as methamphetamine), thereby disrupting normal communication between brain cells and producing euphoria and, as a result, increasing the risk for a substance use disorder (NIDA, 2014). This chapter discusses stimulant use, including illicit compounds such as methamphetamine, cocaine, and synthetic cathinones, which are often referred to as "bath salts."

Stimulant use disorder is a new term in the *Diagnostic and Statistical Manual of Mental Disorders,* fifth edition (*DSM-5;* American

Psychiatric Association [APA], 2013). The terms substance abuse and substance dependence are no longer used and have been replaced with this new term. Substance use disorders are defined as mild, moderate, or severe to indicate the level of severity, which is determined by the number of diagnostic criteria met by an individual:

- Mild – two to three criteria
- Moderate – four to five criteria
- Severe – six or more criteria

Substance use disorders are present when the recurrent use of alcohol and/or drugs causes clinically and functionally significant impairment, such as health problems, disability, and failure to meet major responsibilities at work, school, or home. According to the *DSM-5,* a diagnosis of substance use disorder is based on evidence of impaired control, social impairment, risky use, and pharmacological criteria (APA, 2013; Hasin et al., 2013; Substance Abuse and Mental Health Services Administration [SAMHSA], 2017).

The most commonly misused stimulants are amphetamines, methamphetamine, and cocaine. Stimulants can be synthetic (such as amphetamines) or can be plant derived (such as cocaine). They are usually administered orally, intranasally, or intravenously (SAMHSA, 2017).

EPIDEMIOLOGY

In 2014, almost 569,000 people in the United States ages 12 and older reported using methamphetamine in the past month. That same year, an estimated 913,000 people ages 12 and older had a stimulant use disorder because of cocaine use, and an estimated 476,000 people had a stimulant use disorder as a result of using stimulants other than methamphetamine (SAMHSA, 2017).

According to the 2014 National Survey on Drug Use and Health (Center for Behavioral Health Statistics and Quality [CBHSQ], 2015), there were an estimated 1.5 million current (past-month) cocaine users aged 12 or older. Adults aged 18 to 25 years have a higher rate of current cocaine use than any other age group. The 2015 Monitoring the Future survey, which annually surveys teen attitudes and drug use, reported a significant decline in the 30-day prevalence of use of powdered cocaine among 8th, 10th, and 12th graders from the peak level of use in the late 1990s. Repeated use of stimulants can produce addiction and other adverse health consequences (NIDA, 2016a). Data from the 2011 Drug Abuse Warning Network report indicated that cocaine was involved in 505,224 of the nearly 1.3 million visits to emergency departments for drug misuse (NIDA, 2016a).

TYPES OF STIMULANTS

Methylphenidate

Methylphenidate is a stimulant that affects the central nervous system. It has been classified by the U.S. Drug Enforcement Administration (DEA) as a Schedule II stimulant. All stimulants work by increasing dopamine levels in the brain. Methylphenidate blocks the reuptake of dopamine, a neurotransmitter associated with pleasure, movement, and attention. The therapeutic effect of stimulants is achieved by slow and steady increases of dopamine, which is similar to the way dopamine is naturally produced in the brain. There are various formulations of methylphenidate, including tablets, caplets, liquid, chewable tablets, and patches. Stimulants can increase blood pressure, heart rate, and body temperature and decrease sleep and appetite. When they are misused, medical problems such as malnutrition, feelings of hostility, paranoia, and serious cardiovascular complications, including stroke, may occur (NIDA, 2014).

Amphetamines

Some forms of amphetamines are licensed for ADHD. Two other categories of amphetamines do not currently have licensed use: (1) anorectic drugs, which were formerly licensed for weight loss and (2) the natural amphetamines khat and ephedra, which are primarily consumed in East Africa, the Arabian Peninsula, and China, and are also available in synthetic forms (Haslam, 2016). Table 9-1 lists street names for amphetamines.

TABLE 9-1: SELECTED STREET NAMES FOR AMPHETAMINES

- Bennies
- Black beauties
- Crosses
- Hearts
- LA turnaround
- Speed
- Truck drivers
- Uppers

Note. Adapted from National Institute on Drug Abuse. (2017b). *Commonly abused drugs charts: Prescription stimulants.* Retrieved from https://www.drugabuse.gov/drugs-abuse/commonly-abused-drugs-charts#prescription-stimulants

Anorectics

Anorectics are either Schedule III or IV drugs, meaning they have a lower abuse potential compared with methylphenidate (U.S. Department of Justice [DOJ], n.d.). Anorectics such as phentermine are licensed as appetite suppressants. Anorectics have amphetamine-like effects, but they are less intense. Phentermine was used with fenfluramine and dexfenfluramine as a widely prescribed combination for weight loss, but the latter two were removed from the market because of their tendency to cause heart-valve problems (DEA, n.d.; Haslam, 2016).

Natural Amphetamines and Their Synthetic Counterparts

Khat is found in the young leaves of the *Catha edulis* shrub native to East Africa and the Arabian Peninsula. Used for hundreds of years and legal in parts of its native region, khat may be smuggled into other countries. Khat leaves contain cathine and cathinone and are used in a manner similar to coffee elsewhere in the world (NIDA, 2016b).

Cathinone is the component of khat with more potent amphetamine effects. As the leaves dry and age, cathinone is changed to cathine and norephedrine (very similar to phenylpropanolamine), resulting in lessened stimulatory effects. The most intoxicating effects are experienced when the leaves are consumed within 48 hours from the time they are picked. Although fresh leaves are not readily available in the United States, cathinone, used intranasally or orally, may be used in their place.

Khat leaves are chewed to alleviate fatigue or suppress appetite and, in small to moderate doses, are associated with minimal adverse effects. Dried leaves can also be used to make a tea or paste. Unlike the other amphetamines, khat has some anesthetic effects. Compulsive use is associated with mania, delusions, and paranoia, similar to other types of amphetamines (NIDA, 2016b).

Synthetic cathinones are commonly known as "bath salts." They are chemically related to the natural substance cathinone but are made in a laboratory. Synthetic cathinones can be much stronger than the natural product and, in some cases, very dangerous (NIDA, 2016b). The mechanism of action of cathinones is similar to that of methamphetamine. Cathinones block the reuptake of dopamine, norepinephrine, and serotonin and stimulate the release of dopamine (Prosser & Nelson, 2012).

Ephedra is a natural herb used in China for asthma, hay fever, and nasal congestion. Its principal active ingredients are ephedrine and pseudoephedrine which, when chemically synthesized, are regulated as drugs by the U.S. Food and Drug Administration (FDA). It is available in the United States as ephedrine in over-the-counter asthma medications and as pseudoephedrine in nasal decongestants. In the past, it was commonly used in appetite suppressants and performance-enhancing drugs. Although pseudoephedrine is still an over-the-counter medication, it is now necessary in the United States to request this product directly from the pharmacist because of its illegal use in making methamphetamine. With chronic use, tolerance can develop; in 2004, the FDA prohibited the sale of dietary supplements containing ephedra (National Center for Complementary and Integrative Health, 2016).

Methamphetamine

Methamphetamine is a highly addictive stimulant that affects the central nervous system (CNS). Methamphetamine can be smoked, inhaled (snorted), injected, or orally ingested. Smoking or injecting methamphetamine is a rapid method for the drug to enter the bloodstream and brain, causing an immediate rush. The effects last a few minutes and have been described as being very pleasurable. This drug is often misused in a binge-and-crash pattern where the individual continues to take the drug for up to several days without the need to sleep or eat (NIDA, 2013).

Cocaine

Cocaine is found naturally in the leaves of *Erythroxylon coca,* a shrub native to western South America. It was used frequently in the Inca civilization, primarily in religious ceremonies but also by farmers to lessen fatigue. By the latter half of the 19th century, coca extract was used in multiple products, including soft drinks (such as Coca-Cola) and lozenges. With the development of hypodermic syringes, cocaine was also extracted for use as the first local anesthetic for eye, ear, and throat surgeries and briefly recommended as a treatment for such diverse illnesses as asthma and depression (NIDA, 2016a). A paste made from *E. coca* leaves is the basis for commonly used cocaine preparations. Cocaine hydrochloride in powdered form is readily water soluble and is used intranasally (referred to as snorting or sniffing) or intravenously (called mainlining). The powdered form can be inhaled (i.e., smoked) if it is extracted into a volatile organic solvent (such as ether) and heated, a process called freebasing. Freebasing became less common when it was discovered that a mixture of cocaine, baking soda (or ammonia), and water will harden, and the subsequent rock, known as crack, can be heated and the resulting vapors inhaled. As a street drug, cocaine appears as a fine, white, crystalline powder and is also known as coke, C, snow, powder, or blow (NIDA, 2016a). See Table 9-2 for other street names for powdered and crack cocaine (NIDA, 2016a).

Cocaine's effects are influenced by its purity. Dealers often dilute cocaine to increase their profits. Purity is also affected by the substances drug dealers use to dilute the cocaine. These diluents range from inactive substances, such as sugar or talcum powder, to baking soda. Dealers may alter cocaine with other drugs, such as procaine or amphetamines. Some users combine cocaine with heroin, known as a speedball (NIDA, 2016a).

THE BIOCHEMISTRY OF COMMON STIMULANTS

There are only two distinct groups of stimulants available on the market for treatment of medical disorders such as ADHD:

TABLE 9-2: SELECTED STREET NAMES FOR COCAINE

- Blow
- Bump
- C
- Candy
- Charlie
- Coke
- Crack
- Flake
- Rock
- Snow
- Toot

Note. Adapted from National Institute on Drug Abuse. (2017a). *Commonly abused drugs charts: Cocaine.* Retrieved from https://www.drugabuse.gov/drugs-abuse/commonly-abused-drugs-charts#cocaine

methylphenidate and amphetamines. They are considered Schedule II drugs, meaning they are prescribed for medical reasons but have a high misuse potential (DOJ, n.d.). All stimulants work by inhibiting the reuptake of dopamine, norepinephrine, and serotonin, thereby increasing the level of these neurotransmitters. Methamphetamine and cocaine are also stimulants but are not commonly used to treat medical conditions due to their highly addictive CNS effects (NIDA, 2014).

Methylphenidate

Although methylphenidate is principally used to increase concentration and focus in people with ADHD, methylphenidate is also used to treat narcolepsy. Students in particular misuse this drug for its ability to increase concentration and alertness, leading to potential improvements in academic performance (NIDA, 2014).

Methylphenidate tablets can be crushed and used intranasally or mixed with water and injected intravenously. In addition to the well-known adverse effects of needle sharing, a dan-

ger of intravenous (IV) use is that the fillers in tablets can be insoluble. These insoluble fillers can block small blood vessels, causing potentially lethal damage to the lungs, heart, and brain. Formulations include immediate and sustained release; the latter form is commonly preferred by individuals who misuse methylphenidate because crushing the tablet immediately releases the entire dose (NIDA, 2014).

Amphetamines

Amphetamines are similar to methylphenidate and exert their effects by interfering with dopamine reuptake. In high doses, amphetamines also inhibit the monoamine transporter, further preventing dopamine and norepinephrine reuptake. In addition to the resulting dopamine excess, amphetamines release stores of norepinephrine, epinephrine, and serotonin from nerve endings, which is unlike the effect of methylphenidate (Heal et al., 2013).

Amphetamines have a slow onset of action and a long half-life; therefore, they produce a long duration of effects. The half-life of amphetamines is from 4 to 8 hours, contributing to prolonged stimulatory effects. Amphetamines can be used orally or intravenously (Heal et al., 2013).

Methamphetamine

The methamphetamine molecule is similar to that of amphetamines and acts on the neurotransmitter dopamine, which plays an important role in the regulation of reward. It has a long duration of action and essentially remains unchanged in the body, allowing it to remain in the brain longer and prolong its stimulant effects. Most methamphetamine is manufactured in superlabs, using pseudoephedrine and other chemicals that can be toxic to humans and the environment (NIDA, 2013).

Cocaine

Cocaine is a powerfully addictive stimulant. It is classified in the United States as a Schedule II drug, meaning that medical indications exist, but there is a very high potential of abuse (DOJ, n.d.). Cocaine can be administered through oral, intranasal, IV, or inhalation routes. The oral route, or chewing, has the slowest rate of absorption, with peak effects taking up to 60 minutes. Furthermore, the bioavailability (the amount of drug available for the body to use) using the oral route is only 20% to 30% because the liver metabolizes 70% to 80% of the cocaine dose. The slower rate of absorption and lower bioavailability are thought to be the reasons the oral route is associated with lower rates of addiction (NIDA, 2016a)

Cocaine is also poorly absorbed by the nasal mucosa. Because cocaine is a potent vasoconstrictor, the blood vessels rapidly become less able to absorb cocaine through the nasal mucosa; this is compounded by the relatively small area available. The bioavailability of intranasal cocaine is equal to the oral route at 20% to 30%. However, unlike with oral use, the effects of cocaine through the nasal mucosa are much quicker, with effects felt in 3 to 5 minutes and then disappearing in 60 minutes, when peak effects from the oral route occur (NIDA, 2016a; University of Arizona, n.d.).

In contrast, after IV injection, the entire dose of cocaine directly enters the bloodstream. With a bioavailability of 100%, effects are felt within 30 seconds and last for 10 to 20 minutes. But the intense high delivered by this route is accompanied by the risks of needle use. Cocaine through inhalation is almost as rapid as injecting cocaine into the venous system (NIDA, 2016a; University of Arizona, n.d.).

Compared with amphetamines, cocaine has a faster onset of action and a shorter half-life (about 30 minutes for cocaine versus 4 to 8 hours for amphetamines). Cocaine affects the body in three ways. It acts as a vasoconstrictor, it prevents reuptake of neurotransmitters in the brain, and it modifies gene expression (University of Arizona, n.d.).

Cocaine exerts direct effects on the blood vessels and gene expression and indirect effects through excessive neurotransmitter activity. Vasoconstriction means that upon cocaine exposure, blood-vessel diameter gets smaller. Neurotransmitters affected by cocaine include dopamine, norepinephrine, and serotonin. Dopamine is involved in the brain's reward system and is the key transmitter responsible for cocaine's effects. Norepinephrine is integral to the body's regulation of arousal, and serotonin has a central role in the regulation of hunger. To maintain the body's equilibrium, cells must be able to recycle (i.e., reuptake) excess neurotransmitters, a task accomplished by special transporting proteins. It is the buildup of excess neurotransmitters that results in the receptor cells' overactivity that is responsible for cocaine's effects. Although it does not change the basic function of genes, cocaine, like other psychoactive drugs, can change the level of a cell's activity, meaning that cocaine can change gene expression. Although a separate and specific gene has not been identified, researchers believe that about 42% to 79% of an individual's risk for cocaine addiction is attributed to his or her genetic makeup (NIDA, 2016a).

Areas of the brain with high concentrations of dopaminergic cells include the nucleus accumbens, hippocampus, amygdala, and frontal cortex – all parts of the limbic system. Together, these areas, when exposed to cocaine, are responsible for the intense feelings of pleasure, drug cravings, and compulsive drug-seeking behaviors. The greater number of areas in the brain where dopamine is active may be central to the strong feelings of euphoria compared with the effects of the other neurotransmitters (NIDA, 2016a). Table 9-3 summarizes the location and function of each neurotransmitter and the basic effects of cocaine on the neurotransmitter receptors.

THE EFFECTS OF STIMULANTS ON THE BODY

The effects of methylphenidate, amphetamines, methamphetamine, and cocaine on the body are caused by excessive amounts of dopamine, norepinephrine, and epinephrine that stimulate the CNS. The effects may be short or long term.

Short-Term Effects

Desirable short-term effects of methylphenidates, amphetamines, and methamphetamine include an increased concentration and alertness, increased confidence, and weight loss. These effects may also be accompanied by hurried speech; rapid, irregular heart rate; high blood pressure; hyperactivity; nystagmus; confusion; paranoid delusions; hallucinations; depression; and loss of rapid eye movement (REM) sleep. Additional effects indicative of intoxication include hypervigilance, anxiety, tension, impaired judgment, and stereotypical, repetitive behaviors that may include hand wringing or foot tapping. These effects manifest within minutes to 1 hour after taking the drug (NIDA, 2013).

The short-term effects of cocaine that users frequently seek include euphoria, heightened alertness and libido, and a decreased need for food and sleep. Undesirable effects that may occur include pain, headaches, anxiety, and increased blood pressure. See Table 9-4 for a more detailed list of cocaine's effects organized by body system (NIDA, 2016a).

Typically, after intense stimulant use (such as a binge), individuals crash and experience withdrawal that includes such symptoms as dysphoria, fatigue, unpleasant dreams, agitation, insomnia or hypersomnia, increased appetite, and consequent craving for more of the stimulant. Withdrawal symptoms may last a few hours to a few days. It is not unusual for these people to use other drugs, such as alcohol, opiates, or benzodiazepines, to decrease the nervous feelings from amphetamine use or to combat the withdrawal symptoms from cocaine or other stimulants (NIDA, 2013).

TABLE 9-3: BRAIN NEUROTRANSMITTERS: LOCATION, FUNCTION, AND COCAINE'S EFFECTS

Neurotransmitter	Location in Brain	Function	Cocaine's Effects on Neurotransmitter
Dopamine	Limbic system: • Hippocampus • Amygdala • Frontal cortex	Reward system	Euphoria Increased feelings of pleasure
Norepinephrine	Brain stem: • Locus coeruleus	Level of arousal and attentiveness	Increased wakefulness Increased alertness
Serotonin	Brain stem: • Raphe nuclei	Hunger control	Decreased food intake and weight loss

Note. Adapted from National Institute on Drug Abuse. (2016a). *Cocaine.* Retrieved from https://www.drugabuse.gov/publications/research-reports/cocaine

TABLE 9-4: COCAINE'S EFFECTS BY BODY SYSTEM	
Body System	**Effects**
General	• Decreased appetite and weight loss • Insomnia • Fever, chills, and sweating
Gastrointestinal	• Nausea and vomiting • Abdominal pain
Respiratory	• Nasal congestion • Hoarseness • Shortness of breath • Productive cough with black sputum
Nervous	• Euphoria • Increased alertness • Headache • Dizziness • Tremor • Dilated pupils • Anxiety
Cardiovascular	• Palpitations • Increased heart rate • Increased blood pressure
Musculoskeletal	• Weakness • Back pain • Muscle pain
Genitourinary	• Increased libido

Note. Adapted from National Institute on Drug Abuse. (2016a). *Cocaine.* Retrieved from https://www.drugabuse.gov/publications/research-reports/cocaine

Long-Term Effects

Long-term effects that represent chronic misuse of stimulants include tolerance, dependence, insomnia, heart failure, psychosis, and aggressive behavior. The likelihood of psychosis is greater for those misusing amphetamines than for misusing cocaine, perhaps due to the longer drug duration. Amphetamines stay in the body for 8 to 24 hours, whereas cocaine remains in the body for 30 minutes to 2 hours (NIDA, 2013).

Amphetamines

Symptoms of amphetamine psychosis include delusions, auditory and visual hallucinations, preoccupation with the individual's own thoughts, and violent, erratic behavior – symptoms not unlike those of schizophrenia. These neurotoxic symptoms can persist for months or years. Cardiotoxic effects include myocardial infarction and death. Another major cause of death is a substantially elevated body temperature, which may also lead to stroke, convulsions, and coma (NIDA, 2013).

Methamphetamine

Evidence suggests that chronic methamphetamine misuse clearly damages the neurocognitive ability of the user and that the severity of the damage is related to the duration and amount of use. What is most troubling is that these neurocognitive deficits persist well into abstinence (NIDA, 2013). Human data suggest that deficits in memory, learning, psychomotor speed, and information processing persist after 2 years of abstinence (NIDA, 2013).

Clinical indicators of methamphetamine misuse include anorexia; weight loss; itching and tickling under the skin; scratching and picking at the skin; severe dental problems ("meth mouth"); paranoia and hallucinations; jerky, rapid body movements; and sexual dysfunction. Renal failure, dehydration, seizures, hyperthermia, myocardial infarction, and stroke also occur with methamphetamine use (NIDA, 2013). Table 9-5 lists some of the effects of methamphetamine use (NIDA, 2013).

Use of methamphetamine places the patient at high risk for sexually transmitted infections and HIV. IV use of methamphetamine increases the risk of transmission of hepatitis B and C and HIV. High-risk sexual practices, men having sex with men, and

TABLE 9-5: EFFECTS OF METHAMPHETAMINE DEPENDENCE

Short-term effects:

- Increased attention and decreased fatigue
- Increased activity and wakefulness
- Decreased appetite
- Euphoria and rush
- Increased respiration
- Rapid or irregular heartbeat
- Hyperthermia

Long-term effects:

- Addiction
- Psychosis
  - Paranoia
  - Hallucinations
  - Repetitive motor activity
- Changes in brain structure and function
- Memory loss
- Aggressive or violent behavior
- Mood disturbances
- Severe dental problems
- Weight loss

Note. Adapted from National Institute on Drug Abuse. (2017c). *Methamphetamine.* Retrieved from https://www.drugabuse.gov/publications/drugfacts/methamphetamine

the exchange of sex for drugs increase the risk of transmission of HIV, hepatitis B, and other sexually transmitted infections (NIDA, 2013).

Cocaine

Long-term effects of cocaine exposure involve physical changes in the nerve cells in the nucleus accumbens. New offshoots from the cell's dendrites occur with cocaine exposure, postulated to permit the collection of more nerve signals from other parts of the brain, such as the hippocampus and amygdala. Tolerance, dependence, and withdrawal syndrome are likely outcomes of long-term use (NIDA, 2016a).

Tolerance occurs when increasing cocaine doses are needed to obtain the same level of euphoria. This occurs when the brain adapts to cocaine's effect. The user then increases the amount of cocaine by increasing the dose or frequency or changing the route of administration in attempts to recapture the euphoria experienced with the first use. Meanwhile, there is an increased likelihood for adverse effects, acute toxicity, and death (NIDA, 2016a). Escalating use of cocaine can cause a depressed mood as well as respiratory, neurological, gastrointestinal and cardiovascular problems.

Individuals who have been misusing cocaine and then abstain may experience the following symptoms:

- Insomnia or hypersomnia
- Unpleasant dreams
- Fatigue
- Increased appetite
- Psychomotor retardation or agitation

Withdrawal symptoms from chronic cocaine use are self-limited and usually resolve in 1 to 2 weeks. Symptoms of depression, anxiety, anhedonia, cocaine craving, and increased sleep are the most common (NIDA, 2016a).

Medical Complications

Most toxicity attributed to cocaine involves the central nervous and cardiovascular systems. Seizures are the most common significant complication of the CNS. Seizures occur as a direct result of cocaine reducing the seizure threshold. Cardiac complications include heart failure, irregular heart rhythm, and myocardial infarction. Chronic use of cocaine is also linked with a more rapid progression of high blood pressure (NIDA, 2016a). Cocaine toxicity can also cause hallucinations and delusions, contributing to psychosis that is commonly accompanied by paranoia. Paradoxically, the body may become more sensitive to the adverse effects of continued cocaine use despite tolerance to its euphoric effects. Death has been documented in the context of seemingly low cocaine doses (NIDA, 2016a). See Table 9-6 for a more detailed list of medical complications resulting from cocaine use.

Cocaine and Alcohol

Although individuals frequently use other drugs in addition to cocaine, simultaneous alcohol use is particularly common. Initially, alcohol may be used to address the anxiety and insomnia caused by cocaine use. Yet when individuals use alcohol and cocaine simultaneously, the body produces a third product, cocaethylene. Effects observed include those from cocaethylene and the independent effects from each drug – the largest impact may be on the cardiovascular system. For example, chest pain is the presenting complaint for 16% of emergency department cocaine-related visits. Individually, cocaine and alcohol are vasoconstrictors and impair cardiac function. However, use of both drugs simultaneously appears to have additive effects. Additionally, cocaethylene has a longer half-life – about 2 hours compared with about 30 minutes for cocaine. Consequently, the effects on the heart, such as cocaine-precipitated increases in blood pressure, are prolonged, with increased chances for lethal heart attacks and strokes. Further complicating this scenario is that alcohol magnifies cocaine's pleasurable effects, leading to an increase in cocaine use and thereby creating a vicious cycle in which abstaining from cocaine is more difficult (Pereira, Andrade, & Valentão, 2015).

TABLE 9-6: MEDICAL COMPLICATIONS FROM COCAINE USE	
Body System	**Medical Complications**
Brain	Disrupts normal brain communication
	Irritability
	Paranoia
	Violent behavior
Central nervous	Seizures
	Stroke
	Psychosis
	Coma
Cardiovascular	Myocardial infarction
	Heart failure
	Irregular heart rhythm
	Aortic dissection
	Accelerated hypertension
	Coronary atherosclerosis
Genitourinary	Kidney failure
Respiratory	Necrosis of the nasal septum

Note. Adapted from National Institute on Drug Abuse. (2016a). *Cocaine.* Retrieved from https://www.drugabuse.gov/publications/drugfacts/cocaine

DIAGNOSTIC CRITERIA

The *DSM-5* criteria for stimulant use disorder, which includes the use of methylphenidate, amphetamine, methamphetamine, or cocaine, involve a problematic pattern of use leading to clinically significant impairment or distress, as manifested by two or more of the following within a 12-month period (APA, 2013):

- The stimulant is often taken in larger amounts or over a longer period than was intended.

- There is persistent desire or unsuccessful efforts to cut down or control stimulant use.

- A great deal of time is spent in activities necessary to obtain stimulant, use stimulant, or recover from its effects.

- The patient has a craving, or a strong desire or urge, to use the stimulant.

- Recurrent stimulant use results in a failure to fulfill major role obligations at work, school, or home.

- Stimulant use continues despite having persistent or recurrent social or interpersonal problems caused or exacerbated by the effects of the stimulant.

- Important social, occupational, or recreational activities are given up or reduced because of stimulant use.

- Stimulant use is recurrent in situations in which it is physically hazardous.

- Stimulant use continues despite knowledge of having a persistent or recurrent physical or psychological problem that is likely to have been caused or exacerbated by the stimulant.

- Tolerance develops.

- Withdrawal occurs.

These criteria are not considered to be met for those patients taking a stimulant solely under appropriate medical supervision, such as for ADHD or narcolepsy.

Specifiers for the diagnosis of stimulant use disorder include the following (APA, 2013):

- In early remission – After full criteria for stimulant use disorder were previously met, none of the criteria for stimulant use disorder has been met (with the exception of craving) for at least 3 months but less than 12 months.

- In sustained remission – After full criteria for stimulant use disorder were previously met, none of the criteria for stimulant use disorder has been met (with the exception of craving) during a period of 12 months or longer.

- In a controlled environment – The individual is in an environment where access to the stimulant is restricted.

As noted earlier, the severity of stimulant use disorder at the time of diagnosis can be specified as a subtype based on the number of symptoms present (APA, 2013):

- Mild – two to three symptoms
- Moderate – four to five symptoms
- Severe – six or more symptoms

TREATMENT

The number of individuals receiving treatment for amphetamines decreased from 8.1% in 2005 to 5.6% in 2011. In 2013, cocaine accounted for almost 6% of all admissions to substance use treatment facilities. The vast majority of admissions were due to the use of smoked cocaine. The majority of individuals who received treatment for cocaine use smoked crack and were more likely to be polydrug users (NIDA, 2016a).

Stimulant treatment begins with a comprehensive health history and physical assessment that includes drug testing to support the diagnosis for stimulant use disorder. All patients should also be explicitly asked about their use of other drugs and medications (NIDA, 2013). If possible, historical data should include information from the patient's family or significant others because the patient may not be the most reliable source.

Laboratory Assessments

Screening for amphetamines is usually done with urine testing. Amphetamines are typically detected in the urine from 1 to 2 days after last use. Because many of these substances are legal, test results show a greater rate of false positives. This poses a challenge in distinguishing between legal and illegal amphetamine use (NIDA, 2013).

When cocaine use is suspected, the physical examination should target the cardiovascular and neurological systems because they are the systems most frequently affected by the use of this drug. A chest X-ray and an electrocardiogram should be included.

Laboratory evaluation in the form of testing for the presence of cocaine is vital. In addition to cocaine itself, cocaine metabolites may also be screened by testing for benzoylecgonine (the primary metabolite) and ecgonine methyl ester. Although urine testing is probably the most common approach, the type of testing administered (such as blood testing) is dependent on the rationale for use. For example, if it is most important to determine if cocaine is in the system at the time of the examination, blood testing would be the best choice. If determining history of use beyond 1 week ago, hair analysis is useful. Specifically, each half inch of hair represents about 1 month of substance use history (SAMHSA, 2006). Saliva testing is increasingly used because of the ease of supervision when compared with urine testing and the difficulty of blood testing. Cocaine levels in saliva have been observed to be similar to cocaine levels observed in plasma.

If urine testing for cocaine is used, the collection should be witnessed to avoid the patient altering the sample (such as diluting with water) to mask the presence of cocaine. With shorter-term cocaine use, urine tests may be positive for cocaine metabolites from 2 to 3 days after use. With longer-term cocaine use, positive tests may be noted up to 2 weeks after use (NIDA, 2012b).

Essentials of Treatment

Treatment can be viewed on a continuum that guides and tracks a patient over time through a comprehensive array of health services that is individualized to address the patient's need. Acute stabilization and withdrawal management includes intervention aimed at managing the physical and emotional symptoms that occur after a patient stops using a substance. Addressing the patient's life-threatening and severe conditions resulting from stimulant toxicity is usually conducted in an inpatient setting. After the patient is stabilized, withdrawal symptoms should be addressed. If there is not a life-threatening condition, withdrawal management may be the first phase of treatment. Although intensely uncomfortable, stimulant withdrawal is not life threatening. Even so, unless these symptoms are addressed and treated appropriately, the likelihood of relapse to stimulant use is extremely high and can often lead to future overdose (U.S. Department of Health and Human Services [HHS], 2016).

Transitioning and engaging the patient from inpatient to outpatient services is critical for future success. Craving should be addressed at this time, and continuing care (also known as aftercare) in the community setting must be in place upon discharge from the formal treatment setting to reduce the likelihood of relapse (HHS, 2016). Patients with stimulant use disorder can be treated in a full range of settings, including inpatient, outpatient, residential, and community-based care. The correct level of placement considers data obtained from the comprehensive assessment.

The American Society of Addiction Medicine (ASAM, 2013) developed adult and adolescent criteria that can be used as a guide for appropriate treatment placement. Six dimensions are considered to determine the recommendation for placement in one of five levels of care depending on the acuity of the patient's problems: (1) acute intoxication and/or withdrawal potential; (2) biomedical conditions and complications; (3) emotional, behavioral, or cognitive conditions and complications; (4) readiness to change; (5) relapse, continued use, or continued problem potential; and (6) recovery environment. The five levels of care are early intervention, outpatient treatment, intensive outpatient or partial hospitalization, residential or inpatient, and medically managed intensive inpatient treatment.

Basic principles of treatment for substance use problems include the following:

- It will likely take more than one treatment episode.

- The longer the patient can remain in active treatment followed by aftercare, the more likely he or she will achieve successful abstinence.

- Aftercare and active treatment should include a 12-step program.

- A slip in drug use does not mean the same as a relapse.

- Treatment at appropriate levels is ongoing and likely lifelong.

(ASAM, 2013)

Generally, treatment is directed toward management of withdrawal symptoms, reversal of post-abstinence craving, and/or prevention of or decreasing the likelihood of relapse.

Pharmacotherapy

The goal of pharmacotherapy is a reversal of the brain changes caused by chronic stimulant use. One of the challenges of treating patients using methamphetamine and cocaine is that the altered neurocognitive abilities associated with stimulant use (deficits in memory, learning, psychomotor speed, and information processing) affect the patient's ability to adhere to and benefit from behavioral treatments. Currently, there are no FDA-approved medications for the treatment of amphetamine, methamphetamine, or cocaine use (HHS, 2016; NIDA, 2013).

Instead, the pharmacologic approach is targeted to withdrawal symptoms. Many patients find the symptoms of withdrawal so intensely dysphoric that they are driven to continue using cocaine to fend off the symptoms. Therefore, any medical treatment that helps relieve withdrawal symptoms improves the prospects of recovery. If medications are used, they should not include phenothiazines, especially chlorpromazine or haloperidol, because these drugs may lower the seizure threshold. Antidepressant medications are also helpful in combating the depressive symptoms that occur in patients using methamphetamine and cocaine (HHS, 2016; NIDA, 2013).

Treating stimulant misuse remains an active area of pharmaceutical research (HHS, 2016). The majority of the medications currently under clinical investigation already have an FDA-approved indication for another condition or focus on antibody-based treatments. Due to substantial numbers of cocaine users who are also opioid dependent, treatment with methadone or buprenorphine has also been investigated. The approved indications tend to reflect such adverse consequences as seizures and cardiovascular complications that occur with cocaine toxicity (HHS, 2016).

Disulfiram (Antabuse) has been well researched and is approved for alcohol use disorder. This drug was initially intended for patients with coexisting cocaine and alcohol dependence. Scientists do not know exactly how disulfiram reduces cocaine use. Disulfiram may work by inhibiting an enzyme that converts dopamine to norepinephrine. However, disulfiram is not effective for everyone. Pharmacogenetic studies show variants in the gene encoding the enzyme that influences disulfiram's effectiveness in reducing cocaine use (NIDA, 2016a).

Another option is antibody-based immunotherapy, in which antibodies are developed to bind with the cocaine to block or degrade the substance so that it is less psychoactive. Cocaine is a simple molecule but can be attached to a complex molecule, which triggers the immune system. This treatment method is used to develop antibodies to cocaine. When the individual uses cocaine, the antibodies bind to the cocaine in the bloodstream, and the drug never reaches the brain or crosses the blood-brain barrier. This is a promising new immunotherapy but has not received FDA approval at this time (Maoz et al., 2013).

Behavioral Therapies

Behavioral therapies such as contingency management, cognitive-behavioral therapy, 12-step support programs, motivational interviewing or enhancement, and combination interventions remain the most effective treatments for stimulant use disorder. All treatments may be provided on an individual or group basis and singly or in combination with one another. Some approaches, such as motivational interviewing and contingency management, are more suited to the individual because these approaches require some degree of tailoring to the individual patient (NIDA, 2016c).

The cornerstone of cocaine addiction treatment is behavioral therapy, and studies suggest that methamphetamine and cocaine users have similar outcomes when exposed to the same treatments (University of California at Los Angeles [UCLA], 2013). Overall, the strongest evidence-based support for stimulant use disorder treatment has been noted for contingency management and cognitive-behavioral therapy (CBT; HHS, 2016). Unless there is a complication such as cardiac arrest, most treatment is delivered in the outpatient setting. Currently, there are two treatment approaches that have evidence to support their efficacy in the treatment of methamphetamine use: contingency management and a combination therapy known as the Matrix Model (UCLA, 2013).

Contingency Management

Research has demonstrated that contingency management is an effective treatment for stimulant use disorder, including methamphetamine and cocaine use. Contingency management is an approach that emphasizes rewards for positive behavior versus punishment for negative behavior. It is based on principles that involve giving patients tangible rewards to reinforce positive behaviors such as abstinence (HHS, 2016).

Cognitive-Behavioral Therapy

CBT is based on social learning theory and emphasizes modification of the patient's thoughts and behaviors. It identifies thoughts that trigger thoughts of using drugs and behaviors that can be used in lieu of drug use whenever these thoughts arise. CBT was initially developed as a method to prevent relapse for alcohol use disorder but was later adapted for substance use. Specific techniques include anticipating problems and enhancing coping strategies, for example, learning how to recognize cravings early and identify situations that might put one at risk for use (HHS, 2016).

Cocaine Anonymous

Cocaine Anonymous, first adapted from but not affiliated with Alcoholics Anonymous, initially began in Los Angeles in 1982 and is now available in the United States, Canada, and Europe (Cocaine Anonymous, 2015). As a 12-step mutual-help group, it does not rely on professional personnel to guide recovery.

Twelve-step groups usually follow the same format and guidelines of working through the steps, commonly encouraging service to others as part of recovery. The goal is to cease using cocaine and other mind-altering substances (Cocaine Anonymous, 2015). Groups involve individuals with similar problems who meet regularly to share their experiences and offer support and encouragement to other group members. Family and friends desiring similar support can contact a Co-Anon Family Group.

Motivational Interventions

Motivational interventions use a nonconfrontational approach and identify contradictions between what an individual is saying and what is happening in his or her life. They use the concept of "rolling with the resistance" and have been helpful in getting individuals to consider initiating change. The results of motivational interventions have been mixed for individuals using substances other than alcohol (NIDA, 2012a). These interventions have not been a commonly researched approach for cocaine use disorder.

Combination Therapy

One combination model that has shown effectiveness is the Matrix Model, a 16-week comprehensive behavioral treatment approach. The Matrix Model was developed in the 1980s in response to the lack of effective treatment for patients with stimulant use disorder (Obert et al., 2000). The Matrix Model is designed to be delivered in the outpatient setting and includes groups for relapse prevention, education, and social support, in addition to individual counseling, family education, drug testing, and encouragement for non-drug-related activities. The clinician is supportive of the patient and uses a direct (rather than a confrontational) approach.

The Matrix Model has been effective in reducing cocaine use (NIDA, 2012a). Patients with methamphetamine use disorders who participated in Matrix Model treatment programs were found to remain in treatment longer, gave more methamphetamine-negative urine samples, and completed treatment at higher rates than those patients who received other treatment (UCLA, 2013). An interesting finding in this study was that patients who were ordered to treatment via the court system demonstrated superior results, suggesting that drug-ordered court treatment programs were beneficial (UCLA, 2013). Additional information about the Matrix Model may be found at http://www.hazelden.org or http://www.samhsa.gov.

CASE STUDY 9-1

A 26-year-old white male patient comes to the emergency department with a 4- to 5-hour onset of nontraumatic chest pain. The patient's chest pain radiates to his left arm, and the patient also reports tingling sensations in his left arm. The patient is having difficulty breathing as well.

The patient appears in moderate discomfort, describing a substernal chest pain he rates as "10 out of 10." He states that while he was spending time with some friends, he suddenly noticed the pain. He explains that he became anxious that the pain may be related to his heart. Because he describes himself as a "type A personality," he wanted to make sure that he took care of the pain right away.

The patient also describes the development, over the last couple of days, of a constant pressure, which increased with exertion and was associated with radiation to his left arm, dyspnea, mild lightheadedness, nausea, and diaphoresis. The patient states he does not have a previously diagnosed history of any cardiovascular condition. He does not give a previous history of chest pain (including chest pain from heart disease, heartburn, or anxiety). However, he does report that on previous visits to his doctor, he has been told he needs to "do more or he will get heart problems." He does not specify what he interprets the doctor meant by this.

The nurse practitioner in the emergency department begins her initial assessment of the patient and documents the following information in the patient's health record:

Surgical history: No history of any surgeries.

Psychological history: Positive history of depression and anxiety. The patient has been prescribed medications for this; however, he is not taking these medications as prescribed.

Allergies: No known drug or food allergies.

Medications: None that he is taking.

Social history: The patient is single and working full time as a broker; he states that his job is stressful. He reports an approximately 10-pack per year smoking history. He drinks alcohol socially on weekends with his friends. He also said he used drugs in the past but swears he has not used drugs recently.

General presentation: Adult man who appears anxious, slightly agitated, and in moderate distress secondary to pain.

Vitals: blood pressure (BP) = 170/98 mmHg; heart rate (HR) = 112 beats per minute (BPM); temperature = 36.1°C; respiratory rate (RR) = 24 breaths per minute; O$_2$ saturation of 90% on room air.

Height: 164 cm

Weight: 64 kg

Skin: Several small, 5- to 8-mm areas of excoriation on left forearm.

Head, eyes, ears, nose, and throat: Anicteric, dilated pupils bilaterally; dry mucous membranes and jugular venous pressure of 6 cm.

Chest: Lungs clear bilaterally, without any rales or rhonchi.

Cardiovascular: Normal S$_1$, S$_2$; no murmurs, rubs, or gallops.

Abdomen: Active bowel sounds; no rebound or guarding.

Back: Examination normal.

Rectal: Heme-negative stools.

Extremities: No clubbing or cyanosis.

Questions

1. Which laboratory test does the emergency nurse practitioner consider ordering? What is another diagnostic test the nurse may order?

2. What is the priority medical diagnosis for this patient?

3. What is the next best course of action for this patient?

Answers

1. The nurse practitioner considers ordering a urine drug screening test, which should detect amphetamines in the urine from 1 to 2 days after last use. Based on the patient's cardiac symptoms, the nurse suspects that the patient may be using amphetamines. To rule out cardiotoxic effects, the nurse may also order an electrocardiogram for the patient.

2. The priority medical diagnosis for this patient is acute chest pain related to possible vasoconstriction of the coronary arteries. Once the patient's acute chest pain is stabilized, the relevant causes of the patient's chest pain, including possible amphetamine use, will require further assessment and management.

3. Referring the patient to outpatient treatment that incorporates components of the Matrix Model has better outcomes for treatment of stimulant use disorders.

CASE STUDY 9-2

After he was discharged from the military, Jason began working nights as an emergency medical technician. He needed to work this shift so that he could attend nursing school during the day. He has a family of three children under the ages of 3 and needs to support his family while going to school.

Jason has developed posttraumatic stress disorder and is scheduled to see a psychiatric provider for treatment, but he missed his initial appointment because he was so busy. His wife is concerned that he never sleeps or sleeps poorly, and even his friends have stated that he seems more irritable. The only time that Jason does not seem irritable is when he gets together with a group of friends that he sometimes hangs out with on weekends.

One evening on his way home from attending classes at the local university, he falls asleep and is involved in a car accident that requires being transported to the emergency department. He is fortunate that he does not sustain any injuries except some contusions and lacerations.

Jason's past medical history is significant for substance use as a teenager; otherwise, he has had no chronic illnesses. On examination in the emergency department, Jason appears anxious and nervous. His blood pressure is elevated at 180/98 mmHg, and his heart rate is 115 beats/min. He confesses to the nurse in the emergency room that he used crack, which he recently has begun doing on occasion, to make him feel better and help alleviate his stress from all of his responsibilities. He reports using crack because it gives him energy and takes away the stress but then confesses that he uses alcohol to bring him down so he can sleep.

Questions

1. What is the nurse's assessment of Jason's substance use at this point?

2. Which laboratory test does the nurse anticipate that Jason will need?

3. What information about using crack and alcohol in combination does the nurse review with Jason?

4. Which treatment and follow-up options are appropriate to begin discussing with Jason and his wife?

Answers

1. This patient has confessed to using cocaine in the form of crack in combination with alcohol. The nurse documents that Jason has a substance use disorder involving both cocaine and alcohol.

2. The type of testing administered depends on the rationale for its use. Although urine testing is most commonly used, this patient has been involved in a motor vehicle accident; therefore, blood testing may be the best route to obtain a screening of current use.

3. Cocaine and alcohol both impair cardiac function, and simultaneous use appears to have additive effects that may lead to elevated blood pressure, heart attack, and stroke. The pleasurable effects, leading to increased use of cocaine, are magnified by alcohol, making it more difficult to stop using the drug.

4. There are no approved pharmacological treatments for cocaine use disorder. Behavioral interventions have been shown to be effective. Contingency management, CBT, motivational interviewing, or the combined Matrix Model may be appropriate treatment options for Jason. Explaining the effects of drug use on the family system and involving family members in treatment can provide support and help in monitoring drug use and cravings. The dynamics of group therapy, self-help or counselor-led, are helpful in supporting the individual's strengths against further use of drugs. In addition, the nurse should refer Jason for intensive outpatient follow-up.

SUMMARY

Stimulant use disorder comprises a group of drugs that are similar from the standpoint of pharmacological structure but have unique implications on the body when misused. Cocaine is the third most commonly used illicit drug, but it is the most frequently mentioned substance documented in drug-related emergency department admissions. Use of methamphetamine is the fourth most common illicit drug use reported in emergency department visits.

Patients who use these stimulants experience euphoria and heightened alertness, which is frequently accompanied by irritability and anxiety. The intensity and duration of effects vary with the form and route of administration used. Both stimulants are highly potent and addictive.

Unfortunately, the development of tolerance requires the patient who is using stimulants to increase the dose used to experience the same effects. Adverse effects include seizures and chest pain. Currently, there are no FDA-approved drugs for cocaine use disorder, but new treatments, including immunotherapies, are in development. The foundation of effective treatment for stimulant use disorders is behavioral therapy. In the future, the best outcomes will probably be realized with a combination of pharmacological and behavioral interventions.

In 2014, an estimated 913,000 people aged 12 and older had a stimulant use disorder because of cocaine use (SAMHSA, 2017). Unlike cocaine, amphetamines have licensed medical indications, and with the exception of methylphenidate and similar drugs, several types have less potential for misuse. As stimulants, both amphetamines and cocaine interfere with dopamine reuptake and have similar health effects. However, a critical difference is that amphetamines have a much longer half-life; therefore, their effects are prolonged.

EXAM QUESTIONS

CHAPTER 9
Questions 46–53

Note: Choose the one option that BEST answers each question.

46. The age group with the highest rate of current cocaine use is

    a. 14- to 17-year-olds.
    b. 18- to 25-year-olds.
    c. 26- to 32-year-olds.
    d. 33- to 38-year-olds.

47. The neurotransmitters that are responsible for the effects of stimulants are dopamine, norepinephrine, and

    a. serotonin.
    b. acetylcholine.
    c. glutamate.
    d. gamma aminobutyric acid.

48. The bioavailability of cocaine is highest by the

    a. oral route of administration.
    b. intravenous route of administration.
    c. intranasal route of administration.
    d. inhalation route of administration.

49. A difference between the mechanisms of action of cocaine and those of amphetamines is that cocaine has a

    a. faster stimulatory effect.
    b. longer duration of effect.
    c. faster onset of action.
    d. longer half-life.

50. Desirable short-term effects of stimulants on the body include increased concentration and

    a. weight gain.
    b. alertness.
    c. low blood pressure.
    d. irregular heart rhythm.

51. Methamphetamine use clearly affects the user's

    a. liver function.
    b. respiratory function.
    c. immunologic function.
    d. neurocognitive function.

52. Which health effect is more associated with methamphetamine use than other stimulants?

    a. Seeing flashes of light
    b. Feeling crawling sensations under the skin
    c. Feeling one's heart beating hard
    d. Hearing voices that other people do not

53. The strongest evidence-based support for the treatment of stimulant use disorder has been noted for contingency management and

    a. cognitive-behavioral therapy.
    b. electroshock therapy.
    c. pharmaceutical therapy.
    d. acupuncture therapy.

REFERENCES

American Psychiatric Association. (2013). *Diagnostic and statistical manual of mental disorders* (5th ed.). Arlington, VA: Author.

American Society of Addiction Medicine. (2013). *The ASAM criteria: Treatment criteria for addictive, substance related and co-occurring conditions.* North Bethesda, MD: Author. Retrieved from http://www.asam.org/quality-practice/guidelines-and-consensus-documents/the-asam-criteria/text

Center for Behavioral Health Statistics and Quality. (2015). *Behavioral health trends in the United States: Results from the 2014 National Survey on Drug Use and Health* (HHS Publication No. [SMA] 15-4927, NSDUH Series H-50). Retrieved from http://www.samhsa.gov/data/

Cocaine Anonymous. (2015). *Cocaine Anonymous world services.* Retrieved from http://ca.org/

Hasin, D. S., O'Brien, C. P., Auriacombe, M., Borges, G., Bucholz, K., Budney, A., ... Grant, B. F. (2013). *DSM-5* criteria for substance use disorders: Recommendations and rationale. *American Journal of Psychiatry, 170*(8), 834-851. doi:10.1176/appi.ajp.2013.12060782

Haslam, D. (2016). Weight management in obesity – Past and present. *International Journal of Clinical Practice, 70*(3), 206-217. doi:10.1111/ijcp.12771

Heal, D. J., Smith, S. L., Gosden, J., & Nutt, D. J. (2013). Amphetamine, past and present – A pharmacological and clinical perspective. *Journal of Psychopharmacology, 27*(6), 479-496. doi:10.1177/0269881113482532

Maoz, A., Hicks, M., Vallabhjosula, S., Synana, M., Kothari, P., Dyke, J., ... Crystal, R. (2013). Adenovirus capsid-based anti-cocaine vaccine prevents cocaine from binding to the nonhuman primate CNS dopamine transporter. *Neuropsychopharmacology, 38,* 2170-2178. Retrieved from https://www.nature.com/npp/journal/v38/n11/pdf/npp2013114a.pdf

National Center for Complementary and Integrative Health. (2016). *Ephedra* (NCCIH Publication No. D336). Retrieved from https://nccih.nih.gov/health/ephedra

National Institute on Drug Abuse. (2012a). *Principles of drug addiction treatment: A research-based guide* (3rd ed.). Retrieved from https://www.drugabuse.gov/publications/principles-drug-addiction-treatment-research-based-guide-third-edition

National Institute on Drug Abuse. (2012b). *Resource guide: Screening for drug use in general medical settings.* Retrieved from https://www.drugabuse.gov/publications/resource-guide-screening-drug-use-in-general-medical-settings

National Institute on Drug Abuse. (2013). *Methamphetamine.* Retrieved from https://www.drugabuse.gov/publications/research-reports/methamphetamine

National Institute on Drug Abuse. (2014). *Stimulant ADHD medications: Methylphenidate and amphetamines.* Retrieved from https://www.drugabuse.gov/publications/drugfacts/stimulant-adhd-medications-methylphenidate-amphetamines

National Institute on Drug Abuse. (2016a). *Cocaine*. Retrieved from https://www.drug abuse.gov/publications/research-reports/ cocaine

National Institute on Drug Abuse. (2016b). *Synthetic cathinones ("bath salts")*. Retrieved from https://www.drugabuse.gov/publications/ drugfacts/synthetic-cathinones-bath-salts

National Institute on Drug Abuse. (2016c). *Treatment approaches for drug addiction*. Retrieved from https://www.drugabuse.gov/ publications/drugfacts/treatment-approaches-drug-addiction

National Institute on Drug Abuse. (2017a). *Commonly abused drugs charts: Cocaine*. Retrieved from https://www.drugabuse. gov/drugs-abuse/commonly-abused-drugs-charts#cocaine

National Institute on Drug Abuse (2017b). *Commonly abused drugs charts: Prescription stimulants*. Retrieved from https://www.drug abuse.gov/drugs-abuse/commonly-abused-drugs-charts#prescription-stimulants

National Institute on Drug Abuse. (2017c). *Methamphetamine*. Retrieved from https:// www.drugabuse.gov/publications/drugfacts/ methamphetamine

Obert, J. L., McCann, M. J., Marinelli-Casey, P., Weiner, A., Minsky, S., Brethen, P., & Rawson, R. (2000). The Matrix Model of outpatient stimulant abuse treatment: History and description. *Journal of Psychoactive Drugs, 32*(2), 157-164.

Pereira, R. B., Andrade, P. B., & Valentão, P. (2015). A comprehensive view of the neurotoxicity mechanisms of cocaine and ethanol. *Neurotoxicity Research, 28*(3), 253-267. doi:10.1007/s12640-015-9536-x

Prosser, J. M., & Nelson, L. S. (2012). The toxicology of bath salts: A review of synthetic cathinones. *Journal of Medical Toxicology, 8*(1), 33-42.

Substance Abuse and Mental Health Services Administration. (2006). *Substance abuse: Clinical issues in intensive outpatient treatment*. Rockville, MD: Author.

Substance Abuse and Mental Health Services Administration. (2017). *Behavioral health treatments and services*. Retrieved from http://www.samhsa.gov/treatment

University of Arizona. (n.d.). *Methoide: Methamphetamine and other illicit drug education*. Retrieved from http://methoide.fcm. arizona.edu/infocenter/index.cfm?stid=170

University of California at Los Angeles, Integrated Substance Abuse Programs. (2013). *Methamphetamine treatment*. Retrieved from http://www.methamphetamine.org/html/treat ment.html

U.S. Department of Health and Human Services, Office of the Surgeon General. (2016). *Facing addiction in America: The surgeon general's report on alcohol, drugs, and health*. Washington, DC: Author. Retrieved from https://www.surgeongeneral.gov/ library/reports/index.html

U.S. Department of Justice. (n.d.). *Title 21 Code of Federal Regulations: Part 1308 – Schedules of controlled substances*. Retrieved from http://www.deadiversion. usdoj.gov/21cfr/cfr/2108cfrt

U.S. Drug Enforcement Administration. (n.d.). *Drug fact sheets: Anorectic drugs*. Retrieved from https://www.dea.gov/dru ginfo/concerns.shtml#anorectic

CHAPTER 10

OPIOIDS

LEARNING OUTCOME

After completing this chapter, the learner will be able to describe the effects of opioid use disorder on the body and current treatment approaches for this disorder.

CHAPTER OBJECTIVES

After completing this chapter, the learner will be able to:

1. Describe the biochemistry of opioid use disorder (dependence).

2. Identify the major classifications and formulations of opioids.

3. Relate appropriate prescription opioid use to factors associated with the development of opioid use disorders.

4. Discuss the short- and long-term health effects and adverse effects of opioid use.

5. Discuss the assessment and treatment of patients with opioid use disorder.

INTRODUCTION

Opioids include drugs naturally derived from opium and morphine-like drugs synthesized in the laboratory. All drugs in this class either stimulate or inhibit the activity of specialized receptors in the brain. Morphine is the primary active ingredient in most of these drugs. Opioids are also referred to as narcotics and are defined as drugs with morphine-like properties. Opioids are used medically for anesthetic purposes, to relieve pain and diarrhea, and as cough suppressants. In accordance with the U.S. Controlled Substances Act, most opioids are classified as Schedule II drugs, meaning that they have medical indications but also a high potential for misuse (U.S. Drug Enforcement Administration [DEA], n.d.).

Opioids are highly addictive, and their use in the United States has risen sharply over the past 15 years (Rudd, Seth, David, & Scholl, 2016). The increased use of opioids has led to a near quadrupling of the death rate from opioid overdose over the same time period. Additionally, there have been alarming increases in visits to emergency departments for nonmedical use of prescription opioids and rates of neonatal abstinence syndrome (NAS) in babies born to addicted mothers. These trends have led the Centers for Disease Control and Prevention (CDC) to describe current opioid use as the worst drug epidemic in U.S. history (Kolodny et al., 2015).

HISTORY

Morphine occurs naturally in opium, which is found in the seed pod of Asian poppy plants native to the Mediterranean region. Documentation of the use of opium dates back 5,000 years, and it was described as the "plant of joy" in ancient writings (Savage, 2014). Opium is the source of the natural opioids: morphine, codeine, and thebaine. In addition to relieving pain, opioids have been used historically to treat headaches, cough, and melancholy since the era of Hippocrates. In the United States, problems resulting from compulsive opium use became increasingly apparent in the early 1900s and even more so after the invention of the hypodermic needle in 1953 and the ensuing use of intravenous (IV) drugs (Savage, 2014).

Morphine, first separated from opium in 1804, preceded heroin as one of the most commonly misused drugs. Heroin was first synthesized from morphine in 1874 and, by 1895, was being sold over the counter for the treatment of numerous maladies (Savage, 2014). But it was soon discovered that all heroin was converted into morphine in the body, and thus the use of heroin, along with that of other opioids, was restricted to medicinal purposes under the Harrison Narcotics Act of 1914. As a result of additional legal measures in the 1920s, patients who were heroin-dependent were no longer permitted to secure prescriptions for narcotics unless they were hospitalized. As a result, prescription opioid use fell to historic lows by the 1960s (Savage, 2014). This view of opioids changed in the 1990s, based on a perception that the benefit they offered in the treatment of pain outweighed the risk of possible addiction and based on the development of extended-release opioid preparations. Another factor influencing the rise of opioid use in the management of pain was the American Pain Society's campaign to assess pain as a "fifth vital sign" (Kolodny et al., 2015). A bias toward minimizing the risks associated with opioid use for pain management spread through the medical profession, resulting in a fourfold increase in prescription opioids from 1999 to 2010 (Savage, 2014).

Unfortunately, during roughly the same time period, from 2000 to 2010, drug-seeking behavior in emergency departments and overdose deaths related to opioid use also rose significantly (Savage, 2014). Regional differences in prescribing patterns were noted, with most prescriptions being written by a relatively small subset of providers (Paulozzi, Mack, & Hockenberry, 2014). Increasingly, opioid diversion was recognized, with around 70% of individuals misusing opioids obtaining them from family or friends (Savage, 2014).

EPIDEMIOLOGY

In the United States, opioid use and opioid-related deaths are rising at alarming rates. According to statistics from the CDC, 91 Americans die every day from an opioid-related overdose, and opioids (including heroin) account for 6 out of 10 overdose deaths (Rudd et al., 2016). In 2016, drug overdose deaths were the leading cause of accidental death in the United States. According to data compiled by the American Society of Addiction Medicine (ASAM, 2016), it is estimated that in the United States, 2 million persons aged 12 years and over have a substance use disorder associated with prescription painkillers, with nearly 600,000 using heroin. There has been a 200% increase in opioid overdoses since 2000, with heroin overdose deaths tripling over a recent 4-year period (Rudd et al., 2016).

The United States is the leading prescriber of opioids for pain management. Prescription opioid use is the main driver of opioid addiction, and the highest use rates are in the United States, with a prevalence rate more than twice that of Canada, the second-leading prescriber of these medications (Paulozzi et al., 2014). An estimated 259 million prescriptions for opioids were written in the United States in 2012, enough for one bottle of pills for every American (Paulozzi et al., 2014). Four out of five heroin users first started using prescription pain medications for either medical or non-medical reasons, with most making the switch to heroin due to lower cost and ease of access (ASAM, 2016).

Rates of prescription opioid use were 6.9% among adults in 2012 (Frenk, Porter, & Paulozzi, 2015) and 4.8% among adolescents in 2015, the latter representing a steady decline since 2011 (National Institute on Drug Abuse [NIDA], 2016b). Adolescents often misuse prescription opioids received from a family member or friend, and one study found that drug-naïve youth who were prescribed opioids before the 12th grade were 33% more likely to misuse opioids by the age of 23 years (Miech, Johnston, O'Malley, Keyes, & Heard, 2015). Heroin use among adolescents in 2015 was estimated to be around 0.3%, 21,000 of whom tried the drug and 5,000 of whom were current users (ASAM, 2016). For adults, heroin use has been increasing steadily, with the highest use rates in males, persons 18 to 25 years old, and those with low income; however, increases have been seen across nearly all demographics in recent years (Jones, Logan, Gladden, & Bohm, 2015).

BIOCHEMISTRY

Opioids are a class of substances, which can be natural, synthetic, and endogenous, that affect the brain and other body systems, including the hypothalamic-pituitary-adrenal axis and the immune, gastrointestinal (GI), and pulmonary systems. To understand a given opioid's mechanism of action, it is necessary to consider the type of receptor the opioid has an affinity for (mu, delta, or kappa) and whether it is an agonist, antagonist, or mixed agonist-antagonist.

Opioids are agonists to three main families of peptides that are found endogenously (naturally produced by the body): beta-endorphins, dynorphins, and enkephalins (Borg et al., 2014).

The mu-opioid receptors (MOPrs) are the most predominant receptor type affected by opioids seen in clinical settings and are responsible for most of their effects. Although all three of the peptide families play a role in the physiologic effects of opioids, the beta-endorphins and enkephalins have the greatest affinity for mu and delta receptors. Dynorphins are primarily selective for kappa receptors and less so for mu or delta receptors. Activation of the mu receptors affects mood, respiration, pain, blood pressure, GI motility, and the endocrine system. The delta and kappa receptors influence pain in the spinal area. Additionally, stimulation of the kappa receptors may be associated with dysphoria (i.e., anxiety, irritability, and depression; Stahl, 2013).

Physiologically, endogenous opioids are released in the brain and nerve endings to ease pain. When the body is exposed to external opioids, the endogenous opioid levels are decreased. With continued external exposure, fewer endogenous neurotransmitters are produced, and the body becomes dependent on that external opioid. This partly explains why users experience pain without a clearly discernable cause when opioids are withdrawn. Negative reinforcing effects are then observed when the user repeatedly self-administers drugs to alleviate the physical pain or dysphoria associated with withdrawal (Tetrault & O'Connor, 2014).

Agonist opioids attach to and activate their specific receptors (e.g., the mu receptor), whereas antagonist opioids attach to those same receptors but do not activate them but inhibit or block the physiologic response. Furthermore, agonist opioids can completely or partially activate receptors referred to as full or partial agonists. Partial agonists demonstrate ceiling effects, which means that as the dose of the partial agonist increases, effects at that receptor site also increase to a limit beyond which further drug increases do not yield increased effects. In contrast, full agonists continue to respond to an escalation in dose beyond the dose limits of partial agonists. Opioids of misuse are usually full agonists with preferential binding at the MOPr (Borg et al., 2014).

Opioids can cause both neurochemical and molecular changes in the brain with chronic use. Typically, short-acting opioids have a relatively short elimination half-life (how long it takes for the body to eliminate half of the drug from the bloodstream), ranging from 2 to 5 hours, with the duration of effects lasting 4 to 5 hours. Long-acting, sustained-release opioids and transdermal preparations are designed to provide more stable levels of medication, which can work to prevent breakthrough symptoms. However, due to the increased risk of misuse and mortality, long-acting preparations are currently recommended for use only in those who have severe, daily pain not responsive to other therapies (Dowell, Haegerich, & Chou, 2016). Additionally, sustained-release preparations are often tampered with to access the short-acting opioid. Work is being done to develop improved tamper-resistant formulations, but there is no current evidence that these technologies will have a significant impact on the morbidity and mortality that are associated with opioid misuse (Dowell et al., 2016).

Opioids can be administered via and absorbed from a variety of routes: oral, nasal, parenteral, rectal, inhalation (smoked), and transdermal. The bioavailability (i.e., amount of drug available for the body to use) of short-acting opioids can range from 30% to 92% and even up to 100% with IV administration because all of the opioid is immediately available to the body. Oral administration causes uneven absorption in the GI tract, making opioid levels more variable because the drug passes through the liver before it reaches the brain. Morphine and hydromorphone are effective analgesics because they are rapidly absorbed into

the central nervous system (CNS) and have high thresholds for adverse effects. Generally, opioids with greater pharmacodynamic efficiency, or the ability to rapidly stimulate desirable effects such as analgesia and euphoria, are the most likely to be misused (Borg et al., 2014).

OPIOID CLASSIFICATIONS AND FORMULATIONS

Natural Opioids

Opium

Opium is extracted from the poppy plant and is highly addictive. Its primary effects are euphoria and analgesia, but physical effects, particularly on the GI system (constipation) and CNS (respiratory depression), are also common. Opium is the key source for morphine, codeine, and heroin. The most common preparation is a dried powder, but it can also be found in liquid and solid forms. It is frequently misused along with other substances, such as marijuana and methamphetamine. Opium is a Schedule II drug, although some drugs derived from it, such as heroin, are Schedule I (DEA, 2015). See Table 10-1 for a description of narcotics scheduling.

Morphine

Morphine is the primary active alkaloid in opium and is the prototype of an MOPr agonist. It is the standard drug against which all opioids are measured. Dosages of opioids are based on a conversion ratio to morphine milligram equivalents (MME) per day (see Table 10-2). Morphine is available in tablets and oral solution, as well as in suppository and parenteral (IV) forms. Its bioavailability is about 35% to 75%. IV use is preferred by those misusing the drug due to the more rapid onset of action. The relative safety of morphine is based on a short half-life (2 to 3.5 hours) and a longer duration of the analgesic effect (4 to 6 hours), which

TABLE 10-1: DEA CONTROLLED SUBSTANCE CLASSIFICATION

DEA Schedule	Abuse Potential	Description
I	High	No medically accepted use in the United States; effects unpredictable. Use can lead to severe dependence or death. Heroin is Schedule I.
II	High	Accepted use with restrictions. Can lead to severe dependence. Hydromorphone, methadone, oxycodone, fentanyl, morphine, opium, codeine, and hydrocodone are Schedule II.
III	Moderate	Accepted uses. May lead to low to moderate dependence. Products containing not more than 90 milligrams of codeine per dosage and buprenorphine are Schedule III.
IV	Low	Accepted uses. May have limited ability to cause dependence. No commonly used opioids are Schedule IV.
V	Lowest	Accepted uses. Generally found in preparations (such as cough syrups or antidiarrheal medications) containing limited quantities of certain narcotics. May lead to limited dependence. Cough preparations containing not more than 200 milligrams of codeine per 100 milliliters or per 100 grams are Schedule V.

DEA = Drug Enforcement Agency.

Note. Adapted from U.S. Drug Enforcement Administration. (2017). *Controlled substance schedules.* Retrieved from https://www.deadiversion.usdoj.gov/schedules/#define

TABLE 10-2: CALCULATING MORPHINE EQUIVALENCY

Opioid (doses in mg/day except where noted)	Conversion Factor
Codeine	0.15
Fentanyl transdermal (in µg/hr)	2.4
Hydrocodone	1
Hydromorphone	4
Methadone	
1 to 20 mg/day	4
21 to 40 mg/day	8
41 to 60 mg/day	10
≥61 to 80 mg/day	12
Morphine	1
Oxycodone	1.5
Oxymorphone	3

These dose conversions are estimated and cannot account for all individual differences in genetics and pharmacokinetics.

Note. From Centers for Disease Control and Prevention. (n.d.). *Calculating total daily dose of opioids for safer dosage.* Retrieved from https://www.cdc.gov/drugoverdose/pdf/calculating_total_daily_dose-a.pdf

reduces the risk of accumulation of the drug in the circulation leading to untoward effects (Borg et al., 2014). For this reason, it is commonly the drug of choice for treating cancer pain. Morphine is a Schedule II narcotic.

Codeine

Codeine is widely used for moderate pain relief and cough suppression. It has a low affinity for opioid receptors and is less potent than morphine. However, it is highly lipophilic, leading to rapid transport to the brain, and it has a lower first-pass metabolism in the liver, making the oral formulations highly bioavailable. Up to 11% of codeine metabolizes into hydrocodone (Borg et al., 2014). Analgesic formulations with acetaminophen are Schedule III, and cough preparations are Schedule V.

Thebaine

Thebaine is a minor component of opium and is not used therapeutically by itself. It has a stimulant rather than depressive effect on the CNS. It is the natural compound that is used to make semisynthetic opioids, such as oxycodone, oxymorphone, nalbuphine, naloxone, naltrexone, and buprenorphine (DEA, 2015).

Semisynthetic Opioids

Heroin

Heroin is a powerful mu-opioid agonist classified as a Schedule I drug, meaning it has a high potential for abuse and no licensed medical indications for use in the United States. It is synthetically derived from morphine and has a short half-life and rapid onset, leading to a surge of euphoria, or "rush." It is the most rapid acting of all the opioids (DEA, 2015). Currently, most of the heroin illegally imported into the United States comes from Mexico and Colombia, South America, although other regions, including Southeast and Southwest Asia, also export the drug (DEA, 2015). Heroin on the streets is in either a powder (white or brown) or tar form ("black tar"). Black tar heroin originates from Mexico (DEA, 2015). Heroin is often mixed with other substances, from those that are relatively benign (e.g., sugar, starch, powdered milk, or baking soda) to those that are harmful (e.g., fentanyl or carfentanil), with potentially deadly results (U.S. Department of Justice [DOJ], 2016). Heroin is commonly injected; however, with purer forms, it can be used intranasally and inhaled or smoked (freebase form) delivering rapid-onset euphoric effects without the risks of infectious disease associated with IV use (Borg et al., 2014).

The sole difference between heroin and morphine is the addition of two acetyl groups to the morphine molecule (thus the chemical name for heroin, *diacetylmorphine*). This change makes heroin more lipid soluble than morphine, enabling faster crossing of the blood-brain barrier. This difference is also responsible for heroin being two to three times more potent than morphine. Once ingested, heroin is con-

verted in the brain to morphine, making heroin a prodrug, which means that heroin is inactive until metabolized (in this case, into morphine) in the body (Borg et al., 2014). In the brain, it is the morphine molecule that attaches to the opioid receptors to produce its effects. Heroin has a very short half-life of about 3 to 30 minutes (Borg et al., 2014).

Hydromorphone, Hydrocodone, and Oxycodone

Hydromorphone, hydrocodone, and oxycodone are mu-opioid agonists and are legally manufactured analgesic pharmaceuticals. Hydromorphone has the same half-life as morphine but is five (when given orally) to eight (when given IV) times more potent. Tablets can be dissolved and injected like heroin. Hydrocodone is typically prescribed in combination with acetaminophen for minor pain and is found in cough suppressants. Oxycodone has a relatively high bioavailability of about 60 to 87%. These opioids have a relatively quick onset of action and a short half-life of 3 to 4 hours. Sustained-release forms are particularly desirable for misuse because they contain large amounts of the drug, which can be converted to immediate release by crushing and then administering intravenously or intranasally, resulting in increased potency and onset of action and greater bioavailability (Borg et al., 2014). They are all (including hydrocodone cough preparations) Schedule II medications. Due to their high rates of diversion and misuse, some states have additional prescribing requirements specifically for hydromorphone and oxycodone.

Synthetic Opioids

Meperidine

Meperidine is a mu-opioid agonist primarily prescribed for short-term use to treat moderate to severe pain. Its bioavailability is variable when given intramuscularly, but it has a rapid onset (15 minutes) and peak (1 to 2 hours) when given orally. Because it is more lipid soluble than morphine, it has a more rapid onset of action. Severe adverse effects from meperidine use, such as convulsions and hallucinations, are principally due to its metabolite norpethidine. Because of toxicity concerns, it is not used for more than brief (48-hour) periods for the management of chronic pain (Borg et al., 2014). Unfortunately, meperidine's adverse effects cannot be reversed with the antagonist naloxone or naltrexone, unlike those for other opioids. Meperidine is a Schedule II medication.

Methadone

Methadone is a long-acting, highly potent mu agonist. As such, it has a greater risk of respiratory depression with use, particularly in patients who are opioid naïve. Originally developed as a synthetic alternative to morphine during World War II to cover a shortage of morphine, it has been used to treat heroin addiction and also for the management of chronic pain (DEA, 2015). It is highly bioavailable (approximately 90%), has a long half-life, and slows tolerance development. Peak levels are achieved in 2 to 4 hours and sustained over 24 hours (Borg et al., 2014). These properties make it an important medication for the treatment of opioid addiction, which is discussed later in the chapter. Methadone undergoes extensive metabolism by cytochrome P450 enzymes in the liver, and multiple, complex drug interactions, including with alcohol, have been noted. Methadone is a Schedule II medication.

Fentanyl

Fentanyl is a mu-opioid agonist used as an IV anesthetic. For chronic pain management, it is available as a patch, lozenge, and effervescent tablet for absorption through the buccal mucosa. Compared with heroin, it produces less euphoria but more analgesia because it is about 80 times more potent than morphine. Fentanyl has been responsible for an increasing number of deaths because users have started combining it with heroin to augment its potency. The transdermal form has a bioavailability of 92%, and the oral form has a bioavailability of 50%. Its half-life ranges from 3 to 12 hours (NIDA, 2016a).

Other Synthetic Opioids

Pentazocine is a mixed agonist-antagonist created to effectively treat mild to moderate pain but with a lower potential for misuse. Butorphanol is a mixed agonist-antagonist administered in the nose to treat migraine headaches and parenterally for anesthesia. Both drugs can produce an abstinence syndrome when given to an opiate-dependent patient and are categorized as Schedule IV drugs (Borg et al., 2014).

Table 10-3 lists opioid classifications; Table 10-4 details the elimination half-life, bioavailability, and duration of effects of opioids.

TABLE 10-3: CLASSIFICATION OF NARCOTICS (OPIOIDS)	
Classification	**Opioid**
Natural	Opium
	Morphine
	Codeine
	Thebaine
Semisynthetic	Heroin
	Hydromorphone
	Oxycodone
	Hydrocodone
Synthetic	Meperidine
	Methadone
	Fentanyl
	Pentazocine
	Butorphanol

Note. Adapted from Pathan, H., & Williams, J. (2012). Basic opioid pharmacology: An update. *British Journal of Pain, 6*(1), 11-16. Retrieved from http://doi.org/10.1177/2049463712438493

TABLE 10-4: OPIOID PHARMACOKINETICS

Drug Name		Half-Life (hr)	Bioavailability (%)	Duration of Effects (hr)
Morphine		2 to 3.5	35 to 75	4 to 6
Codeine		2 to 3	50	4 to 6
Heroin		0.5	35	4 to 5
Hydromorphone		2 to 3	30 to 40	3 to 5
Oxycodone		3 to 4	60 to 87	4 to 6 (12 for controlled release)
Hydrocodone		2 to 4	Varies	3 to 4
Meperidine		3	50	4 to 6
Fentanyl	Buccal	2	50	2 to 3
	Transdermal	12 to 18	92	72
Pentazocine		2 to 3	10	3 to 6
Methadone		24 to 36	90	24
Buprenorphine		24 to 42	29 (varies)	24 to 48

Note. Adapted from Borg, L., Buonora, M., Butelman, E. R., Ducat, E., Ray, B. M., & Kreek, M. J. (2014). The pharmacology of opioids. In R. K Reis (Ed.), *The ASAM principles of addiction medicine* (5th ed., pp. 135-150). Philadelphia, PA: Wolters Kluwer.

PRESCRIPTION OPIOIDS

Misuse of prescription opioids differs from that of heroin in that it typically begins secondary to ineffective management and inappropriate prescribing of opioids for acute and chronic pain (Dowell et al., 2016; Morone & Weiner, 2013). There has been increased emphasis on appropriate pain management, which is often attributed to changes in the assessment of pain proposed by The Joint Commission. Yet the increased use of opioids, the presumption that pain levels can reach zero, and the idea that pain should be considered a vital sign have been misattributed to Joint Commission standards (The Joint Commission, 2016). Although initially promoted, the routine use of opioids as first-line agents in the treatment of chronic pain is no longer considered best practice, except for those patients receiving cancer, palliative, and end-of-life care (Dowell et al., 2016).

In the chronic pain setting, the term misuse is commonly used instead of abuse. Misuse includes the clinician's behavior – for example, prescribing opiates for an inappropriate health problem, at an excessive dose, or for a longer duration than necessary. It has been found that opioid prescribing patterns vary widely and, in general, that a small number of providers prescribe large numbers of opiates (Paulozzi et al., 2014). These increased levels of prescribing have resulted in a higher prevalence of opioid use and addiction in the general population, affecting a wider demographic. It had been assumed that measures taken by states to restrict prescribing of opioids led to an increase in heroin use, but this is not the case; heroin-related deaths have continued to increase with prescription opioid use and co-occurring polysubstance use, which puts persons at increased risk for heroin-related death (Jones et al., 2015).

In response to the increased opioid misuse, the CDC developed guidelines for the use of prescription opioids for pain (Dowell et al., 2016). These guidelines reviewed the evidence for the use of opioids in pain and concluded the following:

- Evidence does not clearly support the use of long-term opioid therapy for chronic pain.

- Evidence does support small to moderate benefits of opioid therapy for short-term pain management, although evidence is inconsistent for improving function.

- Evidence is insufficient to support the use of opioids to produce long-term benefits in low-back pain, headache, and fibromyalgia.

Additionally, the guidelines noted specific factors for which the risk outweighs the benefit of the use of opioids in adults with chronic pain. These include the following:

- Illegal drug use

- Prescription drug use for nonmedical reasons

- A history of substance use disorder or overdose

- Mental health conditions (e.g., depression, anxiety)

- Sleep-disordered breathing

- Concurrent benzodiazepine use

To curb drug diversion, the guidelines (Dowell et al., 2016) recommend the use of drug-monitoring protocols, which have been codified into legislation in several states. Monitoring requirements should include periodic urine drug testing to ensure the presence of the prescribed opioid and the use of a prescription drug-monitoring system, such as the Kentucky All Schedule Prescription Electronic Reporting (KASPER) program, to determine whether opioid prescriptions are being obtained from multiple providers.

Further complicating the issue is the evidence that chronic opioid use leads to increased sensitivity to pain when the drug is withdrawn (Gallagher, Koob, & Popescu, 2014). Chabal and colleagues (quoted in Ling, Wesson, & Smith, 2005) suggest that prescription drug misuse is indicated in patients by the following:

- An overemphasis on opioid issues during pain clinic visits that persists beyond the third treatment session

- A pattern of early refills (three or more) or dose escalation in the absence of acute changes in medical condition

- Multiple phone calls or visits to request more opioids or refills or to discuss problems associated with opioid prescription

- A pattern of reporting lost, spilled, or stolen medication

- Evidence of supplemental sources of opioids, such as other providers, emergency departments, or illegal sources

At least three of these criteria should be met to qualify for misuse. However, having a history of substance use disorder alone should not preclude access to adequate pain management. Appropriate prescribing involves the use of short-acting opioids, if needed, in the lowest effective dose for the shortest interval needed, generally no more than 3 to 7 days (Dowell et al., 2016). Evidence demonstrates that 80% of persons using heroin had a history of misusing prescription opioids (NIDA, 2017b).

HEALTH EFFECTS OF OPIOIDS

Short-Term Effects

At first, the user experiences euphoria, which may be accompanied by dry mouth, a feeling of heaviness in the extremities, and nausea and vomiting. With the initial nausea and vomiting, some individuals may report dysphoria rather than euphoria. Histamine release can occur, which leads to dilation of the peripheral blood vessels, a warm flushing of the skin, and severe itching. Peristalsis is slowed in the GI tract, causing constipation. At the same time, the urinary bladder contracts, resulting in perceptions of urinary urgency.

After experiencing these initial effects, users are often drowsy for several hours, and mental function is clouded. Vomiting, observed initially, ceases to the extent that even emetic agents usually do not succeed in inducing it. Blood pressure and the heart and respiratory rates decrease, sometimes fatally.

Long-Term Effects

Tolerance

As the body adapts to opioids, the user must consume increasingly greater amounts to achieve the same level of euphoria or analgesia, a process known as tolerance. Tolerance is the outcome of the adjustments made at the opioid receptors to the almost continuous binding to external opioids rather than the body's internal opioid substances. To overcome tolerance, the user must increase the drug dose. Tolerance to additional opioids, such as morphine and heroin, also occurs, which is an effect known as cross-tolerance. Consequently, the user requires greater-than-normal doses of other opioids to achieve a substantial analgesic effect.

There is a form of tolerance that is unique to opioids resulting in not just a reduced drug effect, but also a reduced ability to attain pain relief (analgesic tolerance). This effect is called opioid-induced hyperalgesia (OIH) and can occur with both acute and chronic opioid use. The cause of OIH is thought to be related to complex interactions between opioid receptors and other systems that essentially counteract the effects of opioids, resulting in decreased analgesia. This is an important consideration when treating acute pain in patients with a current or past opioid disorder (Gallagher et al., 2014).

Dependence

Patients who are opioid dependent have escalated their dose of the drug in response to tolerance and are physically dependent on the drug. Among patients from various clinical settings, opioid withdrawal occurred in 60% of those who had used heroin at least once in the prior 12 months (American Psychiatric Association [APA], 2013). These patients can exhibit substantial psychosocial and physical problems.

Opioid Withdrawal

Symptoms of withdrawal result when the opioid is stopped or an antagonist is administered. In both circumstances, a typical abstinence syndrome begins. The degree of physical dependence and tolerance varies on a continuum rather than being absolutely present or absent. The severity of withdrawal depends on the specific opioid used, dose, and duration of use. The rate at which the external opioid is removed from its receptor site also affects the withdrawal severity. A more sudden removal results in a more intense abstinence syndrome.

Symptoms of withdrawal are secondary to rebound of the sympathetic nervous system, which results in hyperactivity. Because these symptoms represent sympathetic nervous system hyperactivity, they are too numerous to name in total. These symptoms tend to occur sequentially and typically begin with anxiety and drug craving, progressing to yawning, muscle aches, and runny nose, and then to vomiting and diarrhea. Treatment is generally supportive.

The most rapid removal of opioid from its receptor site is accomplished by opioid antagonists, which selectively compete for the site but have no agonist properties. Shorter-acting opioids exit the receptor site more promptly than do opioids with longer half-lives. Thus, heroin and morphine produce intense abstinence syndromes with relatively rapid onset and progression. With heroin, withdrawal symptoms usually peak between 36 and 72 hours after the last dose and can last about 7 to 14 days (Tetrault & O'Connor, 2014).

After resolution of the acute abstinence syndrome, a more subtle abstinence syndrome may be present for many months, causing the risk of relapse to heroin use to be high during this period. Symptoms include drug craving, anxiety, irritability, difficulty sleeping, increased sensitivity to pain, loss of pleasure (anhedonia), and a reduced ability to endure stress. Protracted abstinence syndromes consisting of prolonged periods of persistent physiologic symptoms, have been observed and cited as a trigger for relapse (Tetrault & O'Connor, 2014).

Intoxication, Overdose, and Medical Complications

Opioid intoxication is defined as "the presence of clinically significant maladaptive behavioral or psychological changes that develop during, or shortly after, opioid use" (APA, 2013, p. 546). It can occur with the first dose or after chronic use, and the symptoms are the same ones described previously as short-term effects but are more intense. Opioid intoxication begins with euphoria and progresses to irritability, anxiety, depression, restlessness or decreased activity, and impaired judgment and social or occupational functioning. These psychological symptoms are accompanied by pupillary constriction and decreased consciousness, which varies from lethargy to coma. These symptoms usually last for several hours, a time frame consistent with the half-life of most opioid drugs.

Opioids' strong depressant effect on the respiratory system is usually the cause of acute overdose and death. Rates of mortality as a result of heroin use have risen sharply in the past decade, primarily due to increased use of the synthetic opioid fentanyl in combination with heroin, with much of the increase in fentanyl use attributed to illicit manufacturing (Rudd et al., 2016). Other common causes of death include drug-related infections (such as from needle use or overall depressed immune function), suicide, homicide, and accidental death.

Endocrine (including thyroid, adrenal, and gonadotropin) activity is reduced through heroin's effects on the pituitary gland and tends to be evident after chronic heroin use. Examples of pituitary dysfunction include erectile dysfunction and irregular menstrual periods. Other complications may be noted as a result of chronic or short-term use. For example, medical complications include hepatitis and HIV infection, which may be direct complications of IV use, particularly with shared needles. Risky behaviors, such as unprotected sex with multiple partners, also contribute to HIV and other sexually transmitted infections. Over half of new hepatitis C infections that occur annually in the United States are among IV drug users, and up to 20 persons are estimated to contract the disease from each infected user (NIDA, 2017b). Furthermore, the likelihood of contracting an infection is augmented by the impaired immune function observed among chronic opioid users.

Selected medical complications of chronic heroin use are included in Table 10-5.

TREATMENT

Overall, the percentage of patients 12 and older hospitalized for opioid-related diagnoses increased significantly in the 10-year period from 2004 to 2014. In 2014, 30% of the total admissions for substance use disorder treatment were opioid related, for which heroin was the primary drug of misuse, constituting 73% of all opioid admissions. In 2004, 18% of total admissions for patients 12 and older

TABLE 10-5: COMPLICATIONS OF HEROIN USE

Short-Term Effects
- "Rush"
- Depressed respiration
- Clouded mental functioning
- Nausea and vomiting
- Suppression of pain
- Spontaneous abortion

Long-Term Effects
- Addiction
- Injection use leading to
  - scarred or collapsed veins,
  - bacterial infections of blood vessels and heart valves,
  - septic emboli, and
  - abscesses or soft tissue infections/ osteomyelitis.
- Infectious disease: HIV, hepatitis B or C, tuberculosis
- Liver disease
- Kidney disease
- Arthritis and other rheumatologic disease

Note. Adapted from National Institute on Drug Abuse. (2014). *What are the medical complications of chronic heroin use?* Retrieved from https://www.drugabuse.gov/publications/ research-reports/heroin/what-are-medical-complications- chronic-heroin-use

were opioid-related, with heroin accounting for 81% of these admissions (Substance Abuse and Mental Health Services Administration [SAMHSA], 2016c). Also notable is that the admission rate for patients 12 years and older increased from 3% to 8% for nonheroin opioids. Males make up the majority of patients hospitalized for opioid treatment, including nearly two-thirds of heroin admissions and 53% of admissions for nonheroin opioids. Non-Hispanic Whites accounted for 69% of heroin admissions and 84% of admissions for other opioids. Most heroin users admitted for treat-

ment reported injecting the drug (77%); fewer patients primarily using nonheroin opioids reported IV use (17%). The proportion of IV users among heroin users aged 20 to 34 years increased from 28% in 2004 to 46% in 2014. Nearly three-fourths of all those admitted for treatment of opioid misuse reported using multiple substances in 2014. Overall, the majority (69%) of those admitted for substance use treatment in 2014 were between the ages of 18 and 44 years. The proportion of admissions of those aged 12 to 17 years declined from 8% in 2004 to 5% in 2014 (SAMHSA, 2016c).

General Considerations

Treatment for opioid dependence can include drug or behavioral therapies or both. Drug therapy may include medications to treat withdrawal, an opioid agonist to substitute for heroin, an opioid antagonist for relapse prevention, or a combination of these. A comprehensive history, physical, and laboratory assessment should be completed before making treatment decisions. If possible, historical data should be corroborated with the user's family or significant others because the patient may not be the most reliable historian. All patients should be asked about their use of other drugs, using the evidence-based screening tools discussed in Chapter 3. Laboratory testing for the presence of hepatitis B and C and HIV with informed consent should also be considered (Saitz, 2014).

It is important to know which opioids you are screening for because all tests may not detect all opioid use. General screening tests for opiates can detect those drugs that are metabolized to morphine, such as heroin and codeine. The reliability of these screening tests is reduced in the detection of semisynthetic opioids (hydromorphone, hydrocodone, oxycodone) and generally will not detect synthetic drugs such as fentanyl and methadone.

More specialized immunoassay tests are needed specifically to detect the synthetics. Detection times can range from 1 to 3 days for most opioids and synthetics (Warner & Lorch, 2014).

Phases of treatment can be viewed on a continuum from acute to long-term treatment. The acute phase addresses life-threatening and severe conditions that can result from opioid toxicity, for which rapid reversal and supportive care are given in the hospital setting. After a patient is stabilized, the patient's withdrawal symptoms will need to be managed. If there is not a life-threatening condition present, withdrawal treatment can be the initial phase. Although intensely uncomfortable, opioid withdrawal is generally not life threatening if the patient is otherwise healthy. However, even if the patient is healthy, unless these symptoms are addressed and treated appropriately, the likelihood of relapse to opioid use is extremely high. This phase may occur in an outpatient setting, and it should ideally include medication and behavioral support. Despite recommendations supporting the use of medications to treat opioid misuse, those receiving medication-assisted therapy decreased from 31% in 2004 to 28% in 2014 (SAMHSA, 2016c).

Measures to ensure continuing care (also known as aftercare) in the community setting must be in place on discharge from the formal treatment setting to reduce the likelihood of relapse to opioid use. Treatment may need to be extended or potentially even lifelong because substance use disorders are chronic conditions, like diabetes and hypertension, and generally require ongoing treatment.

Although these phases are discussed separately, recovery does not occur in distinct phases. There is substantial overlap, for which drug combinations and behavioral therapy can accommodate individual patient needs.

Acute Opioid Intoxication and Overdose

Individuals who have overdosed on opioids usually have severe respiratory depression and may be comatose. The first priority in this situation is to reverse these effects and reestablish adequate respiration by immediately giving an opioid antagonist such as naloxone, preferably by IV. Naloxone is also available in an intranasal spray, which is increasingly available in nonclinical settings and among first responders (SAMHSA, 2016a). A rapid response should be observed within 1 to 2 minutes; if not, other causes should be considered. After a sufficient improvement is noted, monitoring must continue because the relatively short half-life of naloxone means that additional doses may be required, depending on the half-life of the opioid responsible for the overdose. If an inadequate response to naloxone is noted, the possibility of other substances contributing to the overdose should be considered because polysubstance use is relatively common in those misusing opioids (Tetrault & O'Connor, 2014). Naloxone is capable of precipitating severe withdrawal symptoms. When life-threatening events have been resolved, users have four basic treatment options: detoxification, drug substitution, behavioral therapy, or a combination of drug and behavioral therapies.

Opioid Detoxification

The goal of detoxification is to achieve safe withdrawal from opioids with minimal withdrawal symptoms. How a patient is withdrawn from the drug depends in part on the following:

- The degree of withdrawal symptoms tolerated

- The presence of any coexisting medical problems complicating the withdrawal process

- The available treatment settings in which withdrawal can occur (inpatient versus community setting)

Because withdrawal is not inherently dangerous among healthy users, they may opt to withdraw without the support of medications. Otherwise, withdrawal can be treated by substituting another opioid drug and then slowly tapering its dose. Alternatively, withdrawal can be treated with the use of nonopioid medications. Sedatives can help treat the restless sleep and insomnia that often persist for many days or weeks. Sedative use is not recommended as a first-line treatment because patients may develop a physical dependence on them.

The Clinical Opiate Withdrawal Scale (COWS) is used to determine the severity of symptoms and guide the use of pharmacologic interventions, such as methadone, naltrexone, buprenorphine, and clonidine (Tetrault & O'Connor, 2014). Physiologic symptoms such as pulse, sweating, observed restlessness, pupil size, rhinorrhea, GI symptoms, tremors, yawning, generalized irritability, and piloerection and subjective symptoms such as muscle or joint pain are each given a numerically scaled value, resulting in a score that categorizes the withdrawal symptoms as mild, moderate, moderately severe, or severe (Wesson & Ling, 2003; NIDA, n.d.).

Clonidine, a centrally acting alpha-2 agonist used to treat high blood pressure, is useful for the management of withdrawal symptoms without posing a risk for physical dependence. Clonidine acts by dampening parts of the sympathetic nervous system made hyperactive by opioid withdrawal. It suppresses many of the autonomic signs and symptoms of withdrawal, such as nausea, vomiting, perspiration, intestinal cramps, and diarrhea. However, clonidine does not significantly improve the muscle aches, back pain, insomnia, and craving for opioids. The use of clonidine is also limited by its potential to cause sedation and low blood pressure.

A standard approach to opioid detoxification is the use of longer-acting synthetic opioids such as methadone and buprenorphine or buprenorphine/naloxone combination therapy. These drugs are used as a substitution for shorter-acting opioids, thereby stabilizing the patient on a given dose. Doses are then generally titrated based on symptom response and continued for a period of weeks to months. When the patient has withdrawn, the dose is reduced by 20% daily for those in inpatient settings and by 5% daily for those in outpatient settings. Another approach is to switch from methadone to buprenorphine, which allows for less frequent dosing, an improved side effect profile, and ease of transition to outpatient treatment. Facilities are required to be specially licensed to prescribe these medications (Tetrault & O'Connor, 2014).

Alternatively, rapid and ultrarapid detoxification protocols have been developed for use in a monitored hospital setting; these use an antagonist, such as naloxone or naltrexone, to precipitate opioid withdrawal while the patient is heavily sedated. These approaches can produce complete withdrawal in as long as 8 days and as short as 48 to 72 hours. Because of concerns regarding the relative risk and high cost of using heavy sedation for ultrarapid detoxification compared with other methods, this approach is not currently recommended (Stine & Kosten, 2014).

Pharmacotherapy

Drug Substitution

The rationale for drug substitution is that prolonged exposure to opioids induces long-lasting adaptive changes for some individuals. Continued administration of an opioid is then necessary to maintain normal mood states and responses to stress. Goals of drug substitution include minimizing the abstinence syndrome, blocking the euphoric effects of the misused opioid, and relieving opioid craving. Methadone and buprenorphine are commonly used for drug substitution.

Methadone

Methadone has been used for the longest period of time, and it is the most commonly prescribed substitute medication in the treatment setting. Methadone is a synthetic mu-opioid agonist that blocks the euphoric effects of heroin when given at adequate doses while simultaneously eliminating withdrawal symptoms and alleviating the craving for heroin. It is absorbed well when given orally and is neither intoxicating nor sedating at appropriate doses, so its effects do not interfere with activities of daily living. The effects of methadone can last for 24 hours, permitting once-daily dosing that can suppress withdrawal symptoms from heroin for 24 to 36 hours. Methadone has been demonstrated to be safe even when used continuously for many years. Rare instances of QTc prolongation and male hypogonadism have been noted. It is generally recommended that a baseline electrocardiogram be obtained when treatment is initiated, with a follow-up in 30 days (Stine & Kosten, 2014).

Levo-alpha-acetylmethadol is chemically related to methadone but has an even longer duration of effect (48 hours). As such, it had been marketed to treat heroin addiction, but reports of prolonged QT intervals led to a black box warning, and it is not currently marketed in the United States, although the application for use remains active (Borg et al., 2014).

Buprenorphine

Buprenorphine is a mixed agonist-antagonist that has revolutionized opioid treatment. Approved in 2002, it was the first medication approved by the U.S. Food and Drug Administration (FDA) to be prescribed outside of substance use disorder treatment programs (after completing 8 hours of required training). Buprenorphine is a semisynthetic opioid derived from thebaine: a partial mu agonist and a kappa antagonist. Buprenorphine attaches to the same receptors as morphine, but because it is a partial agonist, it yields similar effects but at a reduced intensity. Because buprenorphine is also an antagonist at the kappa receptor, it may inhibit some of the dysphoric effects experienced as part of withdrawal.

Buprenorphine is administered in sublingual tablets that are available in two forms: those containing only buprenorphine and those that contain buprenorphine and naloxone (4:1 ratio) to minimize its potential for misuse. The inclusion of naloxone is intended to minimize the potential for diversion as well, and studies have found that when it is diverted, it is done so to relieve withdrawal symptoms, not primarily for misuse (Martin, Zweben, & Payte, 2014). An implantable form was recently approved for use by the FDA. Buprenorphine is particularly useful for detoxification and can be titrated rapidly over a few days. It can also be administered less frequently than methadone (three or four times per week), which has advantages for supervised treatment settings. It is less likely than methadone to cause QTc prolongation or interactions with other medications (Martin et al., 2014).

Naltrexone

Naltrexone is a long-acting opioid antagonist that can be used to prevent relapse to opioid use. Care should be taken not to confuse it with naloxone, the shorter-acting opioid antagonist. Physical dependence and withdrawal symptoms are not associated with naltrexone, although it can precipitate opioid withdrawal symptoms. Correspondingly, it is not a controlled substance and can be prescribed outside of the drug treatment setting without any additional requirements. Naltrexone has also been found to be effective in combination with clonidine to manage acute withdrawal (Stine & Kosten, 2014).

It is similar to methadone and buprenorphine in that it blocks the euphoric effects of heroin. However, because there are no opioid agonist effects, craving for opioids is not alleviated. Importantly, with naltrexone, any opioid use will precipitate withdrawal symptoms. Abstinence from opioid use reduces tolerance (and therefore physical dependence), but use during relapse at levels that were previously tolerated can lead to overdose – a fact patients should be warned about. Knowledge of this fact is key to the effective use of naltrexone for relapse prevention. Lack of knowledge of this fact is the reason that many individuals do not adhere to its regimen.

Initiation of naltrexone requires that patients have not used short-acting opioids in the previous 5 to 7 days and long-acting opioids in the previous 7 to 10 days to avoid withdrawal symptoms. Naltrexone can also be administered in a long-lasting depot formulation that blocks opioid-induced euphoria for 3 to 5 weeks, which has been found to be associated with higher rates of opioid abstinence at 1-year follow-up (Stine & Kosten, 2014).

Opioid Maintenance Treatment

Opioid maintenance treatment (OMT), also known as medication-assisted treatment, began with the use of methadone in the 1960s and now includes buprenorphine (Martin et al., 2014). Although OMT has been of great benefit in the long-term treatment of opioid use disorders, diversion remains a concern. Over time, participating in methadone maintenance has been shown to reduce mortality, illicit drug use, HIV, and criminal activity and to increase social engagement. The aim of treatment is to prevent and reduce cravings, withdrawal, and relapse and to restore normal physiologic function. Patients enrolled in OMT can progress to monthly visits and home-administered dosing through regulated treatment guidelines for both methadone medical maintenance and buprenorphine (Martin et al., 2014).

Behavioral Therapy

The most effective approach to treatment of opioid use disorders may be the use of both pharmacotherapies and behavioral therapy. The mainstay approaches to behavioral therapy include cognitive-behavioral therapy (CBT), motivational interviewing or enhancement, contingency management, and therapeutic community (TC). All may be provided on an individual or group basis or in combination. Some approaches, such as motivational interviewing and contingency management, are more suited to the individual because these approaches require some degree of tailoring to the individual patient. TC treatment is designed for implementation in a residential setting, relying on treatment through a group approach (Barthwell & Brown, 2014).

Contingency Management

Contingency management (CM) is an approach that emphasizes rewards for positive behavior versus punishment for negative behavior. This approach has four principles:

1. Rapid and accurate detection of drug use

2. Positive reinforcement of abstinence

3. Loss of positive reinforcement on detection of drug use

4. Development of positive reinforcers to compete with drug use

For example, a CM program would include drug testing (e.g., urine), with abstinence being based on these test results. Abstinence is then reinforced with vouchers that can be redeemed for various desirable services or cash. These vouchers increase in value with each consecutive drug-free specimen. Drug-positive tests result in no receipt of vouchers and a reset of the voucher to the initial baseline value (Barthwell & Brown, 2014).

Cognitive-Behavioral Therapy

CBT is based on the social learning theory and emphasizes modification of the patient's thoughts and behaviors. The goal is to encourage abstinence by helping patients learn and master effective coping skills that can help them to believe they can resist returning to substance use. The focus is on the exploration of the positive and negative consequences of substance use. This approach is the foundation for relapse prevention because patients are taught the skills needed to prevent a return to substance misuse after treatment.

Motivational Interventions

Motivational interventions (MIs) focus on meeting patients at their current state rather than presenting treatment options without considering the patient's present readiness to change. Strategies are based on the concept that motivation is the key to changing patients' behavior. This approach can be incorporated into the clinician's interviewing style (in which case it is referred to as motivational interviewing) and used for assessment as well as treatment. MI can be combined with other approaches, such as brief interventions and contingency management (U.S. Department of Health and Human Services, 2016).

Therapeutic Community

TC involves residing in a facility with 24-hour supervision. It uses a structured living environment as an integral part of the patient's treatment plan. These settings may be ideal for patients with a substance use disorder diagnosis that is accompanied by severe psychosocial impairment but who do not meet the clinical criteria for hospitalization. Adherence is reinforced with rewards for responsible social behavior and punishments for nonadherence. Traditionally, the length of stay in TCs ranged from 18 to 24 months, but with the advent of managed care, the typical length of stay is now 12 months or less. Varied individual and group therapy sessions using such approaches as CBT are also implemented within TCs (Barthwell & Brown, 2014).

12-Step Self-Help Groups

Self-help or 12-step groups are widely available and most notably include Narcotics Anonymous. They are unique in that they do not rely on professional personnel to guide recovery. Twelve-step groups usually follow the same format and guidelines of "working through the steps." As a rule, the group's philosophy is highly spiritual but is not associated with a specific denomination or religion. New group members are typically sponsored by another person who is further along in recovery and who acts as a guide to the novice. These support groups are free and typically anonymous and confidential. The goal is total abstinence – a drug-free existence in which use of any medications (including methadone) is not well supported for the long term. Members focus on staying drug-free "one day at a time" and are expected to demonstrate a wish to cease substance use (Nace, 2014).

Harm Reduction

The concept of harm reduction in the treatment of opioid use disorder is controversial and has developed within the context of trying to minimize the significant harms to both individuals and society caused by injection drug use (such as the spread of infectious disease) and the risk of accidental death. Needle exchange programs are increasingly available in which injection drug users can obtain clean syringes and education regarding their risk of contracting hepatitis and HIV. Naloxone, particularly now that is available in a nasal spray, is carried by emergency personnel and given to opioid users who are at risk or to family members to allow for quick reversal of a life-threatening overdose (U.S. Department of Health and Human Services, 2016).

SPECIAL POPULATIONS

Chronic Pain

Chronic nonmalignant pain is common and remains persistent in over 30% of patients on OMT (Martin et al., 2014). Both misuse of prescription opioids and illicit drug use are commonly detected among patients presenting for chronic pain management (Kolodny et al., 2015). Measures to address both primary and secondary prevention of opioid misuse have been developed.

The CDC (2017) has developed guidelines for the prescribing of opioids in chronic pain. These guidelines stress the avoidance of opioids as a first-line treatment for chronic pain and collaborative treatment planning, which includes setting realistic goals for the alleviation or amelioration of pain. An approach of "start low, go slow" is advocated, based on the morphine milligram equivalents (MMEs) needed per day. The concurrent use of benzodiazepines with opioids is strongly discouraged because both medications can cause respiratory depression, and unintentional overdose can lead to death.

As part of the routine history taking and physical (including a record request from previous providers) to evaluate chronic pain, all patients should be explicitly asked about a past or current history of illicit substance use or misuse of prescription opioids. Those patients with a recent history of illicit drug use or prescription opioid misuse should be enrolled in a substance use disorder treatment program or comprehensive pain program, respectively, based on the clinician's evaluation. An agreement or contract clearly detailing the expectations of the patient with set criteria

regarding use and follow-up should be developed and can include the following:

- An agreement not to obtain opioids from other sources

- An understanding that early refills will not be permitted

- A requirement for regular follow-up visits, including urine toxicology screening

- An understanding that the clinician can terminate opioid prescribing if the agreement is broken

Most patients with chronic pain can be stabilized on a daily dose of less than 50 MMEs, and the CDC (2017) recommends specialist consultation for patients needing 90 MMEs or greater. For doses of 50 MME or greater, consider providing naloxone for the treatment of overdose (Dowell et al., 2016). Although methadone is inexpensive and highly effective in the drug treatment setting, it is less desirable for patients with chronic pain. Methadone's long half-life lends itself to once-daily dosing for patients with heroin dependence; however, patients with chronic pain often require more frequent dosing. Concerns have been raised regarding the use of fentanyl patches due to inconsistencies in drug delivery and potency. Most recent recommendations advise limited use of fentanyl patches by prescribers who are very familiar with the medication and who can properly educate their patients regarding correct use (Dowell et al., 2016)

Women Who Are Pregnant

Maternal opioid use has risen dramatically in the past decade, with the greatest increases occurring in rural areas among women receiving Medicaid (Villapiano, Winkelman, Kozhimannil, Davis, & Patrick, 2016). During pregnancy, heroin crosses the placenta and enters into the fetal circulation. Although heroin withdrawal is not fatal to an otherwise healthy woman who is pregnant, withdrawing from heroin (which commonly occurs because heroin is short acting) can result in NAS, which can be fatal to the fetus. It is estimated that in the United States, one baby suffering from opiate withdrawal is born every 25 minutes (Patrick, Davis, Lehman, & Cooper, 2015).

Treating women pharmacologically during pregnancy is controversial but is still used, with the aim being to reduce not only the mother's risk but also the baby's risk of NAS. Methadone and buprenorphine have both been used for OMT in pregnancy and have been shown to reduce NAS, although there is more experience with using methadone (Martin et al., 2014). Women who are pregnant can also undergo detoxification from heroin; however, relapse rates to heroin use are high, and subsequent withdrawal will continue to be a concern until delivery.

NAS prolongs hospitalization for infants and puts them at risk for additional complications. Generally, babies born with NAS are of lower birth weight and are more likely to experience respiratory complications and feeding problems. They may become septic and develop seizures (Patrick et al., 2015). Providing treatment for the mother has been shown to significantly reduce the need for NAS treatment in infants (Martin et al., 2014).

Polysubstance Use

The presence of another substance use disorder and coexisting psychiatric disorder is extremely common for opioid users. Problems with alcohol and benzodiazepines often coexist because these drugs are commonly used to address the adverse effects of heroin. However, combining these substances can pose an increased risk of harm or death when used during opioid agonist treatment (Martin et al., 2014). Alternatively, other drugs may be used to potentiate opioid-induced euphoria. One frequent example is simultaneous cocaine use, called a speedball, which is used to produce a more intense euphoria but less intense adverse effects (Center for Substance Abuse Treatment, 2014).

Recently there has been increasing concern regarding the mixing of heroin and fentanyl or carfentanil, a fentanyl analog that has 10,000 times the potency of morphine, being linked regionally to significant increases in fatal overdoses (NIDA, 2017a). Little is known about how these drugs are currently being distributed. What is known is that the combination of these substances with heroin is deadly.

Psychiatric Comorbidity

Among other mental disorders, depression and personality disorder are frequently identified diagnoses in patients with opioid misuse (Martin et al., 2014). Major depression is the most common mood disorder and occurs more frequently in women than in men, as it does in the general population. Coexisting depression is more strongly associated with a history of concomitant polysubstance use. The dysphoria associated with withdrawal and the impact of stressful life situations increase the risk of relapse during treatment. The use of antidepressant medication has been studied in patients with comorbid opioid use and depression, but results have been inconsistent (Martin et al., 2014).

Of all the personality disorders, antisocial personality disorder is the most commonly diagnosed (mostly among men) in heroin users seeking treatment. Unlike depression, antisocial personality disorder can be diagnosed historically in most individuals because it typically manifests at a young age, before the onset of opioid dependence. However, a cautious approach to diagnosis is warranted because many of the defining characteristics of substance use disorders are very similar (Martin et al., 2014).

The relationship between opioid misuse and antisocial personality is complicated and appears to be influenced by a genetic factor. When antisocial personality and opioid use disorder coexist, the treatment of either problem is challenging. Although this group can have difficulty establishing rapport with a therapist, intensive and tailored approaches to psychotherapy have been found to be effective (Martin et al., 2014).

Anxiety and sleep disorders are also relatively common in patients using opioids. Posttraumatic stress disorder is associated with increased substance use disorder severity, but not with poorer outcomes from treatment. Other disorders, such as schizophrenia or other psychotic disorders, are rarely seen among patients in drug treatment for opioid use (Martin et al., 2014).

CASE STUDY 10-1

John is a 28-year-old male patient who is currently homeless and injecting heroin daily. He comes to the walk-in clinic with symptoms of fever, chills, malaise, and body aches. He last injected heroin this morning, and he shares and reuses needles.

The clinician learns that John started using prescription hydrocodone after having his wisdom teeth extracted at the age of 19 years. His friends at that time were experimenting with drugs and told him about the "rush" he could experience if he crushed and snorted the pills. He tried this and enjoyed the sensation. He started doing this on weekends with friends but quickly progressed to more regular use. He ran out of his prescription but found some oxycodone pills in the family medicine chest. Although outdated, they were still able to provide a good effect. He kept his activities secret from his parents and siblings. He felt guilty about this, as they had always been close.

When those pills ran out, his friend introduced him to a guy he knew who "oxy's." He bought a few pills, but because they were pretty expensive, he quickly ran out of money. The dealer suggested he try injecting heroin to get an even bigger "rush" for less money. John liked this effect very much but soon found he had trouble getting through the day without the drug.

Having spent all of his own money, he started "borrowing" from his siblings first, then his parents. They quickly became suspicious of his addiction, confronted him, and talked to him about getting treatment.

Understanding that treatment would be expensive and feeling like he should be able to kick his use on his own, John tried but found that the withdrawal symptoms he experienced were intolerable. Feeling guilty about his "failure," he left home and headed out of town. He thought this would help him by getting away from his dealer, but found that he remained "obsessed" with getting heroin. He also "almost died" when he again injected after trying to tough through several days of abstinence.

At the clinic, he reports that he initially thought he was just withdrawing but felt much worse than usual, and his symptoms were not relieved at all after injecting heroin a few hours ago.

On examination, he is febrile, with a temperature of 102.5°F, his heart rate is 120 beats/min, and his blood pressure is 80/60 mmHg. His lung sounds are coarse, and his heart sounds demonstrate a loud murmur over the mitral area. He denies any prior history of heart or lung problems. He appears anxious and is having some trouble breathing.

Questions

1. What are the clinician's initial concerns regarding John?

2. What information does the clinician consider when developing a treatment plan for John?

3. What is a good approach to encourage John to follow up for substance use treatment?

4. Which type of substance use treatment should be considered for John once he recovers physically?

Answers

1. John is clearly very ill and needs emergent care. The most likely cause of his illness is a serious infection (sepsis or endocarditis) related to his injection drug use. He will need to be admitted to the hospital for care and should be screened for other infectious diseases such as HIV and hepatitis. He should be told that his current symptoms could be life threatening if not treated.

2. John is likely concerned about his risk of experiencing severe withdrawal symptoms in addition to the symptoms he is already experiencing. He will need to be reassured that his withdrawal can be assessed and treated simultaneously with the management of his infection while hospitalized. The clinician also conducts a thorough assessment of his substance use because polysubstance use is common and may confound or complicate his treatment.

3. This encounter can provide a window of opportunity to promote John's engagement in longer-term substance use treatment. Using principles of motivational counseling, the clinician works with John to facilitate change talk related to the treatment of his addiction. He clearly feels this is something he needed to do on his own based on his patient history. Expressing empathy and including a plan for continuation of care after the resolution of his acute illness should be a priority because relapse posthospitalization is common.

4. John has limited social support at this time and may have financial constraints that affect his access to long-term treatment. Ideally, John would be placed in a residential treatment facility that includes medication treatment and participation in a therapeutic community, which would likely produce the best outcomes for John in this situation. At a minimum, harm reduction education regarding the use of clean needles through needle exchange programs and the use of naloxone for emergent treatment of an overdose is reviewed.

SUMMARY

According to statistics from the CDC, 91 Americans die every day from an opioid-related overdose, and opioids (including heroin) account for 6 out of 10 overdose deaths (Rudd et al., 2016). In 2016, drug overdose deaths were the leading cause of accidental death in the United States. These numbers have risen dramatically and are described as the worst drug epidemic in U.S. history.

Opioids may be naturally derived or semi-synthetic. Their actions demonstrate agonist or antagonist activity depending on their binding to specific opioid receptors.

Opioid effects of euphoria and analgesia may diminish when tolerance occurs, resulting in physical dependence. Abrupt cessation of the opioid produces a distinct withdrawal and may result in a prolonged abstinence syndrome.

Unlike misuse of other substances, there are many pharmacologic approaches to treatment of opioid use disorder, including methadone and buprenorphine. Treatment involving medication combined with behavioral therapies works best, and is used for extended periods of time, even up to a lifetime.

EXAM QUESTIONS

CHAPTER 10
Questions 54–61

Note: Choose the one option that BEST answers each question.

54. What is a major factor contributing to current prescription opioid misuse?

    a. Overregulation of prescribing practices
    b. Routine use of opioids for chronic pain
    c. Periodic urine drug testing
    d. Drug diversion

55. When activated, the type of receptor that is responsible for most of the effects associated with opioid use, including mood, is the

    a. delta opioid receptor.
    b. mu-opioid receptor.
    c. kappa opioid receptor.
    d. alpha opioid receptor.

56. Morphine is classified as a(n)

    a. artificial opioid.
    b. natural opioid.
    c. semisynthetic opioid.
    d. synthetic opioid.

57. The severity of opioid withdrawal symptoms depends on the

    a. specific opioid used, dose, and duration of use.
    b. extent of drug craving.
    c. extent of physical dependence.
    d. number of withdrawal symptoms.

58. In observing for signs of heroin withdrawal, the clinician observes for

    a. a slow pulse and lethargy.
    b. an increase in appetite and constipation.
    c. muscle aches and vomiting.
    d. constricted pupils and low blood pressure.

59. The cause of death from opioids is usually due to

    a. uncontrolled seizures.
    b. HIV.
    c. respiratory depression.
    d. suicide.

60. An advantage of using buprenorphine over methadone is that buprenorphine

    a. attaches to a different receptor.
    b. causes far less respiratory depression.
    c. is a more potent drug.
    d. has less of an effect on the QTc.

61. When used to treat opioid dependence, naltrexone

    a. can have the same euphoric effect as opioids, without addictive potential.
    b. can precipitate severe withdrawal symptoms when opioids are used.
    c. is associated with a severe decrease in blood pressure.
    d. works rapidly to reverse opioid effects.

REFERENCES

American Psychiatric Association. (2013). *Diagnostic and statistical manual of mental disorders* (5th ed.). Washington, DC: American Psychiatric Association.

American Society of Addiction Medicine. (2016). *Opioid addiction 2016 facts and figures*. Retrieved from http://www.asam.org/docs/default-source/advocacy/opioid-addiction-disease-facts-figures.pdf

Barthwell, A. G., & Brown, L. S. (2014). The treatment of drug addiction: An overview. In R. K Reis (Ed.), *The ASAM principles of addiction medicine* (5th ed., pp. 389-402). Philadelphia, PA: Wolters Kluwer.

Borg, L., Buonora, M., Butelman, E. R., Ducat, E., Ray, B. M., & Kreek, M. J. (2014). The pharmacology of opioids. In R. K Reis (Ed.), *The ASAM principles of addiction medicine* (5th ed., pp. 135-150). Philadelphia, PA: Wolters Kluwer.

Center for Substance Abuse Treatment. (2014). *Medication-assisted treatment for opioid addiction in opioid treatment programs* (Treatment Improvement Protocol [TIP] Series 43; HHS Publication No. [SMA] 12-4214). Rockville, MD: Substance Abuse and Mental Health Services Administration.

Centers for Disease Control and Prevention. (n.d.). *Calculating total daily dose of opioids for safer dosage*. Retrieved from https://www.cdc.gov/drugoverdose/pdf/calculating_total_daily_dose-a.pdf

Centers for Disease Control and Prevention. (2017). *CDC guideline for prescribing opioids for chronic pain*. Retrieved from https://www.cdc.gov/drugoverdose/prescribing/guideline.html

Dowell, D., Haegerich, T. M., & Chou, R. (2016). CDC guideline for prescribing opioids for chronic pain – United States, 2016. *MMWR Recommendations and Reports, 65*(RR-1), 1-49. doi:10.15585/mmwr.rr6501e1

Frenk, S. M., Porter, K. S., & Paulozzi, L. J. (2015). Prescription opioid analgesic use among adults: United States, 1999-2012 (NCHS Data Brief No. 189). Hyattsville, MD: National Center for Health Statistics.

Gallagher, R. M., Koob, G. F., & Popescu, A. (2014). The pathophysiology of chronic pain and clinical interfaces with addiction. In R. K Reis (Ed.), *The ASAM principles of addiction medicine* (5th ed., pp. 1435-1456). Philadelphia, PA: Wolters Kluwer.

Jones, C. M., Logan, J., Gladden, R. M., & Bohm, M. (2015). Vital signs: Demographic and substance use trends among heroin users – United States, 2002-2013. *Morbidity and Mortality Weekly Report, 64*(26), 719-725.

Kolodny A., Courtwright, D. T., Hwang, C. S., Kreiner, P., Eadie, J. L., Clark, T. W., & Alexander, G. C. (2015). The prescription opioid and heroin crisis: A public health approach to an epidemic of addiction. *Annual Review of Public Health, 36,* 559-574.

Ling, W., Wesson, D. R., & Smith, D. E. (2005). Prescription opiate abuse. In J. H. Lowinson, P. Ruiz, R. B. Millman, & J. G. Langrod (Eds.), *Substance abuse: A comprehensive textbook* (4th ed., pp. 459-468). Philadelphia, PA: Lippincott Williams & Wilkins.

Martin, J., Zweben, J. E., & Payte. J. T. (2014). Opioid maintenance treatment. In R. K. Reis (Ed.), *The ASAM principles of addiction medicine* (5th ed., pp. 759-777). Philadelphia, PA: Wolters Kluwer.

Miech, R., Johnston, L., O'Malley, P. M., Keyes, K. M., & Heard, K. (2015). Prescription opioids in adolescence and future opioid misuse. *Pediatrics, 136*(5), 1169-1177.

Morone, N. E., & Weiner, D. K. (2013). Pain as the fifth vital sign: Exposing the vital need for pain education. *Clinical Therapeutics, 35*(11), 1728-1732.

Nace, E. P. (2014). Twelve-step programs in addiction recovery. In R. K. Reis (Ed.), *The ASAM principles of addiction medicine* (5th ed., pp. 1033-1042). Philadelphia, PA: Wolters Kluwer.

National Institute on Drug Abuse. (n.d.) *Clinical opiate withdrawal scale.* Retrieved from https://www.drugabuse.gov/sites/default/files/files/ClinicalOpiateWithdrawalScale.pdf

National Institute on Drug Abuse. (2014). *What are the medical complications of chronic heroin use?* Retrieved from https://www.drugabuse.gov/publications/research-reports/heroin/what-are-medical-complications-chronic-heroin-use

National Institute on Drug Abuse. (2016a). *Drug facts: Fentanyl.* Retrieved from https://www.drugabuse.gov/publications/drugfacts/fentanyl#references

National Institute on Drug Abuse. (2016b). *Monitoring the Future survey: High school and youth trends.* Retrieved from https://www.drugabuse.gov/publications/drugfacts/monitoring-future-survey-high-school-youth-trends

National Institute on Drug Abuse. (2017a). *Emerging trends and alerts.* Retrieved from http://www.drugabuse.gov/drugs-abuse/emerging-trends-alerts

National Institute on Drug Abuse. (2017b). *Heroin.* Retrieved from https://www.drugabuse.gov/publications/drugfacts/heroin

Pathan, H., & Williams, J. (2012). Basic opioid pharmacology: An update. *British Journal of Pain, 6*(1), 11-16. Retrieved from http://doi.org/10.1177/2049463712438493

Patrick, S. W., Davis, M. M., Lehman, C. U., & Cooper, W. O. (2015). Increasing incidence and geographic distribution of neonatal abstinence syndrome: United States 2009-2012. *Journal of Perinatology, 35*(8), 650-655.

Paulozzi, L. J., Mack, K. A., & Hockenberry, J. M. (2014). Vital signs: Variation among states in prescribing of opioid pain relievers and benzodiazepines – United States, 2012. *Morbidity and Mortality Weekly Report, 63*(26), 563-568.

Rudd, R. A., Seth, P., David, F., & Scholl, L. (2016). Increases in drug and opioid-involved overdose deaths – United States, 2010-2015. *Morbidity and Mortality Weekly Report, 65*(5051), 1445-1452. doi:10.15585/mmwr.mm6550e1

Saitz, R. (2014). Medical and surgical complications of addiction. In R. K. Reis (Ed.), *The ASAM principles of addiction medicine* (5th ed., pp. 1067-1089). Philadelphia, PA: Wolters Kluwer.

Savage, S. R. (2014). Opioid therapy of pain. In R. K. Reis (Ed.), *The ASAM principles of addiction medicine* (5th ed., pp. 1500-1529). Philadelphia, PA: Wolters Kluwer.

Stahl, S. M. (2013). *Stahl's essential psychopharmacology: Neuroscientific basis and practical applications* (4th ed.). New York, NY: Cambridge University Press.

Stine, S. M., & Kosten, T. R. (2014). Pharmacologic interventions for opioid dependence. In R. K. Reis (Ed.), *The ASAM principles of addiction medicine* (5th ed., 735-758). Philadelphia, PA: Wolters Kluwer.

Substance Abuse and Mental Health Services Administration. (2016a). *Opioid overdose prevention toolkit* (HHS Publication No. [SMA] 16-4742). Rockville, MD: Author.

Substance Abuse and Mental Health Services Administration. (2016b). *Opioids.* Retrieved from http://www.samhsa.gov/atod/opioids

Substance Abuse and Mental Health Services Administration. (2016c). *Treatment episode data set (TEDS): 2004-2014. National admissions to substance abuse treatment services* (BHSIS Series S-84, HHS Publication No. [SMA] 16-4986). Rockville, MD: Author.

Tetrault, J. M., & O'Connor, P. G. (2014). Management of opioid intoxication and withdrawal. In R. K. Reis (Ed.), *The ASAM principles of addiction medicine* (5th ed., pp. 668-684). Philadelphia, PA: Wolters Kluwer.

The Joint Commission. (2016). *Joint Commission statement on pain management.* Retrieved from https://www.jointcommission.org/joint_commission_statement_on_pain_management/

U.S. Department of Health and Human Services, Office of the Surgeon General. (2016). *Facing addiction in America: The surgeon general's report on alcohol, drugs, and health.* Washington, DC: Author.

U.S. Department of Justice. (2016). *Opioid facts.* Retrieved from http://www.justice.gov/opioidawareness/opioid-facts

U.S. Drug Enforcement Administration. (n.d.) *Drug scheduling.* Retrieved from http://www.dea.gov/druginfo/ds.shtml

U.S. Drug Enforcement Administration. (2015). *Drugs of abuse.* Retrieved from https://www.dea.gov/pr/multimedia-library/publications/drug_of_abuse.pdf

U.S. Drug Enforcement Administration. (2017). *Controlled substance schedules.* Retrieved from https://www.deadiversion.usdoj.gov/schedules/#define

Villapiano, N. L. G., Winkelman, T. N. A., Kozhimannil, K. B., Davis, M. M., & Patrick, S. W. (2016). Rural and urban differences in neonatal abstinence syndrome and maternal opioid use, 2004 to 2013. *JAMA Pediatrics, 171*(2), 194-196. doi:10.1001/jamapediatrics.2016.3750

Warner, E., & Lorch, E. (2014). Laboratory diagnosis. In R. K. Reis (Ed.), *The ASAM principles of addiction medicine* (5th ed., pp. 295-361). Philadelphia, PA: Wolters Kluwer.

Wesson, D. R., & Ling, W. (2003). The Clinical Opiate Withdrawal Scale (COWS). *Journal of Psychoactive Drugs, 35*(2), 253-259.

CHAPTER 11

SEDATIVE-HYPNOTICS AND ANXIOLYTICS

LEARNING OUTCOME

After completing this chapter, the learner will be able to describe the biochemical actions, adverse effects, and recommended treatment and nursing care for patients who misuse sedative-hypnotics and anxiolytics.

CHAPTER OBJECTIVES

After completing this chapter, the learner will be able to:

1. Identify populations at risk for misuse of central nervous system (CNS) depressants.

2. Explain the biochemical actions of CNS depressants.

3. Describe the therapeutic actions of the CNS depressants most commonly misused.

4. Discuss adverse health effects related to the misuse of CNS depressants.

5. Select appropriate treatment and nursing care strategies for patients who misuse CNS depressants.

INTRODUCTION

Sedative-hypnotics and anxiolytics, which are often referred to as central nervous system (CNS) depressants, are drugs that alter the function of the central nervous system. CNS depression occurs on a continuum that ranges from mild slowing of the heart and respiratory rates to coma and fatal respiratory depression. Anxiolytic medications are designed to decrease anxiety, whereas sedative-hypnotic medications are designed to induce sleep. The distinction between sedatives and hypnotics is somewhat arbitrary because sedative drugs at higher doses also produce sleep, which is why sedatives and hypnotics are often discussed as a single drug class. CNS depressants are available legally for medical purposes with a prescription, and they are obtained illegally for recreational or non-medical purposes. Most patients use sedatives and hypnotics responsibly, but substantial numbers of patients misuse them. Misuse is defined as taking a prescribed medication at a dose or by a route that was not prescribed (e.g., dissolving a pill in liquid and injecting it); taking someone else's prescribed medication, even if it is for a legitimate medical concern; or taking a medication to feel euphoria ("getting high"; National Institute on Drug Abuse [NIDA], 2016b). Under the Controlled Substances Act, barbiturates are classified according to their abuse potential. For example, secobarbital (Seconal Sodium) is classified as a Schedule II drug (high abuse potential), pentobarbital (Nembutal Sodium) is classified as a Schedule III drug (low abuse potential compared with Schedule II drugs), and methohexital (Brevital Sodium) is classified as a Schedule IV drug (low abuse potential compared with Schedule III drugs; Drug Enforcement

Agency [DEA], Office of Diversion Control, 2017). Anxiolytics such as benzodiazepines are typically classified as Schedule IV drugs (DEA, Office of Diversion Control, 2013).

One of the oldest and most universally used CNS depressants is alcohol. Over the years, hundreds of other substances within the CNS depressant category have been developed. These drugs have been referred to as downers, sedatives, hypnotics, minor tranquilizers, anxiolytics, and anti-anxiety medications. Most of these medications have been developed for legitimate therapeutic uses, but they can be used illegally. This chapter discusses current and common CNS depressants, particularly barbiturates and benzodiazepines.

EPIDEMIOLOGY

Rates of sedative-hypnotic and anxiolytic use have increased in the past few years. In 2015, approximately 446,000 people aged 12 or older reported current nonmedical use of sedatives, compared with 231,000 in 2011, and 1.9 million reported current use of tranquilizers in 2015, compared with 1.8 million in 2011 (Substance Abuse and Mental Health Services Administration [SAMHSA], 2016). Although sedatives and hypnotics are prescribed more often for people ages 60 and older, misuse is most frequent among individuals between the ages of 18 and 25. In 2015, 1.7% of people in this age group reported misuse of tranquilizers, representing an estimated 589,000 people (Center for Behavioral Health Statistics and Quality, 2016).

BIOCHEMISTRY

Sedative-hypnotics and anxiolytics slow normal brain function by stimulating gamma-aminobutyric acid (GABA) activity. When stimulated, GABA, the most widely dispersed inhibitory CNS neurotransmitter, inhibits or depresses neuron discharge in the CNS, thereby decreasing brain activity. CNS depressants such as benzodiazepines work by opening gamma-aminobutyric acid type A ($GABA_A$) complex calcium channels, which inhibits nerve action by causing an influx of calcium ions to create a hyperpolarized state (Varma, 2016). The main effects of this action on $GABA_A$ receptors are reduction of anxiety, sedation, sleep promotion, muscle relaxation, and amnesia (Galarneau & Conrad, 2015; Monti & Pandi-Perumal, 2014; Soyka, 2017). Benzodiazepines also have an anticonvulsant effect (Soyka, 2017).

THERAPEUTIC ACTIONS AND SIDE EFFECTS

Barbiturates

Barbiturates are most commonly used in anesthesia and in the treatment of seizure disorders (NIDA, 2016c). Agents such as methohexital are used as sedatives before outpatient procedures and for sedation in the intensive care unit. Phenobarbital is used in the treatment of generalized tonic-clonic seizures and simple partial seizures and is also used for detoxification from benzodiazepines, especially if the patient has also been using opioids. Pentobarbital and secobarbital were used in the past in the treatment of insomnia but were associated with high abuse potential and narrow therapeutic index, thus increasing the risk for respiratory depression, coma, and death. The use of these drugs in the treatment of insomnia has been replaced by safer medications with less abuse potential, such as zolpidem (Ambien; Sadock, Sadock, & Ruiz, 2015).

Sedating Benzodiazepines

Several sedating benzodiazepines are used in the treatment of insomnia. These include triazolam (Halcion), estazolam (ProSom), temazepam (Restoril), and flurazepam (NIDA, 2016c;

Sadock et al., 2015). These drugs also have a high abuse potential; however, as with barbiturates, their use has diminished because of the availability of safer medications. Midazolam hydrochloride is a short-acting benzodiazepine that reduces anxiety and causes amnesia; it is used preoperatively and in conscious sedation in the intensive care unit (Reade & Finfer, 2014).

Anxiolytic Benzodiazepines

Benzodiazepines that are used as anxiolytics are classified as short and long-acting benzodiazepines. The shorter-acting benzodiazepines include lorazepam (Ativan), alprazolam (Xanax), triazolam, and estazolam. Alprazolam has a short half-life and is more likely to be misused compared with other benzodiazepines (Brett & Murnion, 2015). The longer-acting benzodiazepines include clonazepam (Klonopin), chlordiazepoxide (Librium), and diazepam (Valium). Alprazolam and diazepam are used in the treatment of acute anxiety and panic disorder (NIDA, 2016c). Benzodiazepines are also used in the treatment of alcohol withdrawal.

The evidence base for the use of benzodiazepines in obsessive-compulsive disorder is minimal; therefore, treatment with benzodiazepines is not recommended for this disorder (Brakoulias et al., 2016). In addition, the utility of benzodiazepines in the treatment of post-traumatic stress disorder (PTSD) is unclear. Although pharmacotherapy with benzodiazepines is not currently included in PTSD practice guidelines, benzodiazepine use is estimated at about 25% of veterans diagnosed with PTSD (Krystal et al., 2017).

Practice guidelines recommend that benzodiazepines should be prescribed at the lowest dose for the shortest amount of time possible, optimally no more than 4 weeks (Soyka, 2017; Varma, 2016). Soyka (2017) stresses that the safety of benzodiazepine use beyond 4 weeks is unknown. In addition, patients with substance use disorders should not be prescribed benzodiazepines for any reason (DuPont, 2017). Benzodiazepines should also never be prescribed to patients diagnosed with myasthenia gravis, sleep apnea, chronic respiratory insufficiency (such as chronic obstructive lung disease), angle-closure glaucoma, or acute CNS-depressant intoxication (Soyka, 2017).

Prescribers should be aware that benzodiazepines interact with several other medications. Medications such as cimetidine, estrogen, disulfiram, oral contraceptives, erythromycin, ketoconazole, and some selective serotonin reuptake inhibitors (SSRIs) can increase plasma levels of benzodiazepines, particularly diazepam, chlordiazepoxide, clorazepate, and flurazepam (Sadock et al., 2015; Varma, 2016). Fluvoxamine (an SSRI) can increase the plasma levels of triazolam and alprazolam to toxic levels (Sadock et al., 2015).

Flunitrazepam is a benzodiazepine that is not legally produced or marketed in the United States. Also known as rophies, roach, or roofies, flunitrazepam is a popular club or designer drug. However, it is also known as the date rape drug because it is odorless and tasteless and can be added to a victim's drink without his or her knowledge, causing sedation, confusion, and amnesia (Talbert, 2014). The CNS-depressant effects are enhanced when taken with alcohol and can lead to respiratory depression and arrest (Talbert, 2014).

GABA$_A$ Agonists

GABA$_A$ agonists are the most commonly used medications to aid sleep. These include zolpidem, zaleplon (Sonata), and eszopiclone (Lunesta), which are commonly referred to as Z drugs. GABA$_A$ agonist activity modulates the binding of GABA at the GABA$_A$ site. Z drugs act specifically on the GABA$_A$ α_1 receptor subunit, causing a predominantly sedative effect to promote sleep (Monti & Pandi-Perumal, 2014). In contrast, benzodiazepines act on a broader array of GABA$_A$ receptor subtypes, such as α_2, α_3, and α_5, which cause anxiety reduction, amnesia, and respiratory depression in addition to sedation and sleep promotion (Monti & Pandi-Perumal, 2014; Sutton, 2014). Actions include reduced sleep latency (faster time to fall asleep), improved sleep quality, and improved sleep duration and maintenance (fewer awakenings during the night).

Zolpidem is approved for short-term treatment of insomnia and is one of the most commonly prescribed drugs to treat insomnia (McFarlane, Morin, & Montplaisir, 2014). It is manufactured as an immediate-release formulation (Ambien) and a controlled-release formulation (Ambien CR). Edluar is a sublingual form of zolpidem, and Intermezzo is a sublingual formulation specifically intended to treat awakening in the middle of the night. ZolpiMist is an oral spray formulation of zolpidem.

Rebound insomnia can occur with the use of the Z drugs, in which sleep is worse after stopping use (McFarlane et al., 2014). In addition, clinicians have reported complex sleep-related behaviors with the use of zolpidem, which are referred to as parasomnias in the *Diagnostic and Statistical Manual of Mental Disorders,* 5th edition (American Psychiatric Association, 2013). Parasomnias reported to occur with zolpidem use include sleep conversations (e.g., talking on the phone) and sleep with object manipulation (e.g., cooking and cleaning during sleep), sleepwalking, sleep eating, sleep driving, and sleep shopping (McFarlane et al., 2014). These parasomnias occur most often when higher doses of zolpidem are taken (McFarlane et al., 2014). Problems with next-day psychomotor activities, such as balance, reaction times, and the ability to multitask, can

also occur (Gunja, 2013). In older adults, some research suggests that rates of hip fractures are higher with the use of zolpidem compared with traditional benzodiazepines, such as diazepam or alprazolam (Levy, 2013). Some clinicians have reported that the Z drugs can cause neuroadaptive changes, such as tolerance, dependence, and withdrawal, which appear to be less severe compared with changes that occur with benzodiazepines (Gunja, 2013). Withdrawal symptoms associated with Z drugs include insomnia, delirium, anxiety, tremors, and craving.

ADVERSE EFFECTS OF SEDATIVE-HYPNOTICS AND ANXIOLYTICS

Sedative-hypnotics and anxiolytics are effective drugs that provide therapeutic benefits, but they also have a high abuse potential. Anxiolytics, such as benzodiazepines, are well known for their better safety profiles compared with sedatives, such as barbiturates. Generally, benzodiazepines are much safer than barbiturates and cause significantly less respiratory depression. An excessively high dose of benzodiazepines (2 g) is not lethal; the most serious adverse effects at this dose are drowsiness, lethargy, confusion, and ataxia. In contrast, overdoses of barbiturates can be lethal as a result of induction of coma, respiratory depression, and cardiac arrest (Sadock et al., 2015). However, given the cross-tolerance among barbiturates, benzodiazepines, and alcohol, any combination of these substances can be fatal. In addition, use of opiates or methadone concomitantly with benzodiazepines can cause fatal respiratory depression (Galarneau & Conrad, 2015; Varma, 2016). In 2010, almost 80% of benzodiazepine overdose deaths occurred with the concomitant use of opiates (DuPont, 2017). The health effects of sedatives, hypnotics, and anxiolytics are presented in Table 11-1.

TABLE 11-1: THE HEALTH EFFECTS OF SEDATIVES, HYPNOTICS, AND ANXIOLYTICS				
Prescription Sedatives (Tranquilizers, Depressants)				
Medications that slow brain activity, which makes them useful for treating anxiety and sleep problems				
Street Names	**Commercial Names (Common)**	**Common Forms**	**Common Ways Taken**	**DEA Schedule**
Barbs, phennies, red birds, reds, tooies, yellow jackets, yellows	Barbiturates: pentobarbital (Nembutal), phenobarbital (Luminal)	Pill, capsule, liquid	Swallowed, injected	II, III, IV
Candy, downers, sleeping pills, tranks	Benzodiazepines: alprazolam (Xanax), chlordiazepoxide (Librium), diazepam (Valium), lorazepam (Ativan), triazolam (Halcion)	Pill, capsule, liquid	Swallowed, snorted	IV
Forget-me pill, Mexican valium, R2, roche, roofies, roofinol, rope, rophies	Sleep medications: eszopiclone (Lunesta), zaleplon (Sonata), zolpidem (Ambien)	Pill, capsule, liquid	Swallowed, snorted	IV
Possible Health Effects				
Short-term	Drowsiness, slurred speech, poor concentration, confusion, dizziness, problems with movement and memory, lowered blood pressure, slowed breathing			
Long-term	Unknown			
Other health-related issues	Sleep medications are sometimes used as date rape drugs. Risk of HIV, hepatitis, and other infectious diseases from shared needles			
In combination with alcohol	Further slows heart rate and breathing, which can lead to death			
Withdrawal symptoms	Must be discussed with a healthcare provider; benzodiazepine withdrawal carries serious risk for seizure.			
Treatment options				
Medications	There are no medications approved by the U.S. Food and Drug Administration to treat addiction to prescription sedatives; lowering the dose over time must be done with the help of a healthcare provider.			
Behavioral therapies	More research is needed to find out if behavioral therapies can be used to treat addiction to prescription sedatives.			
DEA = Drug Enforcement Agency.				
Note. Adapted from National Institute on Drug Abuse. (2016a). *Commonly abused drugs.* Retrieved from https://www.drugabuse.gov/drugs-abuse/commonly-abused-drugs-charts#prescription-sedatives-tranquilizers-depressants-				

The onset of action of benzodiazepines depends on the pharmacokinetics of the specific substance. For example, the peak plasma concentration for diazepam occurs 30 minutes to 2 hours after ingestion, whereas the peak plasma concentration for lorazepam occurs 2 to 4 hours after ingestion (Perry, 2014). Effects include drowsiness, reduced anxiety, a calming sensation, and sedation. Anterograde amnesia can also occur (Varma, 2016), defined as loss of new memories during the period of intoxication, whereas past memory remains intact. This effect is intentionally targeted for surgical procedures requiring conscious sedation.

Intoxication

Mild to moderate benzodiazepine intoxication can cause slurred speech, ataxia, incoordination, and behavioral inhibition (Galarneau & Conrad, 2015; Sadock et al., 2015). Severely impaired liver function may interfere with the metabolism of benzodiazepines, resulting in toxic levels of benzodiazepines and fatality (Galarneau & Conrad, 2015).

Barbiturate intoxication is similar to alcohol intoxication and is characterized by slurred speech, sluggishness, disinhibition, argumentativeness, emotional lability, and hostility. Severe benzodiazepine intoxication causes respiratory depression, stupor, and coma. Fatalities from severe benzodiazepine intoxication are rare and may occur in patients with pre-existing pulmonary disease, such as chronic obstructive pulmonary disease (Galarneau & Conrad, 2015).

Tolerance and Dependence

Tolerance is the reduced effect of a medication because of repeated use. Tolerance is thought to occur from the long-term use of sedative-hypnotics that results in downregulation (decreased sensitivity of the GABA receptors; Galarneau & Conrad, 2015). Dependence occurs in about 50% of people who use benzodiazepines for longer than 1 month (Soyka, 2017). Some evidence suggests that benzodiazepines with a shorter half-life, such as temazepam, lorazepam, or alprazolam, present a greater risk for dependence (Soyka, 2017). Psychological dependence or reinforcement is the potential for these medicines to be misused or continued without physical need. Benzodiazepines are not normally primary drugs of misuse, but they are commonly used by addicted patients to increase the effect of heroin, marijuana, or alcohol. In fact, benzodiazepines are indicated to decrease the withdrawal sequelae associated with alcohol use disorder (DuPont, 2017).

Withdrawal

Abrupt discontinuation of benzodiazepines after long-term use can cause withdrawal, serious psychological and physical adverse effects, and death (Turton & Lingford-Hughes, 2016). More severe withdrawal is experienced in those who were treated with higher benzodiazepine doses, with multiple benzodiazepines, or with benzodiazepines with a shorter half-life and in those who have a more rapid taper from benzodiazepines (Puening, Wilson, & Nordstrom, 2017). Psychological effects include re-emergence of anxiety and insomnia, impaired concentration, depression, hallucinations, and delusions (Varma, 2016). Physical effects include gastrointestinal distress, tremors, tachycardia, hypertension, diaphoresis, paresthesias, and visual disturbances. Convulsive status epilepticus can occur among those who are treated with higher doses, have a longer duration of treatment, or have a rapid taper from benzodiazepines (Puening et al., 2017). Rebound symptoms may also occur, which are similar to the original symptoms for which the benzodiazepine was prescribed. However, the rebound symptoms may be more intense compared with the symptoms experienced before treatment with the benzodiazepine (Galarneau & Conrad, 2015).

Benzodiazepines are generally eliminated from the body slowly, depending on the half-life of the medication (Cluver, Wright, & Myrick, 2015; Sadock et al., 2015). The symptoms of withdrawal occur in about 12 to 24 hours for short-acting benzodiazepines. The peak intensity of withdrawal is reached in 1 to 3 days for short-acting benzodiazepines and 4 to 7 days for longer-acting benzodiazepines (grand-mal seizures can occur 1 to 12 days after discontinuation; Brett & Murnion, 2015). Longer use of benzodiazepines and use at higher doses have been linked to more severe withdrawal symptoms (Galarneau & Conrad, 2015).

Galarneau and Conrad (2015) note that withdrawal can be classified into two discontinuation syndromes. Pseudowithdrawal is defined as the overinterpretation of emerging symptoms, in which patient expectations of withdrawal symptoms cause the patient to experience abstinence symptoms. In contrast, true withdrawal symptoms are somatic and psychological symptoms that emerge when a physically dependent patient discontinues use of the benzodiazepine (Galarneau & Conrad, 2015).

TREATMENT OF SEDATIVE-HYPNOTIC MISUSE

Overdose

Flumazenil, a benzodiazepine antagonist, is used in the treatment of benzodiazepine overdose (Sadock et al., 2015). This drug must be used with caution because it may not reverse respiratory depression completely and can provoke withdrawal seizures in patients with benzodiazepine dependence. Benzodiazepine overdose can be fatal when combined with the use of alcohol, other CNS depressants, and opiates (Sadock et al., 2015).

Withdrawal

For emergency department treatment of benzodiazepine withdrawal, the patient is stabilized with long-acting benzodiazepines, either orally or intravenously if the patient is unable to take oral medications (Puening et al., 2017). Haloperidol can be used to treat psychotic symptoms, such as delusions or hallucinations. A blood alcohol screen and a urine toxicology screen are done to evaluate for other substance use (Puening et al., 2017).

Supervised medical treatment for sedative-hypnotic withdrawal is required because the symptoms can be life-threatening. Standard treatment is the gradual withdrawal of the drug of dependence. The benzodiazepine dose should be tapered gradually, typically over 4 to 8 weeks, to avoid seizures and severe withdrawal symptoms (Soyka, 2017). If the patient was taking therapeutic doses, the benzodiazepine dose should be reduced by 10% to 25% initially, and the patient should be evaluated for the emergence of symptoms. The rate of dose reduction is determined by the severity of symptoms and the patient's ability to tolerate them (Sadock et al., 2015; Soyka, 2017). If the patient is withdrawing from a short-acting benzodiazepine, some clinicians recommend switching to a long-acting benzodiazepine, such as clonazepam (Weaver, 2015).

If the patient was taking doses in excess of treatment recommendations (supratherapeutic doses), hospitalization is needed to monitor response to withdrawal. Practice guidelines recommend reducing the dose by 30% and monitoring the response. If the initial dose reduction is tolerated, the dose is gradually reduced by 10% to 25% every few days, depending on the patient's ability to tolerate symptoms (Sadock et al., 2015).

Other evidence-based treatment recommendations for withdrawal include the use of antiepileptics, such as carbamazepine (Sadock et al., 2015), which has the advantage of no abuse potential. The recommended dose of carbamazepine is 200 mg, three times a day, for 7 to 10 days (Cluver et al., 2015). Gabapentin and pregabalin have also been used, although these agents present a risk for misuse (Soyka, 2017). Phenobarbital is used in barbiturate withdrawal as a substitute for a short-acting barbiturate (Sadock et al., 2015). The recommended dose of phenobarbital is 30 mg for every 100 mg of the short-acting barbiturate for at least 2 days to monitor response (Sadock et al., 2015).

Relapse Prevention

When the patient has successfully undergone benzodiazepine withdrawal, relapse prevention strategies are implemented to address the risk of returning to use. Cognitive-behavioral therapy (CBT), which is based on social learning theory and emphasizes modification of the individual's thoughts and behaviors, has been used with supervised withdrawal to prevent relapse. Some research has shown that among patients who received supervised withdrawal combined with psychotherapies such as CBT, the odds of stopping benzodiazepines increased by 5.6 times compared with patients who received control interventions (Gould, Coulson, Patel, Highton-Williamson, & Howard, 2014).

A supportive organization based on the 12-step Alcoholics Anonymous model is Pills Anonymous. A goal of this model is to encourage abstinence by helping individuals learn and master effective coping skills that can help them believe they can resist relapsing to substance misuse. The focus is on the exploration of positive and negative consequences of substance use. Individuals are taught the skills needed to prevent relapse of a substance use disorder after treatment; therefore, Pills Anonymous is the foundation for relapse prevention.

SCREENING AND OTHER STRATEGIES TO ADDRESS SEDATIVE-HYPNOTIC AND ANXIOLYTIC MISUSE

Some patients engage in "doctor shopping" in an attempt to obtain multiple prescriptions simultaneously from several clinicians during a single episode of illness (SAMHSA, 2016, p. 23). Prescribers and law enforcement officials have addressed this issue with the establishment of prescription drug monitoring programs (PDMPs), which are statewide electronic databases that track every prescription that a patient receives for a controlled substance. Goals of PDMPs are to support access to controlled substances that are used legitimately in medical treatment and identify and deter or prevent substance misuse and diversion, which is the sale of prescription medications obtained from a healthcare provider. Additional goals of PDMPs include facilitating the identification of people addicted to prescription drugs, for the purpose of encouraging treatment; informing public health initiatives by tracking trends in the use and misuse of prescribed controlled substances; and educating individuals regarding the consequences of misused prescribed controlled substances and diversion of prescription drugs. As of 2016, 39 states had implemented PDMPs, and the remaining 11 states were in the process of establishing programs (U.S. Department of Justice, 2016).

Other strategies to assess for inappropriate use of benzodiazepines include monitoring the frequency with which patients request refills. Patients who misuse benzodiazepines may tell the prescriber that the prescription was lost or stolen to obtain an early refill. Prescribers should communicate clear guidelines to patients regarding when prescriptions for benzodiazepines, or any controlled substance, will be refilled (Weaver, 2015). Other strategies include pill counts to determine the rate at which patients are taking medications, urine drug toxicity screens, and, if possible, collateral information from family members regarding the frequency of benzodiazepine use in the patient. Benzodiazepines are generally recommended for short-term use. It is also important for the clinician to evaluate contraindications to the use of CNS depressants. These agents should not be used with other substances that cause CNS depression, including the following:

- Alcohol
- Prescription opioid pain medicines
- Some over-the-counter cold and allergy medications

BENZODIAZEPINE USE IN THE GERIATRIC POPULATION

The most common reasons for benzodiazepine use in the elderly are insomnia and anxiety (Markota, Rummans, Bostwick, & Lapid, 2016). Some researchers estimate that about 9% of elderly people in the United States are prescribed benzodiazepines, and over 30% of elderly people who use benzodiazepines are treated long term, defined as over 120 days (Olfson, King, & Schoenbaum, 2015). However, research estimates that only 16% of elderly patients who are prescribed benzodiazepines have a clinical psychiatric diagnosis, and almost none are referred to psychotherapy (Maust, Kales, Wiechers, Blow, & Olfson, 2016). Several treatment issues may be related to patterns of long-term benzodiazepine use among the elderly. Healthcare providers may continue long-term use due to the belief that benzodiazepine use is genuinely helpful to the patient or concerns that stopping benzodiazepines may damage their relationship with the patient (Markota et al., 2016).

Long-term use of benzodiazepines in the elderly population raises serious concerns about adverse effects, such as falls or fractures, impaired ability to drive or motor vehicle crashes, and the risk for developing substance use disorders. In addition, cognitive decline can occur, particularly related to short-term memory, attention and learning, and long-term cognitive deficits (Markota et al., 2016). Consequently, the American Geriatric Association recommends that benzodiazepine use should be avoided in the elderly due to these concerns (Markota et al., 2016). In addition, the Beers Criteria, a practice guideline that identifies inappropriate use of medications in the geriatric population, recommends avoiding both short- and long-acting benzodiazepines in this population (Davidoff et al., 2015).

Elderly patients may also experience more severe withdrawal from benzodiazepines because of the decreased liver function associated with advanced age (Galarneau & Conrad, 2015). A slow-tapering protocol for geriatric patients is recommended. Up to 60% of elderly patients can be tapered off of benzodiazepines in 4 weeks using a protocol that reduces the benzodiazepine dose by 25% every 1 to 2 weeks (Markota et al., 2016); however, some patients may require up to 22 weeks to taper.

Recent research has demonstrated the effectiveness of interventions to reduce benzodiazepine use in the elderly. For example, a randomized controlled trial was conducted to determine the effectiveness of an educational intervention intended to empower geriatric participants by providing them with the evidence base about benzodiazepine use and facilitate participants' questioning about the safety of benzodiazepine overuse (Tannenbaum, Martin, Tamblyn, Benedetti, & Ahmed, 2014). The intervention consisted of a booklet that described the risks of benzodiazepine use, "knowledge statements designed to create cognitive dissonance about the safety of benzodiazepine use" (p. 892), peer narratives to enhance self-efficacy, effective alternative treatments for insomnia and anxiety reduction, and a 21-week tapering schedule. Findings indicated that among participants in the intervention group (*n* = 148), 27% stopped benzodiazepine use, compared with 5% in the control group (*n* = 153). In addition, 11% of participants reduced their benzodiazepine doses (Tannenbaum et al., 2014).

Antidepressants

The first-line pharmacologic treatment for anxiety disorders includes antidepressants, such as SSRIs and serotonin-norepinephrine reuptake inhibitors (SNRIs). SSRIs commonly prescribed for anxiety disorders include fluoxetine (Prozac), sertraline (Zoloft), paroxetine (Paxil), citalopram (Celexa), and escitalopram (Lexapro). Common SNRIs include venlafaxine (Khedezla) and duloxetine (Cymbalta). These first-line antidepressants are effective after about 2 to 4 weeks of treatment. Benzodiazepines are often prescribed to alleviate the acute anxiety associated with these diagnoses, primarily as a "bridge" treatment until the SSRI or SNRI becomes effective (Metzler, Mahoney, & Freedy, 2016, p. 252). Longer-acting benzodiazepines, such as clonazepam, are preferred for bridge therapy because of their longer half-life. This reduces the frequency of dosing and limits the emergence of anxiety symptoms between doses (Metzler et al., 2016).

SUMMARY

CNS depressants substantially slow normal brain function by affecting the neurotransmitter GABA. In lower doses, they act as a sedative; in higher doses, the effect is hypnotic. CNS depressants are commonly prescribed substances that are useful in treating anxiety and sleep disorders, but they also increase a patient's risk for substance misuse and substance use disorders. All medications in the sedative, hypnotic, and anxiolytic class are controlled substances and carry a risk for potential misuse and the development of dependence, tolerance, and withdrawal.

Patients need to be appropriately screened, diagnosed, and managed (i.e., receive appropriate treatment, follow-up, and education) for a substance use disorder involving any CNS depressant, to prevent substance misuse, and clinicians must safely prescribe these medications at the correct dose. With appropriate care and consideration for the patient, these substances are safe and effective medications.

EXAM QUESTIONS

CHAPTER 11
Questions 62–66

Note: Choose the one option that BEST answers each question.

62. Although sedatives and hypnotics are prescribed more often for patients aged 60 and older, misuse is most frequent among individuals

    a. younger than age 18.

    b. between age 18 and age 25.

    c. between age 35 and age 55.

    d. older than age 55.

63. One of the main effects of stimulating gamma-aminobutyric acid A ($GABA_A$) receptors in the brain is

    a. increased sedation.

    b. pronounced drowsiness.

    c. a reduction of anxiety.

    d. a sleep disorder.

64. The class of sedative-hypnotics commonly used in anesthesia and in the treatment of seizure disorders is

    a. anxiolytics.

    b. $GABA_A$ agonists.

    c. benzodiazepines.

    d. barbiturates.

65. The most serious adverse effect associated with the misuse of central nervous system depressants is

    a. death due to coma, respiratory depression, and cardiac arrest.

    b. HIV and other sexually transmitted infections.

    c. liver failure.

    d. cerebral vascular accident (stroke).

66. An appropriate treatment strategy for a patient undergoing benzodiazepine withdrawal is

    a. relapse prevention.

    b. cognitive-behavioral therapy.

    c. stabilization with long-acting benzodiazepines.

    d. monitoring the frequency with which the patient requests refills.

REFERENCES

American Psychiatric Association. (2013). *Diagnostic and statistical manual of mental disorders* (5th ed.). Arlington, VA: Author.

Brakoulias, V., Starcevic, V., Belloch, A., Dell'Osso, L., Ferrao, Y. A., Fontenelle, L. F., ... Viswasam, K. (2016). International prescribing practices in obsessive-compulsive disorder (OCD). *Human Psychopharmacology, 31*(4), 319-324. doi:10.1002/hup.2541

Brett, J., & Murnion, B. (2015). Management of benzodiazepine misuse and dependence. *Australian Prescriber, 38,* 152-155.

Center for Behavioral Health Statistics and Quality. (2016). *Key substance use and mental health indicators in the United States: Results from the 2015 National Survey on Drug Use and Health* (HHS Publication No. SMA 16-4984, NSDUH Series H-51). Retrieved from http://www.samhsa.gov/data/

Cluver, J. S., Wright, T. M., & Myrick, H. (2015). Pharmacologic intervention for sedative-hypnotic addiction. In A. J. Herron & T. K. Brennan (Eds.), *The ASAM essentials of addiction medicine* (2nd ed., pp. 289-293). Philadelphia, PA: Wolters Kluwer.

Davidoff, A. J., Miller, G. E., Sarpong, E. M., Yang, E., Brandt, N., & Fick, D. M. (2015). Prevalence of potentially inappropriate medication use in older adults using the 2012 Beers Criteria. *Journal of the American Geriatric Society, 63,* 486-500.

Drug Enforcement Agency, Office of Diversion Control. (2013). *Benzodiazepines.* Retrieved from https://www.deadiversion.usdoj.gov/drug_chem_info/benzo.pdf

Drug Enforcement Agency, Office of Diversion Control. (2017). *Controlled substances by DEA drug code number.* Retrieved from https://www.deadiversion.usdoj.gov/schedules/orangebook/d_cs_drugcode.pdf

DuPont, R. L. (2017). "Should patients with substance use disorders be prescribed benzodiazepines?" No. *Journal of Addiction Medicine, 11,* 84-86.

Galarneau, D. W., & Conrad, E. J. (2015). Benzodiazepine intoxication and withdrawal: Assessment and management. *Hospital Medicine Clinics, 4,* 513-525.

Gould, R. L., Coulson, M. C., Patel, N., Highton-Williamson, E., & Howard, R. J. (2014). Interventions for reducing benzodiazepine use in older adults: Meta-analysis of randomised controlled trials. *British Journal of Psychiatry, 204,* 98-107.

Gunja, N. (2013). The clinical and forensic toxicology of Z-drugs. *Journal of Medical Toxicology, 9*(2), 155-162.

Krystal, J. H., Davis, L. L., Neylan, T. C., Raskind, M. A., Schnurr, P. P., Stein, M. B., ... Huang, G. D. (2017). It's time to address the crisis in the pharmacotherapy of posttraumatic stress disorder: A consensus statement of the PTSD psychopharmacology working group. *Biological Psychiatry, 82*(7), e51-e59. doi:10.1016/j.biopsych.2017.03.007

Levy, H. (2013). Non-benzodiazepines and older adults: What are we learning about zolpidem? *Expert Review of Clinical Pharmacology, 7*(1), 5-8. doi:10.1586/17512433.2014.864949

Markota, M., Rummans, T. A., Bostwick, J. M., & Lapid, M. I. (2016). Benzodiazepine use in older adults: Dangers, management, and alternative therapies. *Mayo Clinic Proceedings, 91,* 1632-1639.

Maust, D. T., Kales, H. C., Wiechers, I. R., Blow, F. C., & Olfson, M. (2016). No end in sight: Benzodiazepine use in older adults in the United States. *Journal of the American Geriatrics Society, 64*(2), 2546-2553. doi: 10.1111/jgs.14379

McFarlane, J., Morin, C. M., & Montplaisir, J. (2014). Hypnotics in insomnia: The experience of zolpidem. *Clinical Therapeutics, 36* (11), 1676-1701.

Metzler, D. H., Mahoney, D., & Freedy, J. R. (2016). Anxiety disorders in primary care. *Primary Care Clinics and Office Practice, 43,* 245-261.

Monti, J. M., & Pandi-Perumal, S. R. (2014). Role of zolpidem in the management of primary and comorbid insomnia. In W. Vaughn McCall (Ed.), *Advances in the management of primary and secondary insomnia* (pp. 92-103). London, England: Future Medicine Ltd.

National Institute on Drug Abuse. (2016a). *Commonly abused drugs.* Retrieved from https://www.drugabuse.gov/drugs-abuse/commonly-abused-drugs-charts#prescription-sedatives-tranquilizers-depressants-

National Institute on Drug Abuse. (2016b). *Misuse of prescription drugs: Summary.* Retrieved from https://www.drugabuse.gov/publications/research-reports/misuse-prescription-drugs/summary

National Institute on Drug Abuse. (2016c). *Misuse of prescription drugs: What are CNS depressants?* Retrieved from https://www.drugabuse.gov/publications/research-reports/misuse-prescription-drugs/which-classes-prescription-drugs-are-commonly-misused

Olfson, M., King, M., & Schoenbaum, M. (2015). Benzodiazepine use in the United States. *JAMA Psychiatry, 72*(2), 136-142.

Perry, E. C. (2014). Inpatient management of acute alcohol withdrawal syndrome. *CNS Drugs, 28,* 401-410.

Puening, S. E., Wilson, M. P., & Nordstrom, K. (2017). Psychiatric emergencies for clinicians: Emergency department management of benzodiazepine withdrawal. *Journal of Emergency Medicine, 52,* 66-69.

Reade, M. C., & Finfer, S. (2014). Sedation and delirium in the intensive care unit. *New England Journal of Medicine, 370,* 444-454.

Sadock, B. J., Sadock, V. A., & Ruiz, P. (2015). *Synopsis of psychiatry* (11th ed.). Philadelphia, PA: Wolters Kluwer.

Soyka, M. (2017). Treatment of benzodiazepine dependence. *New England Journal of Medicine, 376*(12), 1147-1157.

Substance Abuse and Mental Health Services Administration. (2016). *Preventing prescription drug misuse: Programs and strategies.* Washington, DC: SAMHSA'S Center for the Application of Prevention Technologies. Retrieved from https://www.samhsa.gov/capt/sites/default/files/resources/preventing-prescription-drug-misuse-strategies.pdf

Sutton, E. L. (2014). Insomnia. *Medical Clinics of North America, 98,* 565-581.

Talbert, J. J. (2014). Club drugs: Coming to a patient near you. *The Nurse Practitioner, 39*(3), 20-25.

Tannenbaum, C., Martin, P., Tamblyn, R., Benedetti, A., & Ahmed, S. (2014). Reduction of inappropriate benzodiazepine prescriptions among older adults through direct patient education: The EMPOWER cluster randomized trial. *JAMA Internal Medicine, 174*(6), 890-898.

Turton, S., & Lingford-Hughes, A. (2016). Neurobiology and principles of addiction and tolerance. *Medicine, 44*(12), 693-696.

U.S. Department of Justice, Drug Enforcement Agency, Diversion Control Division. (2016). *State prescription drug monitoring programs.* Retrieved from https://www.deadiversion. usdoj.gov/faq/rx_monitor.htm

Varma, S. (2016). Benzodiazepines and hypnotics. *Medicine, 44*(12), 764-767.

Weaver, M. F. (2015). Prescription sedative misuse and abuse. *Yale Journal of Biology and Medicine, 88,* 247-256.

CHAPTER 12

INHALANTS

LEARNING OUTCOME

After completing this chapter, the learner will be able to describe the characteristics, health effects, diagnosis, and treatment of inhalant use in the U.S. population.

CHAPTER OBJECTIVES

After completing this chapter, the learner will be able to:

1. Explain how inhalants are used and their usage trends and patterns in the U.S. population.

2. Describe the biochemical effects of the four categories of inhalants.

3. List the criteria used to diagnose inhalant-related disorders.

4. Explain the importance of screening for inhalant use.

5. Identify the role of treatment in addressing inhalant use.

INTRODUCTION

Inhalants are volatile solvents and substances that produce chemical vapors, which are inhaled for purposes of producing a euphoric effect. The term inhalant refers to more than a thousand household and commercial products that are generally easily accessible and available at low cost. The substances are inhaled in various ways, including sniffing, snorting, bagging, or huffing. Sniffing or snorting involves inhalation directly from containers or a heated pan. Bagging refers to the inhalation of vapors from plastic bags containing the substance. Huffing is the inhalation of vapors by taking a cloth saturated with the substance and placing the cloth over the nose and mouth or stuffing it in the mouth. Inhaling from balloons filled with nitrous oxide is one method of using this substance. Some common street names for inhalants or using inhalants are laughing gas (nitrous oxide), snappers (amyl nitrite), poppers (amyl nitrite and butyl nitrite), whippets (fluorinated hydrocarbons, found in whipped cream dispensers), bold (nitrites), and rush (nitrites; National Institute on Drug Abuse [NIDA], 2017). The term ocean water refer to combined alcohol and inhalant use, and snotballs refers to balls of rubber cement that are heated before inhalation (Storck, Black, & Liddell, 2016). Other common street terms for inhalants include moon gas, Oz, poor man's pot, Medusa, and hippie crack (Alliance for Consumer Education, 2016).

THE EPIDEMIOLOGY OF INHALANT USE

The National Survey on Drug Use and Health reported that 9.6% of the U.S. population used inhalants at least once in their lives (Center for Behavioral Health Statistics and Quality, 2016). This includes 9.10% of those in the 12-to-17 age group and 13.1% of those aged

13 to 17. Inhalant use in 2016 was reported at 0.7% for ages 12 and up, with 2.7% in the 12-to-17 age group, 4.1% in the 18-to-25 age group, and 0.3% in those 26 and older reporting past-year use. In addition, past-month use was 0.20% for ages 12 and up, with 0.7% in the 12-to-17 age group, 0.9% in the 18-to-25 age group, and 0.1% in those 26 and older.

The peak age of inhalant use is 14 to 15 years, but children as young as 5 or 6 years have been reported as inhalant users (Storck et al., 2016). However, findings from the Monitoring the Future survey, which has been reporting on substance use in 8th, 10th, and 12th graders since 1975, suggest that inhalant use has declined over time in this age group. Among 8th graders, lifetime inhalant use was 7.7% in 2016 compared with 9.4% in 2015. Among 10th graders, lifetime inhalant use was 6.6% in 2016 compared with 7.2% in 2015. Similarly, lifetime inhalant use among 12th graders was 5% in 2016 compared with 6.7% in 2015 (Johnston, O'Malley, Miech, Bachman, & Schulenberg, 2017). The frequency of use in this age group is variable; the majority of youth use inhalants once or twice as an "experiment," but about 20% progress to use that is severe enough to be diagnosed as an inhalant use disorder (Nguyen, O'Brien, & Schapp, 2016).

Although rates of use have declined, they remain a concern due to the young age at which inhalant use is initiated and the risk of sudden death and long-term impairments that can occur. Inhalants are referred to as "kid drugs" (Johnston et al., 2017, p. 15) because of their easy accessibility, lower cost than other substances of abuse, and lack of penalties for possession. A particularly worrisome trend among adolescents is the decreased perceptions of risk from inhalant use. Risk perception was high in this age group between 2001 and 2008 due to a media campaign sponsored by the Partnership

for a Drug-Free America in 1995 and 1996, which focused on the negative health effects of inhalant use. Policymakers have expressed concern about decreased perceptions of risk in the current cohort of 8th, 10th, and 12th graders, who have not been exposed to anti-inhalant messaging in the media (Johnston et al., 2017), and recommend new initiatives to promote anti-inhalant messages for this age group.

Some demographic trends in inhalant use are noteworthy. Some research shows that females in 8th and 10th grades use inhalants more frequently than males in this age group, but this trend appears to reverse by 12th grade. In addition, females are more likely to report recent use, but males are more likely to engage in severe use that requires hospitalization (Halliburton & Bray, 2016). Native Americans, Latinos, and Caucasians are more likely to use inhalants compared with other ethnic groups, and use among Native American adolescents is reported to be up to three times higher compared with adolescents in other ethnic groups. In addition, age at initial use is significantly younger among Native Americans compared with other ethnic groups. Use among rural populations is higher than use in urban populations, particularly in areas plagued by poverty, unemployment, and violence (Nguyen et al., 2016).

THE BIOCHEMICAL EFFECTS AND CATEGORIES OF INHALANTS

The chemicals in inhalants are rapidly absorbed through the lungs into the bloodstream. Inhalants are lipophilic and cross the blood-brain barrier into the lipid-rich organs, such as the central nervous system (CNS), peripheral nervous system, and adipose tissue (Filley, 2013). The onset of inhalant effects is rapid, and effects dissipate quickly. In animal models, inhalant intoxication is evident 20 seconds after use, peak effect occurs at 4 minutes, and return to baseline occurs at 8 minutes (Ford, Sutter, Owen, & Albertson, 2014). Within seconds, users experience an initially pleasurable "high" with euphoria, followed by lightheadedness, impulsivity, excitement, disinhibition, a sensation of floating, and a sense of feeling powerful (Nguyen et al., 2016; Storck et al., 2016). Other common effects include visual, auditory, somatic, and tactile hallucinations (Ford et al., 2014).

There are four general categories of inhalants (see Table 12-1). Volatile solvents are liquids that vaporize at room temperature. These are found in such common household and industrial goods as paint thinners and removers, dry-cleaning fluids, gasoline, correction fluids, and felt-tip markers. Some of the chemicals in these products include trichlorethylene, benzene, methylene chloride, and toluene. A street name for toluene is tolly.

Aerosols are the second category; these are sprays that contain propellants and solvents, such as hair sprays, spray paints, deodorants, and vegetable sprays. The chemicals associated with these products include butane and propane.

The third category is gases. Gases include household and commercial products as well as medical anesthetics. Of the medical anesthetic gases, nitrous oxide is the most frequently abused and can be found in whipped cream dispensers and products that increase octane levels in racing cars. Some common street names for nitrous oxide include whippets, laughing gas, and buzz bombs.

The fourth category, nitrites, includes cyclohexyl nitrite, isoamyl (amyl) nitrite, and isobutyl (butyl) nitrite. Street names include poppers, snappers, bullets, Amys, Ames, or pearl. Although nitrites are prohibited by the Consumer Product Safety Commission, they can still be found in products labeled as video head cleaners, room deodorizers, leather cleaners, or liquid aroma (NIDA, 2017). Nitrites are a special class of inhalants in that they, unlike the other inhalant categories, do not act on the CNS but act directly on the blood vessels and muscles. They dilate the vessels, increase heart rate, create a sensation of heat and excitement, and cause such other effects as dizziness and

TABLE 12-1: CATEGORIES OF INHALANTS		
Categories of Inhalants	**Products Used as Inhalants**	**Chemicals Found in Inhalants**
Volatile solvents	Paint thinners, paint removers, dry-cleaning fluids, gasoline, glue, correction fluids, felt-tip markers, degreasers	Methylene chloride, toluene, benzene, trichlorethylene
Aerosols	Spray paints, deodorant and hair sprays, vegetable oil sprays, fabric protector sprays	Hydrofluorocarbons
Gases	Medical anesthetics, gases in household products (butane lighters, propane tanks, whipped cream dispensers, and refrigerants)	Ether, chloroform, halothane, nitrous oxide, butane, propane, Freon
Nitrites	Video head cleaner, room deodorizers, leather cleaner, liquid aroma	Cyclohexyl nitrite, isoamyl (amyl) nitrite, isobutyl (butyl) nitrite

Note. From National Institute on Drug Abuse. (2012). *Inhalants.* Retrieved from https://www.drugabuse.gov/publications/research-reports/inhalants/what-are-inhalants

headaches. Nitrites are also used to enhance sexual function (NIDA, 2017).

DIAGNOSTIC CRITERIA FOR INHALANT-RELATED DISORDERS

The *Diagnostic and Statistical Manual of Mental Disorders,* fifth edition *(DSM-5;* American Psychiatric Association [APA], 2013) recognizes four inhalant-related disorders: inhalant use disorder, inhalant intoxication, other inhalant-induced disorders, and unspecified inhalant use disorders. Inhalant use disorder is characterized by problematic use leading to clinically significant impairment or distress. Problematic use is evident in the presence of at least two distinctive patterns of use over a 12-month period. These include inhalant use in larger amounts or over a longer period than intended, persistent desire or unsuccessful attempts to cut down on use, spending excessive time on activities to obtain inhalants or recover from inhalant use, craving to use inhalants, failure to fulfill role obligations due to use, continued use despite problems, giving up important activities to use, recurrent use in hazardous situations, continued use despite knowledge of the problems caused by use, and tolerance to inhalant use. As with all substance-related disorders, the *DSM-5* classifies severity of use according to the number of these symptoms seen in the individual. Mild inhalant use disorder is characterized by the presence of two or three symptoms, moderate is characterized by the presence of four or five symptoms, and severe is characterized by six or more symptoms.

Inhalant intoxication results from recent, short-term, high-dose exposure to inhalants. Behavioral symptoms of inhalant intoxication include belligerence, aggressiveness, apathy, and impaired judgment that occur dur-

ing or shortly after use. In addition, two or more of the following signs or symptoms may be seen: dizziness, nystagmus, incoordination, slurred speech, unsteady gait, lethargy, depressed reflexes, psychomotor retardation, tremor, generalized muscle weakness, blurred vision or diplopia, stupor or coma, and euphoria. Inhalant-induced disorders include anxiety and depression resulting from inhalant use, and unspecified inhalant use disorders refer to significant distress and/or impairments in functioning resulting from inhalant use that do not meet the full criteria for an inhalant use disorder (APA, 2013).

THE ADVERSE HEALTH EFFECTS OF INHALANTS

The medical consequences of inhalant use can be severe. The most drastic consequence of use is death; inhalants have a greater fatality rate than any other pharmaceutical or nonpharmaceutical agent (Storck et al., 2016). Fatality rates from inhalant use in the United States are estimated at 100 to 125 deaths per year (Nguyen et al., 2016). The syndrome known as sudden sniffing death can occur in an otherwise healthy patient (Drug Enforcement Agency [DEA], 2015). In this syndrome, sniffing highly concentrated amounts of butane, propane, or aerosols results in acute cardiac toxicity and ventricular arrhythmias, such as ventricular fibrillation (Ford et al., 2014). Immediate death can also occur from suffocation, which may occur when inhaling from a paper or plastic bag in a closed area, convulsions or seizures, coma, choking on vomit after inhalation, or a fatal injury suffered while intoxicated (DEA, 2015). In addition, inhalant use causes motor incoordination, which may result in fatalities in motor vehicle accidents (Woodward & Beckley, 2014).

Chronic abuse can cause severe damage to several body systems. The most significant is damage to the brain and other parts of the CNS. Volatile solvents such as toluene can damage the protective sheath around certain nerve fibers in the brain and peripheral nervous system. Atrophy of the cerebrum, cerebellum, and brain stem can also occur (Filley, 2013). Neurological syndromes will reflect damage to the part of the brain involved, resulting in changes in cognition, movement, vision, or hearing. Major neurotoxic syndromes seen in patients exposed to organic solvents include optic neuropathy with ocular flutter and nystagmus, ototoxicity (damage to the ears, hearing problems), and encephalopathy (Filley, 2013; Ford et al., 2014). Cerebellar ataxic syndrome, mild to severe dementia, parkinsonism, and peripheral neuropathy can also occur (Storck et al., 2016).

Other organs of the body can also be affected by exposure to solvents. Toluene and chlorinated hydrocarbons can cause cardiomyopathy and damage to the liver and kidneys. Methylene chloride can cause a reduction of the oxygen-carrying capacity of the blood and changes to the heart muscle and heartbeat. Nitrous oxide causes megaloblastic anemia, which may clinically resemble pernicious anemia. Benzene, which is found in gasoline, can cause bone marrow injury, impaired immunologic function, an increased risk of leukemia, and reproductive toxicity (Ford et al., 2014). Chronic inhalant use causes death from cardiomyopathy, CNS toxicity, aplastic anemia, leukemia, hepatocellular carcinoma, and renal diseases, such as nephritis, nephrosis, and tubular necrosis (Storck et al., 2016).

Nitrites are a special category. The chemicals in nitrites can cause dangerously low blood pressure, enlarged blood vessels, tachycardia, dizziness, and headaches (NIDA, 2017). Poppers contain isobutyl nitrite, which can cause "pop-per maculopathy" and permanent vision loss (Gruener, Jeffries, El-Housseini, & Whitefield, 2014). Because nitrites are often used to enhance sexual function, research shows that abuse of these drugs is associated with unsafe sexual practices, increasing the risk of sexually transmitted infections. Use of nitrous oxide can cause methemoglobinemia, a condition affecting the function of red blood cells (Ford et al., 2014); in addition, there is a link to the development of other infectious diseases and tumors because of impairment to the immune system and red blood cells (NIDA, 2017).

SCREENING OF SPECIAL POPULATIONS AND RISK IDENTIFICATION

Youth are at particular risk for inhalant use (DEA, 2015). Risk factors associated with inhalant use among youth include delinquency, a history of childhood physical or sexual abuse (Nguyen et al., 2016; Snyder & Howard, 2015), and a history of traumatic brain injury with loss of consciousness (Snyder & Howard, 2015). Other risk factors include parental criminality, low rates of parental oversight or absence of parents in the home, and parental or older sibling drug use. Inhalant users often have comorbid psychiatric disorders, such as conduct disorder and attention-deficit hyperactivity disorder. Use of other substances, including tobacco, cannabis, alcohol, opiates, and benzodiazepines, is also common with inhalant use (Nguyen et al., 2016).

Early identification and intervention are the best public health measures in addressing this problem. Ford and colleagues (2014) stress that urine drug screening is not effective in detecting inhalant use because there are numerous volatile substances that can be used, each with a different metabolite, and biological tests have not been developed to detect each of these metabolites. Therefore, screening for inhalant use involves an assessment of the patient's appearance, along with physical and behavioral signs and symptoms. These include chemical odors on breath or clothing; paint or other stains on face, hands, or clothes; disheveled appearance; hidden empty spray paint or solvent containers found near the patient; chemical-soaked rags or clothing; and drunk or disoriented appearance. Physical signs include dermatitis, a perioral or perinasal rash known as huffer's rash, conjunctivitis, rhinitis, and frequent nose bleeds (Storck et al., 2016). Inhalant users may also have anorexia with weight loss and gastrointestinal problems. Other behavioral symptoms include chronic fatigue, somatization, chronic confusion, poor concentration, depression, irritability, hostility, and paranoia (Nguyen et al., 2016; Storck et al., 2016).

Women who are pregnant are a special population for consideration. There have been some case reports noting abnormalities in newborns and subsequent developmental impairments. Although there is limited research that links exposure to a specific birth defect or developmental problem, some animal studies have found that toluene or trichloroethylene can result in toluene embryopathy (microcephaly and CNS dysfunction), reduced birth weight, and neonatal withdrawal (Ford et al., 2014; Storck et al., 2016).

TREATMENT

Primary prevention of the development of inhalant use disorders involves accessibility issues and education (Nguyen et al., 2016). Ease of access can be curtailed by raising the prices of inhalants to make them unaffordable to adolescents, clearly marking containers of inhalants regarding their abuse potential, and limiting store displays and accessibility in stores. However, these strategies increase the risk of emergence of a black market that can continue to make inhalants easily accessible for users.

Parents also need to be aware of the abuse potential of inhalants and limit the availability of inhalants in the home (Storck et al., 2016). Storck and colleagues (2016) further recommend that parents have a "broad index of suspicion" (p. 505) for use due to the young age in which inhalant use can start. Education via media campaigns is also a primary prevention strategy, particularly regarding the risk of sudden death and long-term cognitive problems that can result from inhalant use.

Secondary prevention targets patients who have preclinical symptoms but have not yet developed a pattern of use consistent with a clinical diagnosis of inhalant use disorder. Treatment involves the use of life skills and communication training to resist peer pressure to use inhalants, along with cognitive therapy to identify, examine, and challenge normative beliefs and positive perceptions about inhalant use (Nguyen et al., 2016).

When inhalant intoxication is suspected, primary attention needs to focus on maintaining the patient's airway, breathing, and circulation through supportive measures. These include intubation, if needed, and oxygen and resuscitation in the event of cardiac arrest. There are no antidotes to reverse the effects of inhalant intoxication (Ford et al., 2014).

If the patient presents with anxiety, depression, or psychosis due to inhalant use, psychopharmacologic treatment is used to address these symptoms. Clinicians who specialize in substance use recommend that benzodiazepines should be avoided in the treatment of anxiety related to inhalant use because "they may enhance the depressant effect of inhalants" (Hassan, Bhatia, & Bhatia, 2017, p. 140)

Some clinicians have proposed that there may be an inhalant withdrawal syndrome that starts about 24 hours after use and may last for several days. Symptoms include irritability, nausea, and dry mouth. It is important to note that inhalants are lipophilic and may remain in the body for an extended period of time, possibly for 2 to 6 weeks (Nguyen et al., 2016). This can cause confusion and interfere with participation in a treatment program after detoxification (Nguyen et al., 2016). Some research suggests that the effects of acute high- and low-level exposure to organic solvents are completely reversible, but chronic neurotoxic injury related to solvents is slowly and incompletely reversible and usually does not progress upon cessation of exposure (Storck et al., 2016).

Treatment of adolescent inhalant use disorders is similar to the treatment approaches for other addictions in this age group (Nguyen et al., 2016). Psychotherapeutic interventions that have shown effectiveness in reducing inhalant use in adolescents include cognitive-behavioral therapy, brief motivational interviewing (Storck et al., 2016), and family therapy. Culturally sensitive therapy can incorporate the social customs of indigenous groups and address the specific cultural identities and norms that predispose youth to inhalant use (Nguyen et al., 2016).

SUMMARY

Inhalant use continues to be an important public health issue. Although use has declined, it continues to present concerns about the potential for sudden death and long-term neurological consequences. Inhalants are unique among substances of abuse because of the lack of control over access, relatively low cost, lack of penalties for possession, and early age of initial use. Pediatric, family practice, and child or adolescent psychiatric providers are challenged to continue screening, prevention, and intervention efforts to reduce use. Parents, teachers, and adolescents need to be aware of the risks and long-term complications of use. Increasing public awareness of the serious and often irreversible effects associated with inhalant use is crucial in these prevention efforts.

EXAM QUESTIONS

CHAPTER 12
Questions 67–71

Note: Choose the one option that BEST answers each question.

67. The peak age of inhalant use is

    a. 10 to 12 years.

    b. 14 to 15 years.

    c. 16 to 18 years.

    d. 20 to 22 years.

68. A class of inhalants that does not act on the central nervous system but instead has a direct effect on the muscles and blood vessels is

    a. volatile solvents.

    b. aerosols.

    c. nitrites.

    d. gases.

69. Inhalant use leading to significant impairment or distress is diagnosed as

    a. inhalant intoxication.

    b. inhalant-induced disorder.

    c. inhalant use disorder.

    d. anxiety and depression.

70. A sign or symptom to note in an inhalant use screening includes

    a. elation.

    b. hyperactivity.

    c. dermatitis.

    d. obesity.

71. When inhalant intoxication is suspected, the primary treatment concern is

    a. assessing for signs of inhalant use, such as skin rashes and conjunctivitis.

    b. brief motivational interviewing.

    c. life skills training.

    d. maintaining airway, breathing, and circulation.

REFERENCES

Alliance for Consumer Education. (2016). *Inhalants.* Retrieved from http://www.con sumered.org/learn/inhalant-abuse

American Psychiatric Association. (2013). *Diagnostic and statistical manual of mental disorders* (5th ed.). Arlington, VA: Author.

Center for Behavioral Health Statistics and Quality. (2016). *Key substance use and mental health indicators in the United States: Results from the 2015 National Survey on Drug Use and Health* (HHS Publication Number [SMA] 16-4984, NSDUH Series H-51). Retrieved from http://samhsa.gov/data

Drug Enforcement Agency. (2015). *Drugs of abuse.* Washington, DC: U.S. Department of Justice.

Filley, C. M. (2013). Toluene abuse and white matter: A model of toxic leukoencephalopathy. *Psychiatric Clinics of North America, 36,* 293-302.

Ford, J. B., Sutter, M. E., Owen, K. P., & Albertson, T. E. (2014). Volatile substance misuse: An updated review of toxicity and treatment. *Clinical Review of Allergies and Immunology, 46,* 19-33.

Gruener, A. M., Jeffries, M. A. R., El-Housseini, Z., & Whitefield, L. (2014). Poppers maculopathy. *Lancet, 384*(9954), 1606.

Halliburton, A. E., & Bray, B. C. (2016). Long-term prevalence and demographic trends in U.S. adolescent inhalant use: Implications for clinicians and prevention scientists. *Substance Use and Misuse, 51,* 343-356.

Hassan, A., Bhatia, S. C., & Bhatia, S. K. (2017). Inhalant use disorder. In S. C. Bhatia, F. Petty, & T. Gabel (Eds.), *Substance and nonsubstance related addiction disorder: Diagnosis and treatment* (pp. 136-142). Potomac, MD: Bentham Science Publishers.

Johnston, L. D., O'Malley, P. M., Miech, R. A., Bachman, J. G., & Schulenberg, J. E. (2017). *Monitoring the Future national survey results on drug use, 1975-2016: Overview, key findings on adolescent drug use.* Ann Arbor, MI: Institute for Social Research, the University of Michigan.

National Institute on Drug Abuse. (2012). *Inhalants.* Retrieved from https://www.drug abuse.gov/publications/research-reports/ inhalants/whatare-inhalants

National Institute on Drug Abuse. (2017). *Commonly abused drug charts: Inhalants.* Retrieved from https://www.drugabuse. gov/drugs-abuse/commonly-abused-drugs- charts#inhalants

Nguyen, J., O'Brien, C., & Schapp, S. (2016). Adolescent inhalant use prevention, assessment, and treatment: A literature synthesis. *International Journal of Drug Policy, 31,* 15-24.

Snyder, S. M., & Howard, M. O. (2015). Patterns of inhalant use among incarcerated youth. *PLoS One, 10*(9), e0135303. doi:10.1371/journal.pone.0135303

Storck, M., Black, L., & Liddell, M. (2016). Inhalant abuse and dextromethorphan. *Child and Adolescent Psychiatric Clinics of North America, 25,* 497-508.

Woodward, J. J., & Beckley, J. (2014). Effects of the abused inhalant toluene on the mesolimbic dopamine system. *Journal of Drug and Alcohol Use, 3,* 1-8. doi:10.4303/jdar/235838

CHAPTER 13

HALLUCINOGENS

LEARNING OUTCOME

After completing this chapter, the learner will be able to discuss the acute effects and health risks related to hallucinogen use disorders.

CHAPTER OBJECTIVES

After completing this chapter, the learner will be able to:

1. Discuss the history of hallucinogenic substances and how their use has evolved.

2. Identify the hallucinogenic substances most commonly used.

3. Describe the physiological and psychological effects of hallucinogens.

4. Identify the health risks associated with hallucinogen use disorders.

5. Select appropriate treatment strategies for hallucinogen use disorders.

INTRODUCTION

Hallucinogens are drugs that cause dramatic alterations in mood and thought. People under the influence of hallucinogenic drugs commonly report seeing images, hearing sounds, and feeling sensations that seem real but do not exist (National Institute on Drug Abuse [NIDA], 2016b). The drug class name "hallucinogens" is somewhat misleading because these substances do not consistently produce hallucinations – defined as false perceptions with no basis in reality – but rather, they cause changes in mood and thought (U.S. Drug Enforcement Agency [DEA], 2013).

HISTORY OF HALLUCINOGENIC SUBSTANCE USE

Hallucinogens include both naturally occurring substances, such as plants and fungi, and synthetically produced substances, such as lysergic acid diethylamide (LSD). Historically, naturally occurring hallucinogens have been used by many different cultures for thousands of years in healing ceremonies and rites of passage (MacLean, Johnson, & Griffiths, 2015). The first synthetic hallucinogen was accidentally discovered in 1938 by researchers in a Sandoz laboratory who were conducting medical research on lysergic acid compounds. These compounds are derived from the fungus ergot, which develops on ryegrass. While searching for a therapeutic ergot-derived analeptic agent, researchers created dozens of lysergic acid compounds. LSD-25 was discovered by a Swiss chemist named Albert Hoffmann. Five years later, in 1943, he accidentally ingested some of the drug and experienced some frightening sensory effects and perceptual distortions, leading to the discovery of the drug's hallucinogenic effects (Liester, 2014; Smith, Raswyck, & Davidson, 2014). He also described the hallucinogenic effects as the perception of a transcendence of time and space and a sense of eternity, with the loss of boundaries between the past, present, and future and beyond three-dimensional space (DeGregorio, Comai, Posa, & Gobbi, 2016). Later, the U.S. Central Intelligence Agency conducted human experiments with LSD, testing its use as an interrogation tool and as a control agent (Smith et al., 2014).

In the early 1960s, Timothy Leary, a psychology instructor at Harvard University, began experimenting with hallucinogens. Leary claimed that LSD provided instant happiness and enhanced creativity in art and music, facilitated problem-solving ability in school and at work, and increased self-awareness, as an aid to psychotherapy (Smith et al., 2014). Leary was not reappointed to the faculty of Harvard and became a self-proclaimed martyr for the LSD cause. In the early years, LSD users banded together, organized their lives around the use of the drug, and ultimately created a subculture. Initially, users were young adults about 21 years of age, and they usually used only LSD.

By the late 1960s, the cultural revolution was actively being influenced by LSD, psychedelics, and other hallucinogenic compounds such as mescaline and psilocybin (Smith et al., 2014). The media publicized the introduction of LSD and indirectly aided in its growth. Musicians, rock music, the hippie lifestyle, and flower children were loosely associated with the Leary philosophy. Eventually, the use of LSD spread through all socioeconomic groups, particularly middle-class and affluent youth. Users of LSD became more involved in poly-drug misuse. Leary's exhortations to "turn on, tune in, and drop out" were interpreted as anti-social messages that encouraged youth to disconnect from their parents' established cultural and social norms, which heightened fear of hallucinogen use among the general population (Haden, Emerson, & Tupper, 2016).

As the popularity and use of hallucinogens increased, so did the reporting of adverse effects. The reporting of "bad trips" and resulting accidents and suicides focused attention on the seriousness of the LSD problem. In late 1966, Sandoz Laboratories stopped distributing the drug, and all existing supplies of the drug were turned over to the government, which made the drug available only for legitimate concerns. In 1967, the federal government classified LSD as a Schedule I drug (no currently accepted medical use and a high potential for misuse), and in 1970, it continued to be classified a Schedule I drug according to the Comprehensive Drug Abuse Prevention and Control Act (DEA, 2013).

Currently, hallucinogens have no established medical use. However, some researchers and clinicians view the restricted availability of hallucinogens since the 1960s as a lost opportunity for research into the pharmacologic properties and potential psychotherapeutic use of these drugs (Smith et al., 2014). Some researchers have advocated for the use of hallucinogens in the treatment of anxiety and depression in terminally ill patients with cancer (Smith et al., 2014).

Hallucinogens are a diverse group of substances that differ in their chemical structures, mechanisms of action, and adverse effects (NIDA, 2015). Most of the naturally occurring hallucinogens can be recreated synthetically, and the synthetics are more potent than their natural forms. The main groups of hallucinogens include lysergamides (LSD, morning glory seeds, or Hawaiian woodrose), indolealkylamines (psilocybin, psilocin, bufotenin, dimethyltryptamine [DMT], 5-MeO-DMT), phenylethylamines (mescaline, methamphetamines, 3,4-methylenedioxy-N-methylamphetamine [MDMA], 3,4-methylenedioxy-N-ethylamphetamine [MDEA], 3-methoxy-4,5-methylenedioxyamphetamine [MMDA], 2,6-dimethoxy-4-methylamphetamine [DOM]), piperidines (ketamine, phencyclidine [PCP]), cannabinols (marijuana, hashish), and dextromethorphan. The best-known and one of the most powerful hallucinogens is LSD. Synthetic hallucinogens include the N-methoxybenzyl (NBOMe) drugs.

EPIDEMIOLOGY

The National Survey on Drug Use and Health (Center for Behavioral Health Statistics and Quality, 2016) reported that in 2015, about 1.2 million people in the United States were current users of hallucinogens, which represents about 0.5% of the population 12 years and older. Among those who reported having used a hallucinogen in the past month, the highest use was among those aged 18 to 25 years, at 1.8%. About 0.2% of those 26 years and older reported past-month use.

Hallucinogen use decreased among younger adolescents (8th through 10th graders) from 2015 to 2016. The Monitoring the Future survey (Johnston, O'Malley, Miech, Bachman, & Schulenberg, 2017) reported that in 2016, 1.9% of 8th graders reported lifetime use of hallucinogens compared with 2.0% in 2015, and in 2016, 4.4% of 10th graders reported lifetime use of hallucinogens compared with 4.6% in 2015. However, rates of hallucinogen use among 12th graders increased from 2015 to 2016. In 2016, 6.7% of 12th graders reported lifetime use of hallucinogens compared with 4.4% in 2015 (Johnston et al., 2017).

BIOCHEMISTRY

LSD is structurally similar to the neurotransmitter serotonin, which modulates mood, pain, sensory perception, personality, sexual activity, and other biological functions. Researchers and clinicians have proposed that the effects of hallucinogens are caused by serotonin receptor agonism on the 5HT1a and 5HT2a receptors (Sutter, Chenoweth, & Albertson, 2014) and possibly dopamine receptors at higher doses (Halberstadt, 2017). The effects occur most commonly in the prefrontal cortex, which regulates mood, cognition, and perception (NIDA, 2015).

TYPES AND CATEGORIES OF HALLUCINOGENS

Lysergamides

Lysergamides include naturally occurring morning glory seeds and LSD. As mentioned previously, LSD was initially produced from the ergot alkaloids from the fungus *Claviceps purpurea,* a contaminant of wheat and rye flour. LSD is now synthesized from lysergic acid and is a clear or white, odorless, water-soluble material. The crystal can be crushed into a powder and mixed with binding agents to produce tablets known as "microdots" or thin squares of gelatin known as "window panes." It is most commonly diluted and applied to paper known as "blotter acid." Today, the typical dose of LSD is 20 to 80 μg. The effects of LSD begin about 30 to 90 minutes after ingestion and continue for about 8 to 12 hours, with the peak effect noted at about 4 hours (Liester, 2014). LSD is known by various street names, usually referring to the pattern printed on the blotter paper, such as *'cid, acid, Bart Simpsons,* and *Sandoz.* Table 13-1 provides a list of LSD street names. LSD is usually taken orally as a pill or liquid or by placing LSD-soaked paper in the buccal or sublingual space (NIDA, 2016b).

The effects of LSD vary dramatically with the amount of the drug ingested and the user's personality, mood, expectations, and surroundings. Users of LSD refer to the effects of the drug as a "trip" (NIDA, 2016b). Initially, users experience

TABLE 13-1: SELECTED STREET NAMES FOR LSD

Acid

Blotter

Blue heaven

Cubes

Microdot

Yellow sunshine

Note. From National Institute on Drug Abuse. (2016a). *Commonly abused drug charts.* Retrieved from https://www.drugabuse.gov/drugs-abuse/commonly-abused-drugs-charts

TABLE 13-2: EFFECTS OF LSD

Physical

Dilated pupils

Higher body temperature

Increased heart rate

Elevated blood pressure

Increased sweating

Loss of appetite or nausea

Dizziness

Sleeplessness

Dry mouth

Tremors

Numbness

Weakness

Psychological

Intense sensory experiences

Mixing of senses (hearing colors, seeing sounds)

Distorted sense of time

Distorted body image

Impulsiveness

Rapid emotional shifts

Fear of

- Losing control
- Insanity
- Death

Flashbacks, which may cause

- Distress
- Impairment of functioning

Paranoia

Confusion

Acute panic (bad trip)

Note. Adapted from National Institute on Drug Abuse. (2015). *Hallucinogens and dissociative drugs.* Retrieved from https://www.drugabuse.gov/publications/research-reports/hallucinogens-dissociative-drugs

dizziness, paresthesias, weakness, and tremors. Later, users experience a marked increase in vision and auditory changes, mood changes, altered time sense, and depersonalization. Sensory input becomes mixed together, and users report "hearing" colors or "seeing" smells. Emotions are often labile and intense, shifting rapidly through a range from fear to euphoria. The sense of touch is significantly magnified (NIDA, 2015).

Symptoms of a transient depression may occur after LSD use. The major physiologic effects of the drug include increased blood pressure and heart rate, dizziness, dilated pupils, loss of appetite, dry mouth, sweating, nausea, numbness, and tremors (NIDA, 2015). Table 13-2 provides a list of the effects of LSD.

During the peak effects of LSD, users usually experience a decrease in the ability to make sensible judgments and avoid common dangers, making them susceptible to personal injury. Occasionally, users experience acute panic reactions, referred to as a "bad trip" (NIDA, 2016b). Some fatal accidents have occurred during states of LSD intoxication, yet no deaths have been reported due to LSD ingestion alone, regardless of the dose.

LSD is not considered a physically or psychologically addictive drug because it does not produce compulsive drug-seeking behavior. LSD does produce tolerance, so users who take the drug repeatedly must take progressively higher doses to achieve their desired level of intoxication (NIDA, 2015). LSD use also creates a cross-tolerance to other hallucinogenic drugs, such as psilocybin and mescaline. Drug tolerance resolves after several days without substance use. Most LSD users usually limit themselves to taking the drug once or twice per week. There are no withdrawal symptoms experienced with stopping LSD use. One of the most dangerous aspects of LSD is its remarkably unpredictable effects, even in experienced users (Das, Barnwal, Ramasamy, Sen, & Mondal, 2016).

Indolealkylamines

Indolealkylamines include the two mushroom-derived substances psilocybin and psilocin, DMT, and bufotenine. Psilocybin and psilocin are obtained from certain mushrooms found in parts of South America, Mexico, and the United States. These substances can produce muscle relaxation or weakness, dilation of pupils, ataxia, altered perception of time, and an inability to discern fantasy from reality (NIDA, 2015). These substances are normally consumed as dried or brewed mushrooms. The effects are not predictable because they depend on the type of mushroom used and the age and preservation of the extract. The mushrooms cause fewer adverse reactions than LSD, although some short-term effects include nervousness, paranoia, and panic reactions (NIDA, 2015). Often, these mushrooms are either accidentally or purposely mis-identified, with only about one third of them being "magic mushrooms," as they are referred to on the street. Many times, the product is simply store-bought mushrooms laced with PCP.

DMT is an indole alkaloid found in various plants and seeds. It can be produced synthetically (Carbonaro & Gatch, 2016; NIDA, 2016b). The drug is ineffective when taken orally. However, shamanic tribes may take it orally as a brewed

tea containing a plant alkaloid known as harmala, which prevents DMT metabolism (DEA, 2016). This allows sufficient DMT absorption to produce a "high" when taken orally. The usual route of administration for this drug is sniffing, smoking, or snorting. It also can be ingested as a tea known as ayahuasca. Ingestion of DMT causes very brief and intense episodes of psychedelic effects, particularly visual hallucinations (Carbonaro & Gatch, 2016). The experience associated with this drug is short (less than 1 hour) and has been nick-named the "businessman's trip."

Bufotenine is a hallucinogenic serotonin that is chemically similar to DMT. It can be found in certain mushrooms and seeds but most notably in frog or toad (*Bufo* genus) skins. The toads produce venom that also has psychoactive properties. Users lick or milk the toads for their venom, which may then be ingested or smoked. Bufotenin (5-OH-DMT) is a tryptamine related to the neurotransmitter serotonin.

Phenylethylamines

A third group of hallucinogens includes phenylethylamine derivatives and other halluci-nogenic amphetamines. The crown of the peyote plant – a small, spineless cactus – consists of disk-shaped buttons that are generally chewed or soaked in water to produce an intoxicating liquid. The effects start about 30 minutes to 2 hours after ingestion and last for up to 12 hours. Mescaline, a psychogenic amphetamine, occurs naturally in the peyote cactus but can also be synthetically produced. Historically, this sub-stance has been ingested during religious cer-emonies by natives of northern Mexico and the southwestern United States, and pre-Colombian Mesoamerican tribes used it for thousands of years (Carod-Artal, 2015). Today some Native American groups use hallucinogens in religious ceremonies; such use has been legally protected by the American Indian Religious Freedom Act since 1994 (Hardaway, Schweitzer, & Suzuki,

2016). Nausea, vomiting, diaphoresis, and ataxia usually precede the hallucinogenic experience. In addition, short-term effects of peyote include hyperthermia, tachycardia, ataxia, profound diaphoresis, and flushing (NIDA, 2015).

Many of the hallucinogenic amphetamines are synthetically produced analogs of mescaline and amphetamine, otherwise known as designer drugs. These drugs include 3,4-methylenedioxy-N-ethylamphetamine (MDEA) and 3,4-methylenedioxy-methamphetamine (MDMA also known as Ecstasy or E), and all have similar psychogenic and stimulant effects (NIDA, 2016c). MDMA is taken orally, usually in the form of a tablet or a capsule. The average reported dose is one to two tablets, and the effects usually last for about 3 to 6 hours. Users of the drug will often take a second dose of the drug as the effects begin to subside. MDMA is rapidly absorbed into the bloodstream, and the drug's metabolites interfere with the body's ability to break down the drug. This can potentially result in dangerously high levels of the drug with repeated dosing in short intervals.

MDMA has become a popular synthetic drug that alters both mood and perception (NIDA, 2016c). Users experience feelings of mental stimulation, increased energy, emotional warmth, empathy toward others, decreased anxiety, and a general sense of well-being. A hallmark of MDMA is enhanced sensory perceptions, especially enjoyment of tactile stimulation. The stimulant effect of this drug allows the users to dance for extended periods, which is associated with dehydration and the potentially fatal adverse effects of severe increases in body temperature (NIDA, 2016c).

The effects of MDMA are caused by altering the activity of many neurotransmitter systems in the brain, including those for serotonin, dopamine, and norepinephrine. The surge in euphoria and energy is caused by the release of dopamine. Norepinephrine release causes physiologic side effects, such as tachycardia and hypertension. The release of serotonin likely causes a sense of empathy and emotional closeness to others (NIDA, 2016c). The drug damages serotonergic axon terminals and causes neuronal cell inflammation and death, which results in long-term impairments in cognitive functioning and mood disorders (Halpin, Collins, & Yamamoto, 2014).

Adverse effects of MDMA include hyperthermia, nausea, muscle spasms and cramping, involuntary teeth clenching, blurred vision, chills, and sweating (NIDA, 2016c). In addition, moderate use of MDMA over the course of a week may cause irritability, impulsiveness, aggression, depression, insomnia, anxiety, and anorexia. MDMA is thought to be less addictive compared with cocaine, but some users report withdrawal symptoms, such as fatigue, anorexia, depression, and difficulty with concentration. The drug markedly decreases the user's ability to process information, making it dangerous for users to perform complex or skilled tasks. Overdose symptoms of MDMA include high blood pressure, faintness, panic attacks, loss of consciousness, and seizures. The half-life of MDMA is 12 to 34 hours, so complications of MDMA toxicity need to be monitored for several days (Woo & Hanley, 2013). NIDA (2016c) stresses that although MDMA is assumed to be "pure" by users, it may contain additives, such as cocaine, ketamine, methamphetamine, over-the-counter (OTC) cough medicine, or synthetic cathinones (bath salts). These additives increase the risk for severe adverse consequences of MDMA use.

NBOMe Drugs

NBOMe drugs are hallucinogens that are synthetic derivatives of phenylethylamines (Lawn, Barrett, Williams, Horne, & Winstock, 2014). The most commonly used NBOMe drugs are 25B-NBOMe, 25C-NBOMe, and 25I-NBOMe.

Common street names include N-Bomb, smiles, legal acid, 25I, 25B, and 25C. These hallucinogens are sold as legal substitutes for LSD and mescaline. They act on serotonin receptors and are much more powerful hallucinogens compared with LSD (NIDA, 2013). They are typically used as powders and liquid solutions that are "laced" on edible items (DEA, 2013, p. 1) and soaked onto blotter papers. The most common routes of use are oral, buccal, and sublingual (Lawn et al., 2014). The DEA (2013) reports that extremely small amounts of these substances can cause seizures and cardiac and respiratory arrest. At least 19 deaths were linked to the use of NBOMe between March 2012 and August 2013 (DEA, 2013).

Dissociative Anesthetics

Dissociative anesthetics include PCP and ketamine, which were developed in the 1950s and 1960s, and dextromethorphan, which has more recently attracted attention from drug awareness groups. These drugs produce sedative and anesthetic effects. The original purpose for these substances was as anesthetic agents. PCP was approved for veterinary use only; however, ketamine, which was developed after PCP, was approved for both human and veterinary uses. Today, much of the legal ketamine is diverted from veterinary offices to be used illegally.

The effects of PCP are extremely unpredictable and dose dependent. Users may appear wild, calm, disoriented, violent, stuporous, or comatose. The dissociative nature of PCP causes users to be at increased risk for trauma because they perceive little or no harm to their bodies. PCP is associated with a higher risk of death than other hallucinogens due to complications related to severe agitation and hyperthermia (NIDA, 2016b).

Ketamine has experienced a resurgence since the 1970s and is a popular drug at all-night dance parties and raves. This drug has a shorter duration than PCP and is much less potent. It is also known as the date rape drug and has been related to the commission of sexual assaults because it produces a sense of detachment and an amnesia effect.

Like PCP and ketamine, dextromethorphan is an N-methyl-D-aspartate (NMDA) antagonist that can produce dissociative effects. Dextromethorphan, also known as DXM or robo, is a cough suppressant found in many OTC medications. The most common source of misused dextromethorphan is extra-strength cough syrup, which typically contains 3 mg of the drug per milliliter of syrup. The drug is generally considered safe and effective in therapeutic doses. The effects are dose related: users experience mild stimulation with ingestion of 100 to 200 mg, euphoria and hallucination at 200 to 400 mg, and distorted visual perceptions and loss of motor coordination at 300 to 600 mg. Users experience dissociative sedation with ingestion of 500 to 1,500 mg of dextromethorphan (DEA, 2017).

Dextromethorphan is commonly used among adolescents due to its availability as an OTC drug, legality, cost, safety, and production of euphoric and hallucinatory effects. Routine urine drug screens do not test for dextromethorphan (Hardaway et al., 2016). Because this is a common OTC drug, most adolescents fail to recognize the health risks associated with high doses. A serious concern related to consuming large amounts of OTC cough medications and cold products is the unintended toxicity from pseudoephedrine, acetaminophen, and antihistamines. High doses of acetaminophen can cause liver toxicity and ultimately liver failure. In addition, about 10% of Caucasians are poor metabolizers of dextromethorphan, which increases their risk of overdose and death with use of dextromethorphan (DEA, 2016). It is important for nurses, primary care providers, pharmacists, educators, counselors, and parents to be aware of this recent trend so that they can help identify potential misuse situations.

Cannabinols

Marijuana contains the psychoactive substance tetrahydrocannabinol (THC), which is found in the leaf or flower of the plant. This substance is grouped with hallucinogens but rarely causes hallucinations. It is available both naturally and synthetically. The leaves of the plant are smoked and create changes in mood and perception, laughter, increased appetite, conjunctival infection, tachycardia, and minimal central nervous system (CNS) depression. Marijuana remains the most commonly misused illegal drug under the federal Controlled Substances Act.

Salvia

Salvia is a plant-based hallucinogen from the perennial mint family that is commonly grown in southern Mexico and Central and South America (NIDA, 2016b). It functions as a kappa opioid agonist (DEA, 2013; Hutton, Kivell, & Boyle, 2016). Common street names include "diviner's sage," "Maria Pastora," "Sally-D," and "magic mint" (NIDA, 2015). The hallucinogenic effects of salvia are very intense and include perceptions of bright lights, vivid colors and shapes, time and space distortions, dissociation, perceptions of changes of bodily forms (such as arms turning into tree branches), and a dream-like state (Hutton et al., 2016). Some users have reported feelings of intense fear, anxiety, and paranoia with use (Hutton et al., 2016). Negative effects include dizziness, mental slowing, and physical exhaustion.

HEALTH EFFECTS

Acute anxiety and panic reactions are the most common problems related to the use of such hallucinogens as LSD or mescaline, which can be addressed with calm reassurance

(Sadock, Sadock, & Ruiz, 2015). The effects of these drugs are extremely unpredictable and vary even in the same patient on different occasions. Someone with a previous pleasant experience on LSD may have an unpleasant experience or bad trip during a subsequent use. The anxiety and paranoia commonly resolve within 24 hours as the drug is metabolized by the body. Deaths from acute overdose of LSD and mescaline are very rare; fatalities most often occur due to dangerous behavior, suicide, accidents, or accidental ingestion of a poisonous mushroom. NBOMe drugs can cause serious renal problems, including acute tubular necrosis due to ischemia (Luciano & Perazella, 2014). PCP or ketamine overdose can cause respiratory depression, coma, seizures, and death due to respiratory arrest (DEA, 2017).

The risk of depression and suicide can last for days after LSD ingestion. A thorough psychiatric examination needs to be conducted with these patients to differentiate among paranoid schizophrenia, LSD psychosis, and other drug-induced psychoses. Toxicology laboratory studies may be helpful, but standard toxicology screens detect only a few hallucinogenic agents. Substances readily identified by standard toxicology screens include MDMA (positive for amphetamines), PCP, and marijuana. Generally, the priority of care is to stabilize the patient and then provide supportive treatment.

Long-term effects of hallucinogens include psychoses, depressive reactions, acting out, paranoid states, and flashbacks (NIDA, 2015). Flashbacks spontaneously occur weeks to months after the original drug experience and may or may not resemble the original drug experience. The experience involves such perceptual and reality distortion as seeing motion on the edges of the field of vision or bright or colored flashes of light. Additionally, psychosis can develop after hallucinogen use, but it remains unclear whether the drugs cause or have a role in precipitating the illness. Chronic personality changes, such as shifts in attitudes and the onset of magical thinking, can occur with the use of hallucinogens.

Common effects of dissociative drugs, such as PCP and ketamine, depend on the dose. Low to moderate doses can cause disorientation, dizziness, nausea, and vomiting, along with increases in blood pressure, heart rate, respiratory rate, and body temperature. High doses can cause dangerously high blood pressure, heart rate, respiratory rate, and body temperature. In addition, high doses of dissociative drugs can cause severe psychological distress, such as extreme panic, fear, anxiety, and paranoia. They can also cause the perception of "invulnerability" (NIDA, 2015, p. 6) and exaggerated strength, as well as aggression. Use of dissociative drugs with alcohol and other CNS depressants can cause respiratory depression and death (NIDA, 2015).

Complications, such as severe hyperthermia, seizures, rhabdomyolysis, myoglobinuric renal failure, and disseminated intravascular coagulation, have been seen with these drugs (Sadock et al., 2015). PCP has also been associated with memory loss and depression that can persist for years after the drug use has stopped.

DIAGNOSTIC CRITERIA

The *Diagnostic and Statistical Manual of Mental Disorders,* fifth edition (*DSM-5*; American Psychiatric Association [APA], 2013) provides the criteria for hallucinogen use disorder, described as a pattern of problematic hallucinogen use that is characterized by two or more of the following in a 12-month period:

- Hallucinogen taken in larger amounts or over a longer period than intended
- Persistent desire to cut down use or unsuccessful attempt to cut down on use

- A great deal of time devoted to obtaining, using, or recovering from use
- Craving
- Failure to fulfill obligations due to use
- Continued use despite persistent problems resulting from use
- Reducing or stopping important activities due to use
- Recurrent use in situations in which it is hazardous to do so
- Continued use despite an awareness of the negative consequences of use

Tolerance also occurs, which is characterized by a diminished effect of the same amount of the hallucinogen over time or the need for increasing amounts of the hallucinogen over time to achieve the original effect (APA, 2013). The *DSM-5* notes that withdrawal syndromes from hallucinogens have not been established (APA, 2013).

Additional *DSM-5* disorders related to hallucinogen use include phencyclidine intoxication, hallucinogen intoxication, and hallucinogen persisting perception disorder (HPPD). Phencyclidine intoxication is diagnosed in a patient with recent PCP use and is associated with clinically significant problematic behavioral changes, such as belligerence, aggression, impulsiveness, unpredictability, psychomotor agitation, and impaired judgment. Within 1 hour of PCP use, two or more of the following signs and symptoms may be evident:

- Vertical or horizontal nystagmus
- Hypertension or tachycardia
- Numbness or diminished response to pain
- Ataxia
- Dysarthria
- Muscle rigidity
- Seizures

- Coma

- Hyperacusis (heightened sensitivity to sound)

The APA (2013) notes that these symptoms emerge very rapidly when PCP is smoked, snorted, or used intravenously.

Hallucinogen intoxication is characterized by the recent use of a hallucinogen, other than PCP, with clinically significant problematic behavioral and psychological changes that occur during or shortly after use (APA, 2013). These changes include anxiety, depression, ideas of reference, paranoid ideation, and impaired judgment. Other symptoms include perceptual changes, depersonalization, illusions, and hallucinations that occur during or shortly after use.

HPPD is characterized by the re-experiencing of one or more of the perceptual symptoms that were experienced during hallucinogen intoxication (APA, 2013). These symptoms can include geometric hallucinations, false perceptions of movement, flashes of color, and intensified colors. They are most commonly identified in people who have used LSD more than 10 times but can even occur after a single use. The prevalence rate of this disorder is about 4.2% of people who use hallucinogens (APA, 2013). The drug-induced psychosis involves a distortion in or disorganization of a patient's capacity to recognize reality, think rationally, and communicate with others. LSD-induced psychosis can last for years and can affect people who have no history or other symptoms of a psychological disorder. Episodes of HPPD, more commonly referred to as flashbacks, are spontaneous, repeated, and sometimes continuous recurrences of some of the sensory distortions originally produced by LSD. Flashbacks can occur for years, normally decreasing in frequency, intensity, and duration over time.

TREATMENT

High schools and colleges are important targets for prevention strategies because adolescents and young adults are the age groups most likely to use hallucinogens. Education continues to be the most promising tool for preventing substance misuse. Clear, accurate dissemination of information regarding the effects of these drugs is essential in treating this problem. Peer-led advocacy programs and drug prevention programs are being used in school systems because they incorporate the importance of social context and networks (Substance Abuse and Mental Health Services Administration, 2012a, 2012b). Most LSD users voluntarily decrease or stop its use over time because it is not an addictive drug. In addition, the experience of using certain hallucinogens, such as salvia, can be intense and negative, which deters people from subsequent use (Hutton et al., 2016).

There are no specific treatments for MDMA or Ecstasy misuse. Generally, cognitive-behavioral therapies (CBTs) and motivational interventions are designed to help modify users' thinking, expectancies, and behaviors; to improve their coping skills; and to enhance their self-efficacy in stopping use (Hardaway et al., 2016). CBT is based on social learning theories and emphasizes modification of the patient's thoughts and behaviors. The goal is to encourage abstinence by helping patients learn and master effective coping skills that can help them believe they can resist relapsing to substance misuse. The focus is on the exploration of positive and negative consequences of substance use. This approach is the foundation for relapse prevention because patients are taught the skills needed to prevent a return to substance misuse. Narcotics Anonymous may be effective when combined with behavioral interventions to create periods of long-term drug-free recovery.

Ketamine is a very addictive drug and has no specific treatments. Current behavioral therapies for chemical addictions such as those mentioned previously are also recommended for patients misusing ketamine. Support groups and recovery networks are helpful to patients in maintaining drug-free periods.

Treatment for acute hallucinogenic intoxication is variable and depends on the purity of the substance, the dose, the setting, and the individual. Emergency department visits are often related to a "bad trip." The primary goal of treatment is harm prevention for the user and those around him or her. The treatment space should be quiet, softly lit, and separated from large groups of people. Calm the user by speaking in a reassuring and confident manner. Always address users by name and remind them often of who they are and who you are. If possible, do not leave someone alone when he or she is experiencing an adverse reaction.

There is no antidote to PCP intoxication, and treatment is supportive (Sadock et al., 2015). Because environmental stimuli can cause unpredictable or violent reactions in patients with PCP intoxication, sensory stimuli should be minimized as much as possible (Sadock et al., 2015). Antipsychotics or benzodiazepines can be used for sedation, but neuroleptic medications with anticholinergic activity should be avoided due to the high anticholinergic activity caused by PCP (Sadock et al., 2015). PCP intoxication can produce seizures and severe hypertension, which should be treated with antiepileptic and antihypertensive medications.

There have been no specific treatments identified for patients with chronic hallucinogen use. However, some evidence suggests that HPPD can be successfully treated with haloperidol, benzodiazepines, and clonidine (Hardaway et al., 2016). Neuroleptics, such as chlorpromazine, phenothiazines, and 5HT2a antagonists, such as risperidone, should be avoided due to the risk of a paradoxical effect and worsening of HPPD symptoms (Hardaway et al., 2016). No one behavioral treatment appears to be more effective than another. (Hardaway et al., 2016). These therapies are usually initiated after the detoxification period. Behavioral therapies are important strategies that assist the patient in preventing relapse to substance misuse.

Behavioral treatment can be delivered at an individual or a group level and can last for a single session (such as a brief intervention) or for 1 year or more. Additional approaches that may complement care include self-help or 12-step groups, family-based treatment, acupuncture, and faith-based groups.

CASE STUDY 13-1

Phil is a 20-year-old college student. He is in his junior year and is majoring in communications. He lives in a fraternity house on his college campus. Phil remembers going to a rave with some friends from his fraternity. The friends report that an acquaintance at the rave gave Phil two capsules, which he ingested. About 1 hour later, he became agitated and fell on the floor due to uncontrollable muscle spasms, at which point his friends brought him to the local hospital. Upon admission to the emergency department, Phil was very agitated and repeatedly stated, "Don't let me die. I don't want to die."

Phil's vital signs upon admission were as follows: blood pressure 156/98 mm Hg; heart rate 152 beats/min; respiratory rate 32 breaths/min; temperature 105.8°F (41.0°C). Phil's laboratory studies were as follows: potassium 6.5 mEq/L; sodium 127 mEq/L; creatine kinase (CK) 5,640 U/L; creatinine 172 μmol/L. In addition, Phil's toxicology screen was positive for marijuana, and his urine MDMA level was 1.3. Phil's urinalysis was positive for proteinuria.

The nurse in the emergency room then conducts a brief past medical history with Phil:

Tobacco: smokes about one pack per day

Substance use: marijuana and alcohol at weekend fraternity parties

Medical diagnoses: none

Medications: none

The nurse then explains to Phil that he is going to be admitted to the intensive care unit (ICU), where he will be closely monitored for severe complications, such as acute kidney injury and heart rhythm disturbances.

Questions

1. What is Phil's most likely diagnosis?

2. What are the treatment priorities for Phil?

3. What are Phil's potential complications that need monitoring in the ICU?

Answers

1. Assessment data support the diagnosis of MDMA intoxication with hyperthermia, hyperkalemia, hyponatremia, and rhabdomyolysis (i.e., a condition characterized by muscle necrosis and the release of intracellular muscle constituents into the circulation). Hyperthermia is supported by a fever of 105.2°F. Hyperkalemia is supported by a potassium level of 6.5 mEq/L (normal range 3.5-4.5 mEq/L). Hyponatremia is supported by a sodium level of 127 mEq/L (normal range 135-145 mmol/L). Rhabdomyolysis is supported by a CK level of 5,640 U/L (normal range 10-200 U/L), creatinine level of 172 μmol/L (normal range 50-95 μmol/L), and the presence of proteinuria.

2. Treatment priorities for Phil include rapid fever reduction, stabilization of potassium and sodium levels, hydration, reduction of muscle spasms, and sedation. Interventions to reduce fever should include cooling blankets or ice packs applied to the neck, groin, and axillary areas. Hydration needs to be maintained with intravenous fluids. Benzodiazepines can be used for sedation and treatment of muscle spasms (Woo & Hanley, 2013).

3. Potential complications include seizures, cardiac arrhythmias, and acute renal failure. Seizure precautions also need to be implemented. In addition, Phil will require continuous cardiac monitoring via telemetry. Rhabdomyolysis can cause acute renal failure due to the release of myoglobin from muscle tissue. Phil's urine output, renal function, and electrolytes will all need to be closely monitored. Because the half-life of MDMA is 12 to 34 hours, Phil will need to be monitored over several days.

SUMMARY

Historically, naturally occurring hallucinogens have been used by many different cultures for medicinal, religious, and recreational purposes. In the late 1930s, synthetic hallucinogens were created.

The rise and decline of LSD use can be documented through the cultural revolution of the 1960s. Although LSD is among the most potent synthetically produced hallucinogens, its use has been consistently decreasing over the past several years, and the DEA does not expect a change in this encouraging pattern.

EXAM QUESTIONS

CHAPTER 13
Questions 72–76

Note: Choose the one option that BEST answers each question.

72. The hallucinogenic effects of LSD were originally identified in

    a. 1943 when Dr. Albert Hoffman accidentally consumed the substance.

    b. the 1950s when the Central Intelligence Agency tested its use as an interrogation tool.

    c. 1950 when synthesized in a Harvard University laboratory.

    d. 1962 when Timothy Leary discovered the compound.

73. A dissociative drug commonly used by adolescents is

    a. dextromethorphan.

    b. ketamine.

    c. peyote.

    d. phencyclidine.

74. High doses of dissociative drugs such as phencyclidine can cause

    a. disorientation and dizziness.

    b. low blood pressure, heart rate, and respiratory rate.

    c. nausea and vomiting.

    d. severe psychological stress, including panic and fear.

75. Use of dissociative drugs with alcohol and other central nervous system depressants can cause

    a. transient depression.

    b. recurring flashbacks.

    c. respiratory depression and death.

    d. phencyclidine and hallucinogen intoxication.

76. Which is a true statement regarding behavioral treatment for patients with chronic hallucinogen use?

    a. Behavioral treatment is most effective when initiated before detoxification.

    b. No one behavioral treatment appears to be more effective than another.

    c. Twelve-step groups are more effective than cognitive-behavioral therapies.

    d. Contingency management is the most effective behavioral treatment for these patients.

REFERENCES

American Psychiatric Association. (2013). *Diagnostic and statistical manual of mental disorders* (5th ed.). Washington, DC: Author.

Carbonaro, T. M., & Gatch, M. B. (2016). Neuropharmacology of N,N-dimethyltryptamine. *Brain Research Bulletin, 126*(Pt. 1), 74-88.

Carod-Artal, F. J. (2015). Hallucinogenic drugs in pre-Colombian Mesoamerican cultures. *Neurologia, 30,* 42-49.

Center for Behavioral Health Statistics and Quality. (2016). *Key substance use and mental health indicators in the United States: Results from the 2015 National Survey on Drug Use and Health* (HHS Publication No. SMA 16-4984, NSDUH Series H-51). Retrieved from http://www.samhsa.gov/data

Das, S., Barnwal, P., Ramasamy, A., Sen, S., & Mondal, S. (2016). Lysergic acid diethylamide: A drug of "use"? *Therapeutic Advances in Psychopharmacology, 6*(3), 214-228. doi: 10.1177/2045125316640440

DeGregorio, D., Comai, S., Posa, L., & Gobbi, G. (2016). D-lysergic acid diethylamide (LSD) as a model of psychosis: Mechanism of action and pharmacology. *International Journal of Molecular Sciences, 17*(11), 1-20. doi:10.3390/ijms17111953

Drug Enforcement Agency (2016). *N,N-dimethyltryptamine (DMT).* Retrieved from https://www.deadiversion.usdoj.gov/drug_chem_info/dmt.pdf

Haden, M., Emerson, B., & Tupper, K. W. (2016). A public-health-based vision for the management and regulation of psychedelics. *Journal of Psychoactive Drugs, 48*(4), 243-252.

Halberstadt, A. L. (2017). Hallucinogenic drugs: A new study answers old questions about LSD. *Current Biology, 27,* R15158.

Halpin, L. E., Collins, S. A., & Yamamoto, B. K. (2014). Neurotoxicity of methamphetamine and 3, 4, methylenedioxymethamphetamine. *Life Sciences, 97* (1), 37-44.

Hardaway, R., Schweitzer, J., & Suzuki, J. (2016). Hallucinogen use disorders. *Child and Adolescent Clinics of North America, 25,* 489-496.

Hutton, F., Kivell, B., & Boyle, O. (2016). "Quite a profoundly strange experience": An analysis of the experiences of *Salvia divinorum* users. *Journal of Psychoactive Drugs, 48*(3), 206-213.

Johnston, L. D., O'Malley, P. M., Miech, R. A., Bachman, J. G., & Schulenberg, J. E. (2017). *Monitoring the Future national survey results on drug use, 1975-2016: Overview, key findings on adolescent drug use.* Ann Arbor, MI: Institute for Social Research, University of Michigan.

Lawn, W., Barrett, M., Williams, M., Horne, A., & Winstock, A. (2014). The NBOMe hallucinogenic drug series: Patterns of use, characteristics of users and self-reported effects in a large international sample. *Journal of Psychopharmacology, 28*(8), 780-788.

Liester, M. (2014). A review of lysergic acid diethylamide (LSD) in the treatment of addictions: Historical perspectives and future prospects. *Current Drug Abuse Reviews, 7,* 146-156.

Luciano, R. L., & Perazella, M. A. (2014). Nephrotoxic effects of designer drugs: Synthetic is not better! *Nature Reviews: Nephrology, 10*(6), 314-324. doi:10.1038/nrneph.2014.44

MacLean, K. A., Johnson, M. W., & Griffiths, R. R. (2015). Hallucinogens and club drugs. In M. Galanter, H. D. Kleber, & K. T. Brady (Eds.), *Textbook of substance abuse treatment* (5th ed., pp. 209-222). Washington, DC: American Psychiatric Publishing.

National Institute on Drug Abuse. (2013). Other drugs: "N-bomb." Retrieved from https://www.drugabuse.gov/drugs-abuse/other-drugs

National Institute on Drug Abuse. (2015). *Hallucinogens and dissociative drugs.* Retrieved from https://www.drugabuse.gov/publications/research-reports/hallucinogens-dissociative-drugs

National Institute on Drug Abuse. (2016a). *Commonly abused drug charts.* Retrieved from https://www.drugabuse.gov/drugs-abuse/commonly-abused-drugs-charts

National Institute on Drug Abuse. (2016b). *Drug facts: Hallucinogens.* Retrieved from https://www.drugabuse.gov/publications/drugfacts/hallucinogens

National Institute on Drug Abuse. (2016c). *Drug facts: MDMA (Molly/Ecstasy).* Retrieved from https://www.drugabuse.gov/publications/drugfacts/mdma-ecstasymolly

Sadock, B. J., Sadock, V. A., & Ruiz, P. (2015). *Kaplan & Sadock's synopsis of psychiatry, behavioral sciences/clinical psychiatry* (11th ed.). Philadelphia, PA: Wolters Kluwer.

Smith, D. E., Raswyck, G. E., & Davidson, L. D. (2014). From Hofmann to the Haight Ashbury, and into the future: The past and potential of lysergic acid diethylamide. *Journal of Psychoactive Drugs, 46*(1), 3-10.

Substance Abuse and Mental Health Services Administration. (2012a). *Results from the 2011 national survey on drug use and health: Summary of national findings* (NSDUH Series H-44, HHS Publication No. SMA 12-4713). Rockville, MD. Retrieved from http://www.samhsa.gov/data/NSDUH/2k11Results/NSDUHresults2011.htm

Substance Abuse and Mental Health Services Administration. (2012b). *Treatment Episode Data Set (TEDS) 2000-2010: National admissions to substance abuse treatment services.* Retrieved from http://www.samhsa.gov/data/2k12/TEDS2010N/TEDS2010NWeb.pdf

Sutter, M. E., Chenoweth, J., & Albertson, T. E. (2014). Alternative drugs of abuse. *Clinical Review of Allergies and Immunology, 46,* 3-18.

U.S. Drug Enforcement Agency. (2013). *Hallucinogens.* Retrieved from https://www.dea.gov/druginfo/drug_data_sheets/Hallucinogens.pdf

U.S. Drug Enforcement Agency. (2016). *N,N dimethyltryptamine (DMT).* Retrieved from https://www.deadiversion.usdoj.gov/drug_chem_info/dmt.pdf

U. S. Drug Enforcement Agency. (2017). *Drugs of abuse: A DEA resource guide (2017 edition).* Retrieved from https://www.dea.gov/pr/multimedia-library/publications/drug_of_abuse.pdf

Woo, T. M., & Hanley, J. R. (2013). "How high do they look?" Identification and treatment of common ingestions in adolescents. *Journal of Pediatric Healthcare, 27*(2), 135-144.

CHAPTER 14

DESIGNER DRUGS

LEARNING OUTCOME

After completing this chapter, the learner will be able to discuss the current use of designer drugs as well as their adverse health risks.

CHAPTER OBJECTIVES

After completing this chapter, the learner will be able to:

1. Identify populations at risk for using designer drugs.

2. Explain the biochemistry and drug effects of the designer drugs most commonly used.

3. List the adverse health risks related to the use of designer drugs.

4. Review effective prevention strategies and treatment interventions for patients using, or at risk for the use of, designer drugs.

INTRODUCTION

Designer drugs are synthetic derivatives of federally controlled substances, created by slightly altering the molecular structure of existing drugs. They are manufactured illegally for illicit use. Today's most frequently used designer drugs are 3,4-methylenedioxy-N-methamphetamine (MDMA; Ecstasy), flunitrazepam (Rohypnol), gamma-hydroxybutyrate (GHB), ketamine, synthetic cathinones (bath salts), synthetic cannabinoids (Spice), and synthetic hallucinogens (National Institute on Drug Abuse [NIDA], 2016a, 2016c, 2016d, 2016e). Lysergic acid diethylamide (LSD) and methamphetamine are also considered designer drugs but are not included here because they have been discussed in depth in previous chapters.

AT-RISK POPULATIONS AND EMERGING DESIGNER DRUG TRENDS

Use of designer drugs is most prevalent among young adults at bars, nightclubs, and concerts (NIDA, 2016a). They are also used during covert dance events known as raves (Joe-Laider, Hunt, & Moloney, 2014), in which young people gather in abandoned buildings or warehouses to listen to electronic dance music that is often accompanied by bright lights and visual effects. Use of MDMA during raves may intensify the experience of the rave environment and provide a sense of euphoria and connectedness with other rave attendees (Joe-Laider et al., 2014). Central nervous system depressants, such as flunitrazepam and GHB, are known as date-rape drugs due to their sedating and amnesic effects; these drugs have been reported as contributing factors in sexual victimization among females on college campuses (Belknap & Sharma, 2014).

The emergence of designer drugs, known as "legal" highs, presents significant challenges to clinicians and drug enforcement officials. The process of synthesizing designer drugs slightly alters the chemical structures of commonly used illicit drugs while retaining their ability to cause alterations in mood and consciousness. Designer drugs can be illegally manufactured by people with no training in chemistry by obtaining the necessary instructions, chemicals, and equipment via the Internet. Therefore, designer drugs are not detectable by standard drug-screening tests due to their altered chemical structure (Weaver, Hopper, & Gunderson, 2015); the chemical structures of these drugs are constantly changed to evade legal regulation and detection.

Substance use clinicians and researchers have expressed concern that the rapid and continuous introduction of new drugs on the market is one of the primary reasons for problems with drug use in the United States, stressing that "the forces of containment are always playing catch-up with the forces of encouragement and exploitation" (Johnston, O'Malley, Miech, Bachman, & Schulenberg, 2017, p. 52). Regulatory legislation regarding designation of these new drugs as controlled substances is often delayed due to the speed with which new drugs appear on the market (Sutter, Chenoweth, & Albertson, 2014). Drug enforcement officials and healthcare providers often become aware of new designer drugs after they have caused significant harm (Patterson, Young, & Vaccarino, 2017). However, the Synthetic Drug Abuse Prevention Act in 2012 included synthetic cannabinoids, which has reduced the availability of some of these drugs (Nelson, Bryant, & Aks, 2014). Table 14-1 provides a list of designer drugs and their most common street names.

Global drug enforcement agencies that provide surveillance for new drug emergence and use are monitoring almost 500 designer drugs, and 98 of these were newly discovered in 2015 (Patterson et al., 2017). Although use is most prevalent in Europe, North America, and Australia, new markets for designer drugs are emerging around the globe (Dolliver & Kuhns, 2016). Global access to new designer drugs is facilitated by websites that serve as "virtual drugstores" (Dolliver & Kuhns, 2016, p. 322). These websites include Silk Road, Evolution, and Pandora. An encrypted website known as Tor allows anonymous drug purchasing and trading transactions that are financed with Bitcoins, which are untraceable (Dolliver & Kuhns, 2016).

EPIDEMIOLOGY

The growing popularity of designer drugs is thought to be related to their relatively low cost and their intoxicating highs. Attempts to measure the prevalence rates of use of designer drugs are difficult due to the rapid emergence of new drugs, unreliable reporting, and the inability of routine drug testing to detect use (Sutter et al., 2014). The annual Monitoring the Future (MTF) survey began to measure the use of synthetic cathinones (bath salts) among 8th, 10th, and 12th graders in 2016. Past-year use of synthetic cathinones was reported by 0.9% of 8th graders, 0.8% of 10th graders, and 0.8% of 12th graders during 2016 (Johnston et al., 2017). The MTF survey also began monitoring the use of GHB among 12th graders in 2016. The survey reported that in 2016, 0.9% of 12th graders reported past-year use of GHB (NIDA, 2016a). Use of MDMA has increased since 2015 among adolescents. According to the MTF survey, 8th graders reported lifetime MDMA use at 1.7% and past-month use at 1.0%, 10th graders reported lifetime use at 2.8% and past-month use at 1.8%, and 12th graders reported lifetime use at 4.9% and past-month use at 2.7% (NIDA, 2016a). Poison control centers monitor reports of poisoning from several designer drugs, including Spice and bath salts. In 2012, poison control centers recorded 5,225 cases

TABLE 14-1: DESIGNER DRUGS – COMMON STREET NAMES

Drug	Common Street Names
3,4-methylenedioxy-N-methamphetamine (MDMA)	Adam Clarity Eve Lover's Speed Peace Uppers Molly Ecstasy X
Gamma hydroxybutyrate or sodium oxybate (GHB)	G Georgia Home Boy Goop Grievous Bodily Harm Liquid Ecstasy Liquid X Soap Scoop
Flunitrazepam (Rohypnol)	Roofies Rophies Roach Rochas Forget-me pill Rope
Ketamine	K Special K Vitamin K Cat valium
Synthetic cathinones	Bath salts (e.g., Ivory Wave, Vanilla Sky)
Synthetic cannabinoids	Spice K2 K9 Aroma Herbal Highs
Synthetic hallucinogens	N-bomb Solaris Smiles

Note. From National Institute on Drug Abuse. (2016b). *Commonly abused drug charts.* Retrieved from https://www.drugabuse.gov/drugs-abuse/commonly-abused-drugs-charts

of Spice exposure, with six deaths reported from synthetic cannabinoid products (Dart et al., 2015). Bath salt use accounted for 6,137 cases of exposure and 31 deaths reported to poison control centers in 2011. However, bath salt use decreased in 2012, with 994 exposures and 16 deaths reported to national poison control centers (Dart et al., 2015).

THE BIOCHEMISTRY AND DRUG EFFECTS OF EMERGING CLASSES OF DESIGNER DRUGS

The exact chemical composition of designer or club drugs is not clear. These illegal drugs are manufactured with uncertain drug sources or pharmacological agents and uncertain contaminants, resulting in uncertain toxicity profiles (NIDA, 2016a; Weaver et al., 2015). For example, product analyses suggest that synthetic cathinones may be adulterated with a variety of other substances, such as lidocaine, procaine, caffeine, cocaine, amphetamines, ketamine, and piperazine compounds (Weaver et al., 2015). This results in inconsistencies in the amounts, purity, and potency of these compounds (Patterson et al., 2017). The varied nature of the designer drugs makes reporting of their effects, symptoms, consequences, and toxicities more difficult.

Synthetic Cannabinoids

Synthetic cannabinoids (SCs) are chemicals that resemble the properties of the naturally occurring cannabinoids in the marijuana plant (NIDA, 2015). SCs are classified in a group of drugs known as "new psychoactive substances" (NIDA, 2015). Common street names for SCs include K2, Spice, fake weed, Joker, Black Mamba, Kush, Kronic, Smashed, Bombay Blue, and Moon Rocks.

Before 2011, SCs were sold in drug paraphernalia stores, head shops, and gas stations, typically marketed as herbal incense or potpourri (Spaderna, Addy, & D'Souza, 2013). SCs are sprayed on plant materials and then smoked in a cannabis pipe, smoked in a water pipe, or rolled in cigarette paper (Spaderna et al., 2013). The onset of action of SCs occurs within minutes when absorbed through the lungs (Woo & Hanley, 2013). Additionally, SCs can be consumed as a vaporized liquid or brewed as a tea (NIDA, 2015). The 2012 Synthetic Drug Abuse Prevention Act classified SCs as Schedule I drugs due to their high misuse potential and lack of medical benefit (NIDA, 2015). SCs are now illegal to sell, buy, or possess (Kemp et al., 2016).

Manufacturers repeatedly change the chemical composition of SCs to avoid detection by drug testing, which presents a risk in that the user does not really know what he or she is consuming. In addition, the dose of active ingredient in an SC is typically unknown due to unregulated manufacturing, and it can be laced with a variety of additives, ranging from flavorings to other substances such as rat poison or embalming fluid (Kemp et al., 2016). It is important to note that SCs such as Spice are chemicals that act on cannabinoid receptor agonists and mimic the action of marijuana. Spice should not be confused with legal synthetic marijuana or cannabis developed for medical purposes, such as nabilone (Cesamet) or dronabinol (Marinol; Kemp et al., 2016).

The psychological effects of synthetic cannabinoids include elevated mood, relaxation, and altered perceptions and awareness of surroundings. Psychosis can also occur, which includes delusional thinking that is not supported by reality. Psychosis is also associated with extreme anxiety, confusion, extreme distrust of others (paranoia), and visual and auditory hallucinations (sensations, sounds, and images that are not perceived by others or supported by reality; NIDA, 2015).

Flunitrazepam (Rohypnol)

Flunitrazepam and GHB are both predominantly central nervous system (CNS) depressants. These drugs have been associated with date rape (Sutter et al., 2014). They are ingested orally, and their effects remain constant for about 8 to 10 hours. The drugs are odorless, tasteless, and colorless, making it relatively simple for them to be added to beverages and ingested without ever being detected. Flunitrazepam is a benzodiazepine that is chemically similar to diazepam (Valium) and alprazolam (Xanax). Short-term effects of flunitrazepam include sedation, confusion, amnesia, and muscle relaxation, as well as impairments in reaction time, motor coordination, mental functioning, and judgment (NIDA, 2016b).

Gamma-Hydroxybutyrate

GHB is a precursor to gamma-aminobutyric acid, and it is known for its euphoric and sedative effects. Bodybuilders have used GHB to improve fat reduction and muscle growth. GHB reaches a high level in the blood 15 to 30 minutes after ingestion, with effects lasting about 3 hours. The neurologic effects of GHB intoxication include depressed consciousness, unresponsiveness, and amnesia at high doses (Sutter et al., 2014). It can also cause disorientation, aggressiveness, and hallucinations. Both flunitrazepam and GHB cause lethal respiratory depression when mixed with alcohol (NIDA, 2016a).

Ketamine

Ketamine is an anesthetic that has been approved for both human and animal use. It is commercially available in the form of a liquid. This drug causes a dissociative, dreamlike state and hallucinations. It is commonly evaporated using a hot plate or microwave oven, which yields a powder that is either snorted, dabbed on the tongue, or smoked (NIDA, 2016c). The onset of the desired dissociative effect is rapid and lasts about 45 to 60 minutes. The molecular function of ketamine is similar to that of phencyclidine (PCP); they both inhibit the neuronal reuptake of serotonin, norepinephrine, and dopamine (Sutter et al., 2014).

Synthetic Cathinones

Synthetic cathinones are chemically similar to a stimulant found in the khat plant (NIDA, 2016e). They are called "bath salts" because they are sold over the counter in head shops as seemingly harmless products, such as incense, jewelry cleaners, and plant food. Use of three synthetic cathinones – mephedrone, methylone, and methylenedioxypyrovalerone (MDPV) – is reported to be widespread (Karch, 2015). Street names for synthetic cathinones include Bloom, Cloud Nine, Cosmic Blast, Flakka, Ivory Wave, Lunar Wave, Scarface, Vanilla Sky, and White Lightening. NIDA (2016e) reports that products marketed as "Molly" (a form of Ecstasy) may contain synthetic cathinones instead of, or in addition to, MDMA.

Synthetic cathinones are part of the class of drugs known as stimulants (Weaver et al., 2015). They are sold as inexpensive substitutes for stimulants such as methamphetamine and cocaine (NIDA, 2016e). Synthetic cathinones alter the action of several neurotransmitters, such as dopamine, norepinephrine, and serotonin. It is believed that they increase the extracellular release and inhibit reuptake of these neurotransmitters (Weaver et al., 2015).

Common forms of these drugs include a white or brown crystalline powder that is swallowed, snorted, or injected. Use of synthetic cathinones causes euphoria and increased sociability, energy, and sex drive, along with rapid thoughts, reduced appetite, and panic attacks.

Excited delirium, characterized by extreme agitation and violent behavior, can also occur (Ashrafioun et al., 2016; NIDA, 2016e). The effect of the synthetic cathinone known as MDPV is similar to cocaine, but it is 10 times more potent (NIDA, 2016e). The short-term effects of synthetic cathinones include agitation, insomnia, tachycardia, hypertension, nausea, vomiting, diaphoresis, and suicidal thoughts (Ashrafioun et al., 2016; NIDA, 2016e). Synthetic cathinones are addictive and trigger intense cravings for repeated use. Symptoms of withdrawal include depression, anxiety, tremors, insomnia, and paranoia (NIDA, 2016e).

THE ADVERSE HEALTH EFFECTS OF DESIGNER DRUGS

Acute toxicity is common among users of designer drugs and often manifests with a constellation of psychiatric and medical effects, which may be severe (e.g., anxiety, agitation, psychosis, tachycardia). Multiple deaths have also been reported with each class of designer drug (Weaver et al., 2015).

Synthetic Cannabinoids

The immediate effects of SCs are similar to marijuana and include elevated mood, a feeling of well-being, calmness, relaxation, mild changes in perception, and mild memory impairments (NIDA, 2015; Spaderna et al., 2013). Nausea and vomiting can also occur, which may help clinicians distinguish between the use of SCs and marijuana (Woo & Hanley, 2013). NIDA stresses that the effects of SC ingestion are unpredictable and can be severe and life-threatening. Serious adverse effects include extreme anxiety, confusion, agitation, aggression, catatonia, and depersonalization. Neurological effects can also include tremor,

ataxia, nystagmus, hypertonicity, hyperflexion, and hyperextension (Spaderna et al., 2013). Some research suggests that Spice is addictive and that users experience withdrawal when use is stopped; symptoms include craving, headache, hypertension, diaphoresis, and nightmares (Kemp et al., 2016).

Psychosis is a common and serious side effect of SC use. Users experience hallucinations and paranoid delusions, characterized by extreme distrust of others (NIDA, 2015). Hallucinations consist of vivid flashes of light, which users refer to as fractals or trails (Spaderna et al., 2013). Most psychotic symptoms resolve in a few hours, but they occasionally may last for several days (Spaderna et al., 2013). Acute symptoms of psychosis and agitation have been treated with antipsychotics, such as haloperidol, risperidone, olanzapine, or quetiapine, and benzodiazepines, such as lorazepam (Papanti et al., 2013). Supportive treatment included monitoring vital signs, ensuring hydration, and maintaining a calm environment (Spaderna et al., 2013).

Flunitrazepam

Flunitrazepam is not manufactured or approved for any medical use in the United States, but it is manufactured in Europe and Latin America and is the number-one sleep medication in the world. This drug belongs to the pharmacological class of benzodiazepines and has been associated with date rape because it can be given without the victim's knowledge. The drug is colorless, odorless, and tasteless and is usually added to a victim's beverage without his or her knowledge. It causes the victim to be incapacitated, preventing him or her from resisting a sexual assault, and then usually causes amnesia (NIDA, 2014).

Flunitrazepam can be fatal when taken with alcohol or other depressants (NIDA, 2016d).

Neurological effects include sedation, dizziness, memory impairment, decreased coordination, muscle relaxation, decreased blood pressure, slurred speech, impaired judgment, amnesia, loss of inhibitions, loss of consciousness, vision disturbances, and nausea.

Gamma-Hydroxybutyrate

GHB is a CNS depressant that is approved under the medication name sodium oxybate for the treatment of narcolepsy. It is tasteless, colorless, and odorless and is usually added to alcohol and other beverages (NIDA, 2016b). During the 1980s and 1990s, GHB was legally available in health-food stores and was marketed as a bodybuilding supplement and growth hormone booster. It is classified as a Schedule I and Schedule III drug due to concerns about its use as a date-rape drug (Sutter et al., 2014). Short-term effects include euphoria, drowsiness, confusion, memory loss, unconsciousness, seizures, decreased heart rate, and suppression of respiratory drive (NIDA, 2016b; Sutter et al., 2014). The depressant effects of GHB are greatly enhanced when it is used with alcohol. The most frequent symptoms of GHB intoxication include ataxia, disinhibition, loss of consciousness, confusion, seizures, dizziness, extreme drowsiness, stupor, coma, agitation, nausea, and hallucinations (Busardo & Jones, 2015). Cardiac and respiratory arrest occur at high doses (Sutter et al., 2014).

Physical dependence can occur with GHB use, and tolerance and withdrawal are likely after prolonged use. Withdrawal symptoms appear within 24 hours after stopping use and can last up to 6 days. Early GHB withdrawal symptoms include insomnia, anxiety, tremors, vomiting, and sweating. At 6 days after the last dose, anxiety, delirium, confusion, insomnia, and visual hallucinations can also occur. However, episodic symptoms of withdrawal, such as anxiety, confusion, insomnia, and visual hallucinations, can occur up to 15 days after the last dose (Busardo & Jones, 2015). GHB withdrawal is treated with benzodiazepines, such as diazepam and lorazepam, for 1 to 7 days (Busardo & Jones, 2015).

Ketamine

Ketamine is an anesthetic used in veterinary and human medicine. This drug causes dream-like states and hallucinations often described as out-of-body experiences. Ketamine has been associated with date rape due to the dissociative effect of the drug (NIDA, 2016c). Some of the more common adverse effects include seizures, nystagmus, nausea and vomiting, respiratory depression, amnesia, depression, high blood pressure, impaired motor function (e.g., problems with balance and coordination), long-term memory and cognition problems, and renal problems (NIDA, 2016c; Sutter et al., 2014).

Ketamine is currently being investigated in clinical trials for the treatment of major depressive disorder in treatment-resistant patients (Murrough et al., 2013). Ketamine is administered intravenously as a single dose over 40 minutes at 0.5 mg/kg. Symptom reduction is rapid, with peak effects seen 24 hours after infusion. Depression symptoms gradually return over a period of 3 days, and a return to preinfusion levels of depression occurs after 7 days. Researchers and clinicians are encouraged by symptom alleviation in previously treatment-resistant patients with major depressive disorder, but they stress that continued research is needed to investigate the safety and long-term efficacy of ketamine (Murrough et al., 2013).

Synthetic Cathinones

Use of three synthetic cathinones – mephedrone, methylone, and MDPV – appears to cause neurotoxicity, which causes seizures, altered mental status, hyperreflexia, and myoclonus. In particular, MDPV can cause an excited delirium syndrome, characterized by hyper-arousal, confusion, and psychosis (Karch, 2015). Other adverse effects can occur in multiple organ systems. Cardiovascular effects include tachycardia, hypertension, myocarditis, and cardiac arrest. Hematologic adverse effects include disseminated intravascular coagulation, thrombocytopenia, and anemia. Rhabdomyolysis is a risk to the musculoskeletal system (Karila, Megarbane, Cottencin, & Lejoyeux, 2015). Intravenous injection of synthetic cathinones can cause vein blockages, abscess formation, gangrene, and skin erosion. Synthetic cathinones are also nephrotoxic and can cause acute tubular ischemia and necrosis, which in turn can cause renal failure (Luciano & Perazella, 2014).

PREVENTIVE STRATEGIES AND TREATMENT

High schools and colleges are important settings for prevention strategies because adolescents and young adults are most likely to take designer drugs. Identification of at-risk age groups and populations is important. Risk factors for experimental and regular use among adolescents include parents who use substances, poor family relationships with high conflict, and involvement in foster care and the criminal justice system (Weaver et al., 2015). Education continues to be the most promising tool for preventing substance use. Prevention efforts need to stress the uncertainty and unpredictability of designer drug use, with an emphasis on serious and potentially lethal effects (Patterson et al., 2017). Dissemination of clear, accurate information regarding the effects of these drugs is essential to target this problem.

Emergency Care

Designer drugs are illicit substances that have usually been adulterated or substituted and should be considered unknown substances during initial treatment. It is important to remember that many patients who use these drugs are polysubstance users. The safety of the patient, other patients in the emergency department, and emergency department staff needs to be ensured due to the potential for agitation, aggressive behaviors, and violence; this may require sedation and isolation from other patients, as well as physical restraints if the potential for physical harm is imminent (Andrabi, Greene, Moukaddam, & Li, 2015).

When a patient arrives in the emergency department, it is important to attempt to identify the illicit substance consumed and, if possible, obtain a sample of the substance used. Initial care includes maintaining adequate cardiorespiratory system function, evaluating basic laboratory values, taking seizure precautions, and minimizing the risk of self-injury. No standard treatment has been developed for designer drug poisoning. For cases of acute toxicity, Rech, Donahey, Dziedzic, Oh, and Greenhalgh (2015) recommend a treatment order based on the mnemonic ABCDEFG: A = airway maintenance; B = breathing; C = circulation; D = decontamination; E = enhanced elimination; F = focused therapy, or antidote administration; and G = "get tox help" from a toxicologist or poison control consultation. The basic management should be supportive, including cardiac monitoring, pulse oximetry, urinalysis, and a comprehensive chemistry panel to check for electrolyte imbalance, renal toxicity, and possible underlying disorders. Intubation and mechanical ventilation may be needed to maintain a patent airway and prevent respiratory failure (Andrabi et al., 2015; Karila et al., 2015). It is always important to institute seizure precautions.

There are no antidotes available for designer drugs; only supportive care is available. Anxiety and agitation are generally managed with rapid-acting benzodiazepines, such as midazolam (Versed). The hypertension and tachycardia are usually resolved with management of anxiety and agitation. Hyperthermia can be treated with tepid-water baths and fanning. A physical examination is performed to assess for sympathomimetic and serotonergic toxicities. Sympathomimetic toxicity is characterized by hypertension, tachycardia, mydriasis, agitation, diaphoresis, and hyperthermia (Andrabi et al., 2015). Serotonin toxicity is characterized by tremor, hyperreflexia, shivering, confusion, and diaphoresis. Excessive psychomotor agitation that occurs with intoxication presents a risk for rhabdomyolysis, which is treated with intravenous fluids. Laboratory testing is conducted to detect metabolic acidosis.

Behavioral Therapy

Behavioral therapy can be used to help the user gain insight into use and foster motivation to abstain. Generally, cognitive-behavioral therapies (CBTs) are designed to help modify the user's thinking, expectancies, and behaviors; improve coping skills; help the user recognize triggers for use; and assist with planning for avoiding high-risk situations that trigger use (Andrabi et al., 2015). In addition, motivational interviewing can be used to enhance perceptions about the importance of abstinence and foster confidence in the user's ability to abstain. No single, specific behavioral therapy appears to have greater efficacy. Although not typically initiated during the detoxification period, if this time is extended, behavioral therapy should be initiated.

Behavioral treatment can be delivered at an individual or a group level and last for a single session, such as a brief intervention, or for more than 1 year. Historically, Narcotics Anonymous has been effective when combined with behav-ioral interventions to create periods of long-term substance-free recovery.

Flunitrazepam and GHB are also treated with CBTs. GHB can cause a physiological dependence that appears similar to alcohol withdrawal. The user will experience anxiety, tremor, insomnia, and feelings of doom. These symptoms usually resolve within a few weeks. Benzodiazepines can be used with caution to control some of the symptoms (Busardo & Jones, 2015).

Ketamine is an addictive drug and has no specific treatments. Current behavioral therapies for chemical addictions are recommended for treating ketamine use. Support groups and recovery networks are helpful in maintaining drug-free periods.

CASE STUDY 14-1

Jeremy is a 17-year-old male patient who was brought to the emergency department by the police. His parents called the police when he barricaded himself in his room. They report that he destroyed his cell phone and the cell phones of his sister and mother the previous day. In the admission clinical interview, Jeremy states that he is being followed and that he destroyed the phones because they are tapped. He appears guarded but is cooperative with the nurse during the interview. Jeremy further describes seeing multiple flashes of color for the past 3 days, which he states are "darts" coming from the people who are following him, and this has caused him to become stiff. A neurologic examination of Jeremy reveals tremor, ataxia with difficulty walking, hypertonicity, and hyperreflexia. His urine toxicology screen is negative for cannabinoids. There was also a lack of detection of other drugs on Jeremy's standard urine drug-screening test.

Jeremy's past medical history reveals no prior psychiatric illnesses or treatment. He had a tonsillectomy at age 6 and a broken arm at age 8 after falling out of a tree. He reports "occasional" alcohol use (12 pack of beer) on weekends and occasional marijuana use on weekends, although he states that he has not "smoked pot" for some time. He is a junior in high school and is on the football team. Jeremy gets As and Bs in his coursework and is currently in the process of applying to colleges and for football scholarships.

Jeremy is admitted to the inpatient psychiatric unit for treatment of psychosis. After 3 days, Jeremy reports no delusions or hallucinations, and his behavior is appropriate and cooperative. Jeremy's demeanor is pleasant and friendly as well.

Questions

1. Which designer drug is likely causing Jeremy's reported symptoms? What is a diagnostic challenge with Jeremy's presentation?

2. What treatment and management approaches are recommended for Jeremy's symptoms?

3. What are some of the long-term psychotic symptoms associated with Jeremy's use of Spice?

Answers

1. Paranoid delusions and hallucinations of vivid, flashing lights are known adverse effects of Spice intoxication. Also, psychosis is a common reason for Spice users to seek treatment in the emergency department (Spaderna et al., 2013). Woo and Hanley (2013) point out that Spice intoxication should always be suspected in a patient with no previous psychiatric illness who presents with new-onset psychosis, agitation, and bizarre behavior.

The diagnostic challenge is to determine whether the presenting symptoms are associated with a psychotic disorder or psychosis related to substance use. Jeremy's mental health assessment reveals delusions (paranoia – people are following him; phones are tapped; people are sending darts into his body to harm him), bizarre behavior (barricading himself in his room; destroying several cell phones), and hallucinations (flashes of colored lights). Jeremy's neurologic examination reveals tremors, ataxia, hypertonicity, and hyperreflexia. These neurologic findings suggest Spice intoxication rather than new-onset psychosis.

Psychotic symptoms related to schizophrenia are typically preceded by a prodromal period, in which the patient displays a decline in function and increasingly bizarre behavior. There are no signs of a prodromal period in Jeremy's case, as evidenced by his high grades in school, sports participation, initiative to attend college, and lack of a history of psychiatric illness.

2. The recommended treatment for Jeremy's symptoms includes benzodiazepines for his agitation and an antipsychotic medication (i.e., haloperidol, risperidone, olanzapine, or quetiapine) for his symptoms of psychosis (Papanti et al., 2013; Spaderna et al., 2013). Supportive measures such as maintaining hydration, monitoring vital signs, and ensuring a calm and nonthreatening treatment environment are also implemented if needed.

3. In most cases, psychotic symptoms resolve after about 5 to 8 days, but they may continue for up to 5 months in some patients (Amsterdam, Brunt, & van den Brink, 2015).

SUMMARY

The dangers and risks associated with the use of designer drugs have been clearly identified. During recent years, some of the nation's best monitoring mechanisms have noted an increase in the popularity of these drugs. The most recent data from the MTF survey indicate a decrease or stabilization in the use of many of these illegal drugs (Johnston et al., 2017), but one concern that should influence future prevention strategies is a significant decrease in the number of high school students who identify a great risk in using designer drugs occasionally.

Clearly, designer drugs are a significant health risk in this country. These drugs are commonly used in combination with alcohol, creating an even more dangerous scenario for the user. The development of prevention and treatment strategies targeting these at-risk populations needs to continue to be a priority.

EXAM QUESTIONS

CHAPTER 14
Questions 77–81

Note: Choose the one option that BEST answers each question.

77. Due to its sedating and amnesic effects, flunitrazepam is highly associated with

    a. young adults with alcohol use disorders.

    b. adolescents aged 12 to 15.

    c. drug use by healthcare professionals.

    d. sexual victimization on college campuses.

78. Synthetic cathinones belong to the class of drugs known as

    a. stimulants.

    b. inhalants.

    c. opioids.

    d. hallucinogens.

79. An adverse health effect of ketamine noted in users is

    a. euphoria.

    b. impulsivity.

    c. hallucinations.

    d. perceptions of empathy.

80. The most promising tool for the prevention of designer drug use among high school and college students is

    a. increased criminal penalties for first-time offenses.

    b. informational material for parents.

    c. training sessions for teachers.

    d. education for adolescents and young adults.

81. When a patient arrives in the emergency department with suspected designer drug use, an initial treatment action is to

    a. administer the available antidote.

    b. attempt to identify the illicit substance consumed.

    c. integrate motivational interviewing in the patient assessment.

    d. apply physical restraints immediately.

REFERENCES

Amsterdam, J., Brunt, T., & van den Brink, W. (2015). The adverse health effects of synthetic cannabinoids with emphasis on psychosis-like effects. *Journal of psychopharmacology (Oxford, England) 29.* doi:10.1177/0269881114565142

Andrabi, S., Greene, S., Moukaddam, N., & Li, B. (2015). New drugs of abuse and withdrawal syndromes. *Emergency Medicine Clinics of North America, 33,* 779-795.

Ashrafioun, L., Bonadio, F. A., Baik, K. D., Bradbury, S. L., Carhart, V. L., Cross, N. A., ... Zaturenskaya, M. (2016). Patterns of use, acute subjective experiences, and motivations for using synthetic cathinones ("bath salts") in recreational users. *Journal of Psychoactive Drugs, 48*(5), 336-343. doi: 10.1080/02791072.2016.1229875

Belknap, J., & Sharma, N. (2014). The significant frequency and impact of stealth (nonviolent) gender-based abuse among college women. *Trauma, Violence and Abuse, 15*(3), 181-190.

Busardo, F. P., & Jones, A. W. (2015). GHB pharmacology and toxicology: Acute intoxication, concentrations in blood and urine in forensic cases and treatment of the withdrawal syndrome. *Current Neuropharmacology, 13,* 47-70.

Dart, R. C., Bronstein, A. C., Spyker, D. A., Cantilena, L. R., Seifert, S. A., Heard, S. E., & Krenzelok, E. P. (2015). Poisoning in the United States: 2012 emergency medicine report of the National Poison Data System. *Annals of Emergency Medicine, 65*(4), 416-422.

Dolliver, D. S., & Kuhns, J. B. (2016). The presence of new psychoactive substances in a Tor network marketplace environment. *Journal of Psychoactive Substances, 48*(5), 321-329. doi:10.1080/02791072.2016.1229877

Joe-Laider, K., Hunt, G., & Moloney, M. (2014). "Tuned out or tuned in": Spirituality and youth drug use in global times. *Past and Present, 222*(9), S61-S80. doi:10.1093/pastj/gtt029

Johnston, L. D., O'Malley, P. M., Miech, R. A., Bachman, J. G., & Schulenberg, J. E. (2017). *Monitoring the Future national survey results on drug use, 1975-2016: Overview, key findings on adolescent drug use.* Ann Arbor, MI: Institute for Social Research, University of Michigan.

Karch, S. B. (2015). Cathinone toxicity ("the 3Ms"). *Current Neuropharmacology, 13*(1), 21-25.

Karila, L., Megarbane, B., Cottencin, O., & Lejoyeux, M. (2015). Synthetic cathinones: A new public health problem. *Current Neuropharmacology, 13,* 12-20.

Kemp, A. M., Clark, M. S., Dobbs, T., Galli, R., Sherman, J., & Cox, R. (2016). Top 10 facts you need to know about synthetic cannabinoids: Not so nice Spice. *American Journal of Medicine, 129,* 240-244.

Luciano, R. L., & Perazella, M. A. (2014). Nephrotoxic effects of designer drugs: Synthetic is not better! *Nature Reviews Nephrology, 10,* 314-324.

Murrough, J. W., Iosifescu, D. V., Chang, L. C., Al Jurdi, R. K., Green, C. M., Perez, A. M., ... Mathew, S. J. (2013). Antidepressant efficacy of ketamine in treatment-resistant major depression: A two-site randomized clinical trial. *American Journal of Psychiatry, 170*(10), 1134-1142.

National Institute on Drug Abuse. (2014). *Drug facts: Club drugs (GHB, ketamine, and Rohypnol).* Retrieved from https://www.drugabuse.gov/sites/default/files/drugfacts_clubdrugs_12_2014.pdf

National Institute on Drug Abuse. (2015). *Drug facts: Synthetic cannabinoids.* Retrieved from https://www.drugabuse.gov/publications/drugfacts/synthetic-cannabinoids

National Institute on Drug Abuse. (2016a). *Club drugs.* Retrieved from https://www.drugabuse.gov/drugs-abuse/club-drugs

National Institute on Drug Abuse. (2016b). *Commonly abused drug charts.* Retrieved from https://www.drugabuse.gov/drugs-abuse/commonly-abused-drugs-charts

National Institute on Drug Abuse. (2016c). *Ketamine.* Retrieved from https://www.drugabuse.gov/drugs-abuse/commonly-abused-drugs-charts#ketamine

National Institute on Drug Abuse. (2016d). *Rohypnol.* Retrieved from https://www.drugabuse.gov/drugs-abuse/commonly-abused-drugs-charts#rohypnol

National Institute on Drug Abuse. (2016e). *Synthetic cathinones.* Retrieved from https://www.drugabuse.gov/publications/drugfacts/synthetic-cathinones-bath-salts

Nelson, M. E., Bryant, S. M., & Aks, S. E. (2014). Emerging drugs of abuse. *Emergency Medical Clinics of North America, 32,* 1-28.

Papanti, D., Schifano, F., Botteon, G., Bertossi, F., Mannix, J., Vidoni, D., ... Bonavigo, T. (2013). "Spiceophrenia": A systematic overview of "Spice"-related psychopathological issues and a case report. *Human Psychopharmacology: Clinical and Experimental, 28*(4), 379-389.

Patterson, Z. R., Young, M. M., & Vaccarino, F. J. (2017). Novel psychoactive substances: What educators need to know. *Clinical Pharmacology & Therapeutics, 101*(2), 173-175. doi:10.1002/cpt.538

Rech, M. A., Donahey, E., Dziedzic, J., Oh, L., & Greenhalgh, E. (2015). New drugs of abuse. *Pharmacotherapy, 35*(2), 189-197.

Spaderna, M., Addy, P. H., & D'Souza, D. C. (2013). Spicing things up: Synthetic cannabinoids. *Psychopharmacology, 228,* 525-540.

Sutter, M. E., Chenoweth, J., & Albertson, T. E. (2014). Alternative drugs of abuse. *Clinical Reviews in Allergy and Immunology, 46,* 3-18.

Weaver, M. F., Hopper, J. A., & Gunderson, E. W. (2015). Designer drugs 2015: Assessment and management. *Addiction Science & Clinical Practice, 10*(8), 1-9. doi:10.1186/s13722-015-0024-7

Woo, T. M., & Hanley, J. R. (2013). "How high do they look?": Identification and treatment of common ingestions in adolescents. *Journal of Pediatric Healthcare, 27*(2), 135-144.

CHAPTER 15

ANABOLIC STEROIDS

LEARNING OUTCOME

After completing this chapter, the learner will be able to discuss the biochemical influences and negative health effects related to anabolic steroid use.

CHAPTER OBJECTIVES

After completing this chapter, the learner will be able to:

1. Review the anabolic steroids that are most commonly misused.

2. Discuss the biochemical changes and patterns of misuse of anabolic steroids among patients.

3. Distinguish among the presenting signs and symptoms of anabolic steroid misuse for male and female patients.

4. Describe the health problems associated with misuse of anabolic steroids.

5. Discuss prevention strategies for patients who misuse anabolic steroids.

INTRODUCTION

The formal scientific term for the class of drugs known as anabolic steroids is anabolic-androgenic steroids (AASs). These drugs are synthetic substances that are similar to the male hormone testosterone. The scientific term anabolic-androgenic can be better understood by reviewing the individual words: anabolic, meaning muscle building, and androgenic, meaning to increase male characteristics (National Institute on Drug Abuse [NIDA], 2016). The most common reason these drugs are used is to promote physical strength, athletic endurance, and muscle size.

The first documented use of anabolic steroids as performance enhancers in the United States was with Bob Hoffman, a World War I veteran, who invented the barbell in 1923. Later, anabolic steroids were used during World War II to help increase the muscle size and strength of German soldiers. After World War II, anabolic steroids were used to promote weight gain in concentration camp survivors (Pietro, 2017). A Maryland healthcare provider, John Zeigler, studied the effects of anabolic steroids on weightlifting athletes, and as a result, in 1958, methandrostenolone was the first mass-produced anabolic steroid. In 1960, U.S. weightlifters started using anabolic steroids, and by 1968, the use of anabolic steroids in the Olympics had become so common that routine urine testing became necessary.

During the 1970s and 1980s, the use of anabolic steroids among athletes continued to grow. In 1991, the Anabolic Steroid Control Act was passed, making anabolic steroids a Schedule III drug requiring a prescription (Drug Enforcement Administration [DEA], n.d.). The Dietary Supplement Health and Education Act of 1994 was responsible for promoting the use of legal nutritional supplements as opposed to illegal anabolic steroids.

In 2010, a bill called the Dietary Supplement Act of 2010 was introduced by Senator John McCain after six players from the National Football League were suspended due to the league's antidoping policy. These players were taking over-the-counter nutritional supplements and were unaware that the ingredients in the supplements were banned substances. Nutritional substances are not required to include the ingredients on a label. This bill was designed to require nutritional supplements to list all ingredients in the drug or supplement. However, the bill did not pass the Senate due to consumer concerns that this would drive up costs for nutritional supplements (Civic Impulse, 2017). Today, anabolic steroid use remains a significant health problem in the United States because anabolic steroids are being misused by consumers, sometimes resulting in sudden or unnatural deaths (Frati, Busardò, Cipolloni, Dominicis, & Fineschi, 2015).

STEROID ADMINISTRATION AND USE

There are many types of anabolic steroids available by prescription in the United States. These drugs come in a variety of formulations, such as intramuscular injections, oral forms, or creams, gels, or patches that can be applied to the skin. There are various therapeutic indications for these medications used in many fields of medicine. Anabolic steroids are prescribed by healthcare providers to treat hormonal issues such as delayed puberty and diseases such as muscle loss, cancers, and AIDS (NIDA, 2016).

Anabolic steroids are synthetic derivatives of testosterone. Anabolic steroids can be administered orally, intramuscularly, or topically. Some of the more common street names for these drugs are listed in Table 15-1 (NIDA, 2016). When administered, anabolic steroids increase mus-

TABLE 15-1: COMMON STREET NAMES FOR STEROIDS

Arnolds

Gear

Gym candy

Juice

Pumpers

Roids

Stackers

Weight gainers

Note. Adapted from National Institute on Drug Abuse. (2017). *Commonly abused drug charts: Steroids (anabolic).* Retrieved from https://www.drugabuse.gov/drugs-abuse/commonly-abused-drugs-charts#steroids-anabolic-

cle size and may affect one's ability to tolerate increased exercise by making the muscles more capable of overload and a quicker recovery (Frati et al., 2015). The most common anabolic steroids used today, which can be taken orally or injected, include oxymetholone, oxandrolone, methyltestosterone, fluoxymesterone, and nandrolone decanoate (Frati et al., 2015).

Individuals who misuse anabolic steroids use extremely high doses of these medications, often 10 to 100 times higher than the prescribed doses (NIDA, 2016). These same individuals also have specific dosing regimens for using the drugs, such as cycling, stacking, and pyramiding. Cycling is a technique of alternating between use and nonuse of anabolic steroids. By cycling, the user is attempting to minimize the unwanted adverse drug effects. Cycling usually involves administering the specific anabolic steroids every 4 to 18 weeks, followed by a drug-free period of 1 month to 1 year. A second technique is called stacking, which is a common practice of using multiple different anabolic steroids to maximize the effect on muscle size. A third dosing technique, pyramiding, involves initially administering a low dose of the anabolic steroid, gradually increasing the dose to the middle of the cycle, and then tapering the dose to complete the cycle. A final dosing alternative, known as stacking the pyramid, combines the dosing techniques of stacking and pyramiding. Steroid users are often extremely exacting in the dosing and timing of their anabolic steroid regimens. The perceived benefits of these techniques have not been scientifically documented (NIDA, 2016).

EPIDEMIOLOGY

The spread of anabolic steroid use has been significant in the United States. The Designer Anabolic Steroid Control Act of 2014 (H.R. 4771) became Public Law 13-260 on December 18, 2014. This bill expanded the list of anabolic steroids regulated by the DEA to include about two dozen new substances and established new crimes relating to false labeling of anabolic steroids.

In 2011, 1.2% of 19- to 30-year-olds reported having used anabolic steroids in their lifetime. The highest rate of annual use was among 12th graders, at 1.2%. Annual and 30-day rates for anabolic steroid use were very low for college students and young adults, at 0.2%. Anabolic steroid use remains higher among males than females. Of the high school students surveyed, 1.2% of 8th graders, 1.4% of 10th graders, and 1.8% of 12th graders indicated that they had used anabolic steroids in their lifetime (Johnston, O'Malley, Bachman, & Schulenberg, 2012).

The incidence of anabolic steroid misuse is especially high among recreational athletes, particularly noncompetitive bodybuilders and weightlifters. Anabolic steroid misuse is also related to a behavioral syndrome called muscle dysmorphia, where the patient has a distorted body image. Some people use anabolic steroids to increase their muscle size after experiencing either sexual or physical abuse. In general, most people who initiate anabolic steroid use have normal psychological functioning when they begin but develop abnormal personality traits and disturbances that can be attributed to anabolic steroid use (Pope, Khalsa, & Bhasin, 2017). There is growing evidence and agreement that performance-enhancing drugs (PEDs) and body-image-enhancing drugs may be better terms to capture the various substances used by individuals to improve performance and body image. There are currently 3 million PED users, and PED use ranks ahead of both type 1 diabetes and HIV infection in prevalence. Most PEDs users are not competitive athletes (Pope et al., 2014).

BIOCHEMISTRY

An androgen is a sex hormone that promotes the development and maintenance of male sexual characteristics. Testosterone is the main sex hormone secreted in males (Pope et al., 2014). Anabolic steroids are synthetic derivatives of the male sex hormone testosterone. Testosterone is a steroid hormone produced in male testes; however, it is also present in females in smaller amounts, produced by the adrenal glands and the ovaries. In females, the testosterone is acted upon in adipose tissue and converted into estrogen. Males maintain plasma concentration levels of 300 to 1,000 ng/dl, whereas females maintain levels between 15 and 70 ng/dl (Rosenfield, Barnes, & Ehrmann, 2016). Testosterone is metabolized extensively in the liver. This hormone promotes the growth of skeletal muscle and the development of male sex characteristics (Pope et al., 2014).

Some steroid supplements can be purchased over the counter in most health food stores and are advertised as supplements. These items are popular with athletes because they advertise their ability to increase muscle mass. The concern is that when these substances are consumed in high doses, there is a significant rise in the body's testosterone level similar to that of prescription anabolic steroids. These products may produce the same type of adverse effects as seen with anabolic steroids. Even after the Food and Drug Administration (FDA) recalled supplements that contained harmful substances such as anabolic steroids, these substances were still found to be present in dietary supplements 6 months later (ScienceDaily, 2014).

Athletes who experience a large increase in muscle mass (greater than 20 lb of muscle) in a relatively short amount of time may be abusing anabolic steroids. Anabolic steroids commonly cause dramatic changes in personality, such as moodiness, aggression, and extreme irritability. Users of anabolic steroids may also experience paranoid jealousy, delusions, and feelings of invincibility, resulting in impaired judgment. Males will have an increase in breast tissue called gynecomastia and a decrease in testicular size (NIDA, 2016). Both males and females may notice stretch marks called cutaneous striae around the breast area. An increased amount of acne on the face, back, and chest is also common. In addition, the face may appear puffy due to fluid retention. Users of anabolic steroids may also have an elevated blood pressure and increased heart rate. Parents who identify at least three of these signs in their child should consult their primary care provider to consider anabolic steroid misuse. Testicular atrophy is a hallmark of anabolic steroid misuse and should always be evaluated by the primary care provider.

Groups at high risk for anabolic steroid misuse include competitive athletes and bodybuilders (Pope et al., 2014). Laboratory drug testing is commonly required for professional athletes during competitive events to ensure fairness. Urine drug testing is reliable when done by a qualified laboratory, but not all laboratories test for all anabolic steroids, and there are new

anabolic steroids on the market all the time. Therefore, a negative laboratory test does not rule out misuse, particularly in cases where body composition indicates otherwise. Many athletes have learned how to avoid a positive test by stopping use for an appropriate amount of time to allow for the drugs to leave their system. Some athletes use combinations of drugs, such as probenecid and diuretics, to decrease the urinary concentrations of anabolic steroids and avoid potential positive tests (Pope et al., 2014). In addition, the detection of testosterone is complicated because it is a naturally occurring hormone, and testing must rely on ratios of testosterone to epitestosterone. If the ratio of testosterone to epitestosterone is greater than 4:1 (i.e., representing a change from the 6:1 normally occurring ratio of testosterone to epitestosterone), it is considered evidence of possible doping and leads to further tests. Some athletes have also been found to self-administer epitestosterone in an attempt to nullify the laboratory tests (Ventura & Segura, 2010).

In general, the amount of time anabolic steroids remain detectable in a patient's system is dependent on the length of use, the doses used, and the individual's ability to clear the drug. Most intramuscular anabolic steroids are detectable for 3 to 4 months after ceasing use, and oral anabolic steroids are detectable for 1 to 4 weeks after the last use (Ventura & Segura, 2010).

MEDICAL PROBLEMS AND CO-OCCURRING DISORDERS

General Effects

Anabolic steroid use has been associated with various health effects that range in severity from abnormal changes in appearance to life-threatening adverse events. Most of these effects are considered reversible after the user stops using the drugs, but some are permanent. Most of the data on long-term adverse effects have been compiled through case reports as opposed to formal epidemiological studies. Medically related problems have been noted in the endocrine, musculoskeletal, cardiovascular, and integumentary systems, as have effects causing liver, psychiatric, and infection problems (NIDA, 2016). Table 15-2 provides a summary of these medical problems.

Endocrine Effects

The endocrine system is seriously altered by the use of anabolic steroids. A decrease in sperm production and atrophy of the testicles are reversible effects noted in male anabolic steroid users. Gynecomastia, or enlargement of male breast tissue, and male-pattern baldness are irreversible effects that occur in male anabolic steroid users more than 50% of the time. It has also been found that male anabolic steroid users complain of breast pain and experience a decrease in naturally occurring gonadotropins, which results in variable effects on sexual interest, erections, the prostate, and fertility (Pope et al., 2014).

In females, anabolic steroids have been used therapeutically to treat osteoporosis and menopause; to date, the role of these drugs in breast growth and development has not been completely determined. Anabolic steroid misuse in females causes masculinization – notably, a decrease in breast size, increase in facial and body hair growth, decrease in scalp hair growth, deepening of the voice, and coarseness of the skin (American College of Obstetricians and Gynecologists, 2015). Females also experience a decrease in body fat, an increase in menstrual irregularities, and clitoral enlargement. In contrast to males, the female adverse effects are usually irreversible.

TABLE 15-2: EFFECTS OF ANABOLIC STEROIDS BY SYSTEM (1 OF 2)

Cardiovascular system

- Myocardial infarctions
- Thrombocytosis
- Lipodystrophy
- Hypertension
- Cerebral vascular accident (i.e., stroke)
- Enlarged heart
- Changes in blood cholesterol

Endocrine system

Male

- Testicular atrophy
- Infertility (i.e., decreased sperm count)
- Gynecomastia
- Increased sex drive
- Increased risk of prostate cancer

Female

- Amenorrhea or menstrual cycle changes
- Masculinization (e.g., voice deepening, breasts shrinking)
- Excessive growth of body and facial hair
- Clitoris enlargement

Both genders

- Male-pattern baldness

Immune system

- Hepatitis B
- Hepatitis C
- HIV
- Bacterial endocarditis
- Abscesses

Digestive system (liver disease)

- Hepatic tumors
- Liver damage

TABLE 15-2: EFFECTS OF ANABOLIC STEROIDS BY SYSTEM (1 OF 2)

Digestive system (liver disease) *cont'd*

Peliosis

Hepatomegaly

Musculoskeletal system

Short stature (i.e., stunted height in teens due to signal to stop bone growth)

Ruptured tendons

Avulsions

Integumentary system

Acne

Cutaneous striae

Increased oily scalp

Nervous system (psychiatric illnesses)

Increased violence and aggression ("roid rage")

Depression/risk of suicide

Mania

Delusions/paranoid jealousy

Major mood swings

Restlessness/irritability

Hallucinations

Impaired judgment

Note. Adapted from National Institute on Drug Abuse. (2016). *DrugFacts: Anabolic steroids.* Retrieved from https://www.drugabuse.gov/publications/drugfacts/anabolic-steroids

Both males and females who use anabolic steroids experience an increase in insulin resistance. Anabolic steroid use can alter fasting blood sugar levels and decrease glucose tolerance. Insulin has also been used as a PED. Injection of insulin increases the transport of glucose and amino acids into the skeletal muscle. The downside is that it can cause weight gain, which can be counterproductive for most athletes (Pope et al., 2014).

Musculoskeletal Effects

The musculoskeletal system responds to rising androgenic steroids by triggering bone growth during puberty and adolescence. In young adults who have not reached this increased state by naturally occurring hormones but instead experience the increase of hormones through anabolic steroid misuse, stunted height may occur due to the increased levels of anabolic steroids signaling the bones to stop growing (NIDA, 2016). Another issue with anabolic steroid misuse is the increase of muscular skeletal injuries. Anabolic steroids cause the muscle to grossly increase in size, resulting in stress on the tendons and ligaments. Tendon rupture (unilaterally and bilaterally) and avulsions can result from bulking due to anabolic steroids (Pope et al., 2014).

Cardiovascular Effects

Cardiomyopathy, myocardial infarction, cerebrovascular accidents, conduction abnormalities, and coagulation abnormalities have been reported in individuals misusing anabolic steroids (Pope et al., 2014). Oral anabolic steroids are known to increase the low-density lipoprotein cholesterol and decrease the high-density lipoprotein cholesterol, which increases the risk of atherosclerosis. Testosterone is known to increase platelet activation in anabolic steroid users and has caused thrombosis (blood clot) in weightlifters with no evidence of atherosclerosis. Anabolic steroids cause an increase in hemoglobin and hematocrit due to the increased synthesis of erythropoietin, which is beneficial in the treatment of anemia but contributes to thrombosis (Pope et al., 2014).

Dermatologic Effects

Dermatologic effects of anabolic steroids are readily apparent. An increase in sebaceous secretions creates noticeably oily hair and skin. Acne is a common effect of anabolic steroid misuse. Cystic acne and pitting scars are significant findings when screening for anabolic steroid use. Anabolic steroids have also been associated with linear keloids; striae; hirsutism; seborrheic dermatitis; baldness, especially in males; and secondary infections (Pope et al., 2014).

Hepatic Effects

Chronic use of an AAS has been associated with several serious changes in the liver. Current studies are not adequate to draw causal relationships between anabolic steroid use and liver disease due to the limitations in research design, such as no controls for muscle damage, alcohol consumption, other illnesses, or medications. There does seem to be an increase in hepatic tumors in individuals with long-term use. Such liver diseases as hepatomegaly, enlarged liver, and peliosis (blood-filled cysts that can rupture, causing hemorrhage and death) have also been seen in the chronic use of anabolic steroids. Other hepatic disorders, such as biliary stasis, jaundice, and hepatorenal syndrome, have been documented with anabolic steroid use. Although liver toxicities are expected to occur with supratherapeutic doses of anabolic steroids, further research needs to be conducted to clearly define the extent of the disease risks (Pope et al., 2014).

Psychiatric Symptoms

There is a growing body of evidence from field studies to describe the psychiatric symptoms associated with the misuse of anabolic steroids. Anabolic steroids work differently from other drugs of misuse. The most important difference is that anabolic steroids do not trigger a rapid increase in the brain chemical dopamine, which causes the "high" that drives people to misuse other substances. However, long-term anabolic steroid misuse can act on dopamine, serotonin, and opioid systems and may result in significant effects on mood and behavior (NIDA,

2016). Some studies have suggested that individuals who are misusing anabolic steroids exhibit hypomanic or manic symptoms during exposure. These episodes include an increase in irritability, aggressiveness, exaggerated self-confidence, hyperactivity, reckless behavior, psychotic symptoms, and depressive symptoms (Pope et al., 2014). Withdrawal symptoms have been reported after the use of higher doses of anabolic steroids. These symptoms include depressed mood, loss of interest in usual activities, hypersomnia, anorexia, loss of libido, and occasional suicidality (Pope et al., 2014).

Dependence on anabolic steroid use has been observed in some individuals. It can occur in about 30% of AAS users. Addiction is a problem seen in some anabolic steroid users; it is identified through continued drug use despite serious physical and behavioral problems. Anabolic steroids are different from other drugs of misuse in that many of their "reinforcing effects" (those effects that keep a person using a drug) are not experienced immediately or rapidly (Pope et al., 2014). The main reason people misuse anabolic steroids is to improve their performance in sports or their appearance (to increase their muscle size and/or reduce their body fat). These effects take time to develop, but once developed, they may be strong incentives for continued anabolic steroid misuse (Pope et al., 2014). Symptoms of anabolic steroid dependence include loss of control, withdrawal symptoms, and interference with other activities.

Muscle dysphoria may be closely associated with AAS use. When AAS use is stopped, the individual may become extremely anxious even over a minimum change in muscle mass. Neuroendocrine factors may also contribute to dependence on AAS use. There may be profound hypogonadism for weeks or months after discontinuing AAS use. Symptoms of fatigue, loss of libido, and depression may prompt reformed users to begin using the AAS again for alleviation of these symptoms (Pope et al., 2014).

Infections

Another health problem related to injected anabolic steroids is infections. People who inject anabolic steroids commonly use nonsterile needles, poor injection techniques, and nonsterile drugs, which can cause risk of serious infection. People who inject anabolic steroids are at risk for such life-threatening infections as HIV, hepatitis B and C, and bacterial endocarditis. Infections at the injection sites due to bacteria could result in serious abscesses (Pope et al., 2014).

PREVENTIVE STRATEGIES AND TREATMENT

Prevention research focused on substance misuse is currently ongoing in this country. A recent report titled *Facing Addiction in America* by the Office of the Surgeon General emphasized the need for evidence-based programs to address our addiction problem. There is strong evidence to support the effectiveness of substance use prevention programs and policies (U.S. Department of Health and Human Services, 2016). One program that has been shown to be effective is Adolescents Training and Learning to Avoid Steroids (ATLAS; Goldberg et al., 2000). This is a universal program that can be delivered in the school.

The ATLAS program is a multifocused approach that promotes nutrition and strength training as alternatives to anabolic steroid misuse and includes drug-refusal role play and an antisteroid media campaign (Goldberg et al., 1996). This program also has a parent component designed to inform, support, and encourage parents in communicating with their susceptible teenagers.

Prevention strategies for amateur and professional athletes have been focused on changes in federal laws, rules, and regulations for professional sports and the regulations of the International Olympic Committee. In 1999, the World Anti-Doping Agency was established to develop standard drug testing protocols, accredit drug testing laboratories, and compile and publish current information on its website (World Anti-Doping Agency, 2017). The World Antidoping Code is the document that brings together antidoping rules, regulations, and policies worldwide. The most recent update of prohibited drugs and substances can be found on the website.

Another policy change occurred in 1995 when the U.S. Supreme Court ruled that drug testing for high school athletes was constitutional. Whenever a governmental agency tests an athlete for drugs, it must comply with the Fourth Amendment, which states:

The right of the people to be secure in their persons, houses, papers and effects against unreasonable searches and seizures, shall not be violated and no Warrants shall issue, but upon probable cause, supported by Oath or affirmation and particularly describing the place to be searched and the persons things to be seized (USLegal, n.d.).

There is controversy around this policy of testing student athletes and its effectiveness. Studies have been mixed and inconclusive, from those reporting no difference in schools that do test regarding drug use and others that have reported a reduced prevalence of drug use in schools that do test athletes (National Center on Addiction and Substance Abuse, 2016).

It is estimated that there are approximately 3 million people who misuse anabolic steroids in this country; only a small percentage of these people seek or receive treatment (NIDA, 2016). Supportive therapy and education programs have been effective in treating some individuals. Interventions that are effective include providing education to patients about what they may experience during withdrawal and close evaluation for co-occurring depression and other psychiatric problems, including suicide. Medications may be needed to treat depression, headaches, and muscle and joint pain. Behavioral therapies are effective in addressing the psychosocial issues related to anabolic steroid use disorders. Peer-led counseling and support groups are excellent methods of reinforcing positive behaviors in stopping use of performance-enhancing drugs (NIDA, 2006).

SUMMARY

Misuse of anabolic steroids and PEDs remains a serious health problem in this country. Misuse of anabolic steroids or PEDs is more prevalent among noncompetitive athletes than the rest of the population. As a society, the message is being sent that physical beauty and athletic accomplishments are valued and worth the physical, psychological, and legal risks to achieve them. Prevention is the key to eliminating misuse of these drugs or supplements. Screening of high school and college athletes and other students raises ethical and constitutional concerns about the rights of individuals. Universal and targeted education and campaigns will assist in educating about the harms of misuse of these substances. Policies and laws surrounding misuse of these drugs or supplements need to be reexamined continually while protecting the privacy and rights of individuals.

EXAM QUESTIONS

CHAPTER 15
Questions 82–88

Note: Choose the one option that BEST answers each question.

82. Street names for commonly misused anabolic steroids include gear, stackers, roids, and

    a. molly.
    b. boom.
    c. juice.
    d. buddha.

83. Stacking is a technique of anabolic steroid misuse that

    a. increases the dose of the anabolic steroid being administered.
    b. uses multiple different anabolic steroids to maximize the desired effects.
    c. varies the dose of the anabolic steroid being administered.
    d. allows the body to have drug-free periods.

84. Testosterone promotes the development of male sex characteristics and

    a. decreases insulin resistance.
    b. decreases heart rate and blood pressure.
    c. promotes excessive fluid loss.
    d. promotes the growth of skeletal muscle.

85. An irreversible symptom that is seen in male patients who misuse anabolic steroids is

    a. testicular atrophy.
    b. increased lipid levels.
    c. infertility.
    d. gynecomastia.

86. Adolescents who misuse anabolic steroids can experience musculoskeletal disorders such as tendon rupture, avulsion injuries, and

    a. osteoarthritis.
    b. fibromyalgia.
    c. stunted bone growth.
    d. bone fractures.

87. Chronic anabolic steroid use is associated with damage to several body organs, including the

    a. lungs.
    b. liver.
    c. stomach.
    d. bladder.

88. Tom, age 16, has been training hard all summer for the school football team and has significantly increased his muscle mass. When his mother overhears him talking on the telephone about "roids," she calls the pediatric nurse who advises which of the following?

    a. "Bring your son to the office for evaluation and education."
    b. "Do not worry about the situation; it is perfectly normal."
    c. "Ask your son's friends if he is using anabolic steroids."
    d. "Search your son's room for evidence of drug use."

REFERENCES

American College of Obstetricians and Gynecologists. (2011). Performance enhancing anabolic steroid abuse in women. Committee Opinion No. 484. American College of Obstetricians and Gynecologists. *Obstetrics and Gynecology, 117,* 1016-1018. [Reaffirmed in 2015]

Civic Impulse. (2017). *S. 3002 – 111th Congress: Dietary Supplement Safety Act of 2010.* Retrieved from https://www.govtrack.us/congress/bills/111/s3002

Drug Enforcement Administration. (n.d.). *Steroids.* Retrieved from http://www.justice.gov/dea/druginfo/drug_data_sheets/Steroids.pdf

Frati, P., Busardò, F. P., Cipolloni, L., Dominicis, E. D., & Fineschi, V. (2015). Anabolic androgenic steroid (AAS) related deaths: Autoptic, histopathological and toxicological findings. *Current Neuropharmacology, 13*(1), 146-159.

Johnston, L. D., O'Malley, P. M., Bachman, J. G., & Schulenberg, J. E. (2012). *Monitoring the Future national survey results on drug use, 1975-2011. Volume I: Secondary school students.* Ann Arbor, MI: Institute for Social Research, University of Michigan.

National Center on Addiction and Substance Abuse. (2016). *Should students be drug tested at school?* http://www.centeronaddiction.org/the-buzz-blog/should-students-be-drug-tested-school

National Institute on Drug Abuse. (2006). *Anabolic steroid abuse: Letter from the director (NIH Publication No. 06-3721).* Retrieved from http://www.nida.nih.gov/ResearchReports/steroids/AnabolicSteroids.html

National Institute on Drug Abuse. (2016). *DrugFacts: Anabolic steroids.* Retrieved from https://www.drugabuse.gov/publications/drugfacts/anabolic-steroids

National Institute on Drug Abuse. (2017). *Commonly abused drug charts: Steroids (anabolic).* Retrieved from https://www.drugabuse.gov/drugs-abuse/commonly-abused-drugs-charts#steroids-anabolic-

Oregon Health and Science University. (2017). *Athletes Training and Learning to Avoid Steroids (ATLAS).* Retrieved from http://www.ohsu.edu/xd/education/schools/school-of-medicine/departments/clinical-departments/medicine/divisions/hpsm/research/atlas.cfm

Pietro, J. (2017). *The history of anabolic steroids.* Retrieved from http://www.steroids.org/History-of-Anabolic-Steroids.php

Pope, H. G., Jr., Khalsa, J. H., & Bhasin, S. (2017). Body image disorders and abuse of anabolic-androgenic steroids among men. *JAMA, 317*(1), 23-24. doi:10.1001/jama.2016.17441

Pope, H. G., Jr., Wood, R. I., Rogol, A., Nyberg, F., Bowers, L., & Bhasin, S. (2014). Adverse health consequences of performance-enhancing drugs: An Endocrine Society scientific statement. *Endocrine Reviews, 35*(3), 341-375. doi:10.1210/er.2013-1058

Rosenfield, R. L., Barnes, R. B., & Ehrmann, D. A. (2016). Hyperandrogenism, hirsutism, and polycystic ovary syndrome. In J. L. Jameson, L. J. De Groot, D. M. de Kretser, L. C. Giudice, A. B. Grossman, S. Melmed, … G. C. Weir (Eds.), *Endocrinology: Adult and pediatric* (7th ed., pp. 2275-2296). Philadelphia, PA: Elsevier Saunders.

ScienceDaily. (2014). *High percentage of recalled dietary supplements still have banned ingredients*. Retrieved from http://www.sciencedaily.com/releases/2014/10/141021162025.htm

U.S. Department of Health and Human Services, Office of the Surgeon General. (2016). *Facing addiction in America: The surgeon general's report on alcohol, drugs, and health*. Washington, DC: Author. Retrieved from https://www.surgeongeneral.gov/library/reports/index.html

USLegal. (n.d.). *Sports law: Drugs and testing*. Retrieved from https://sportslaw.uslegal.com/drugs-and-testing/

Ventura, R., & Segura, T. (2010). Masking and manipulation. In D. Thieme & P. Hemmersbach (Eds.), *Doping in sports: Biochemical principles, effects and analysis* (pp. 324-357). Berlin: Springer. doi:10.1007/978-3-540-79088-4_15

World Anti-Doping Agency. (2017). *Who we are*. Retrieved from https://www.wada-ama.org/en/who-we-are

CHAPTER 16

SUBSTANCE USE ACROSS THE LIFE SPAN

LEARNING OUTCOME

After completing this chapter, the learner will be able to identify the unique challenges of preventing and identifying substance use disorders in patients during the reproductive, adolescent, college-age, and older-adult years.

CHAPTER OBJECTIVES

After completing this chapter, the learner will be able to:

1. Discuss substance use disorders in women and neonates, including their prevalence, screening, and treatment interventions.

2. Discuss substance use disorders in the adolescent population, including their prevalence, screening, and treatment interventions.

3. Discuss substance use disorders in the college-age population, including their prevalence, screening, and treatment interventions.

4. Discuss substance use disorders in the older-adult population, including their prevalence, screening, and treatment interventions.

INTRODUCTION

This chapter discusses special populations that pose unique concerns or challenges to nurses and clinicians when identifying and treating substance use: women of reproductive age, adolescents, college-age students, and older adults. This chapter also discusses the prevalence, screening, and treatment of substance use disorders in these special populations. For women, the highest risk of developing a substance use disorder is during their reproductive years (Forray, 2016). The developing fetus and neonate are especially vulnerable to exposure to toxic substances (National Institute on Drug Abuse [NIDA, 2017]). Adolescents are risk takers, and this may result in early exposure to substance use that may continue into adult life (NIDA, 2014b.) College-age adults have been shown to have high rates of marijuana, alcohol, nicotine, and stimulant use. Lastly, the older adult with chronic health issues and a substance use disorder is more likely to experience a shortened life span and decreased quality of life (Mattson, Lipari, Hays, & Van Horn, 2017).

WOMEN AND NEONATES

Current practice encourages women who are pregnant to abstain from all alcohol, nicotine, and illicit drugs. The most frequently used substance in pregnancy is tobacco, followed by alcohol, cannabis, and other illicit substances (Forray, 2016). The National Survey on Drug Use and Health (NSDUH) showed that from 2009 to 2013, 0.9% of pregnant women met the criteria for opioid use disorder, and 0.2%

met the criteria for heroin use disorder (Center for Behavioral Health Statistics and Quality [CBHSQ], 2013). When women use opioids and other substances while pregnant, their infants may exhibit withdrawal symptoms within the first 24 hours of birth. The neonatal period is defined as birth to 28 days (American Academy of Pediatrics [AAP] Division of Health Care Finance, 2015).

Prevalence

The health of the mother and exposure to toxic substances in utero can influence the behavioral, developmental, and physical health of the neonate (Ross, Graham, Money, & Stanwood, 2015). Women who are pregnant are encouraged to abstain from all alcohol, nicotine, and illicit drugs. The effects of alcohol, for example, on the developing fetus can result in fetal alcohol spectrum disorders (FASDs), which is a term that is used to describe a range of adverse mental and physical effects associated with prenatal alcohol exposure. Maternal alcohol use is evident in fetal alcohol syndrome, which is the most common cause of childhood intellectual disability (Williams, Smith, & Committee on Substance Abuse, 2015). About 9% of women in the United States drink alcohol at least once during pregnancy (Substance Abuse and Mental Health Services Administration [SAMHSA], 2014). FASD is the leading preventable cause of birth defects, intellectual disability, and neuro-developmental disability. No amount of alcohol is considered safe during pregnancy (Williams et al., 2015). Cannabis use during pregnancy has also been shown to have adverse effects on the fetus, such as fetal growth restriction, and can result in learning disabilities and memory impairment (Wu, Jew, & Lu, 2011).

Infants born to mothers who used opioids and other substances while pregnant may exhibit withdrawal symptoms within the first 24 hours of birth. Neonatal abstinence syndrome

(NAS) refers to "a treatable condition that newborns experience after chronic exposures to certain substances, primarily opioids, while in utero" (National Association of State Alcohol and Drug Abuse Directors, 2015, p. 1). Other substances, such as benzodiazepines, barbiturates, and alcohol, that affect the developing fetus are also linked to neonatal withdrawal symptoms; however, chronic opioid use currently is the most common source of NAS (National Association of State Alcohol and Drug Abuse Directors, 2015).

Risk and Protective Factors

Risk factors for women in initiating the use of substances include stress, negative affect, influence of relationships (e.g., boyfriend, family member, or close friend), genetics, and characteristics of the family of origin (e.g., exposure to chaotic, argumentative, and violent households; Center for Substance Abuse Treatment, 2009). Substance use disorders during pregnancy have associated effects on the fetus, as well as an association with a lack of prenatal care, poor nutrition, use of tobacco, and incarceration, which all affect the overall health of the mother as well (AAP, 2012). Untreated heroin use during pregnancy may cause physical effects such as growth issues, placental abruption, preterm labor, and fetal demise. Protective factors in preventing substance use include a positive self-image, self-control, and social competence (SAMHSA, 2015a).

Screening

The American College of Obstetricians and Gynecologists recommends screening women who are pregnant for alcohol and illicit substances at every visit (American College of Obstetricians and Gynecologist [ACOG], 2015). Most screening tools evaluate for the risk associated with the substance and do not directly screen for use (Yonkers et al., 2010). The 4 P's

Plus screen for alcohol and general substances use in pregnancy can be used in the inpatient and outpatient setting during prenatal visits. The first four questions of this tool ask about substance use, followed by two additional questions addressing domestic violence (Yonkers et al., 2010). Substance use disorders and domestic violence often co-occur. When asking women about histories of domestic violence, it is important to do so privately, away from the potential abuser or other people who may inform the abuser. If women reveal a history of or report current domestic violence, the clinician's assessment must address safety concerns and substance use disorders. The patient is advised to keep emergency phone numbers (e.g., police, domestic violence hotline, shelter) and critical items, such as money and birth certificates, on hand to facilitate escape from a dangerous situation. The clinician also guides the patient to establish a code for trusted others so that she can communicate any threat of impending danger.

Treatment for Women and Neonates

The American Society of Addiction Medicine recommends medication-assisted treatment (MAT) for women with an opioid use disorder who are pregnant. The benefits of MAT have been reported to include stabilization of the mother, enhanced prenatal care, and decreased or prevention of withdrawal symptoms, and it may also reduce criminal activity (ACOG Committee on Health Care for Underserved Women & American Society of Addiction Medicine, 2012). There are few existing psychosocial treatments specifically for prenatal substance use in women. Contingency management has shown to be the most effective prevention strategy during the prenatal period (Forray, 2016). Contingency management is based on the principle of positive reinforcement as a means of operant conditioning to influence behavior change. For example, monetary vouchers may be used to modify and reinforce behaviors (Forray, 2016).

Treatment guidelines by the AAP (2012) for the neonate first recommend nonpharmacological measures such as rooming in, breastfeeding, gentle handling, swaddling, and a dark room and quiet environment. These measures, especially breastfeeding, have shown to decrease the severity of NAS. Pharmacological measures are used to treat the infant only after nonpharmacological measures have been unsuccessful. Pharmacologic therapy includes opioids, such as morphine or methadone, followed by phenobarbital (AAP, 2012). The type of drug used by the mother during pregnancy will determine the pharmacological therapy for the treatment of NAS. For opioids (paregoric, tincture of opium, morphine, methadone, and buprenorphine), barbiturates (phenobarbital), benzodiazepines (diazepam and lorazepam), clonidine, and phenothiazines (chlorpromazine) may be prescribed (Siu & Robinson, 2014). A standard scoring method such as the Neonatal Abstinence Scoring Tool is recommended to monitor newborn symptoms (Hudak, Tan, Committee on Drugs, & Committee on Fetus and Newborn, 2012).

Prevention

Educational strategies – such as providing lifestyle guidelines, teaching coping skills, and promoting self-care – to prevent the use of substances that are specifically designed for women of childbearing age have been shown to prevent or reduce substance use and its negative consequences during this critical period in the life of the female and neonate. Public health campaigns targeted to women in the reproductive years may also be beneficial in reducing substance use in this population (SAMHSA, 2016a).

ADOLESCENTS

Alcohol is the most widely misused substance among America's youth and contributes to more than 4,300 annual deaths among youth and accounts for 189,000 emergency department visits by people under age 21 for injuries and other conditions (Centers for Disease Control and Prevention [CDC], 2016). Underage drinking remains a considerable public health challenge. It is not an adolescent rite of passage, and it can cause serious health problems.

Prevalence

In 2014, 22.8% of underage individuals were current alcohol users, 13.8% were binge alcohol users, and 3.4% were heavy alcohol users (SAMHSA, 2015b). For young people between the ages of 12 and 20, the reported rates of alcohol use in the past month in 2014 varied according to race: 13.5% of Asian Americans, 17.3% of African Americans, 21.1% of people reporting two or more races, 21.2% of Hispanics, 21.9% of American Indians or Alaska Natives, and 26% of Whites (SAMHSA, 2015b). Adolescent brains may be particularly susceptible to the long-term negative consequences of alcohol use and other substances. During the adolescent period, the brain is undergoing a maturation and refinement of key neural pathways. This maturation process occurring in the adolescent brain makes the brain more vulnerable to the negative effects of substance use (Asato, Terwilliger, Woo, & Luna, 2010). Alcohol use during adolescence may have lifelong effects and can change brain development. Magnetic resonance imaging studies in those who drank heavily throughout adolescence have demonstrated a decrease in the gray-matter volume of the anterior cingulate cortex and right insula. In addition, heavy use of alcohol may disrupt the maturational process in the frontal areas and cingulate cortex of the brain (Heikkinen et al., 2017).

The adolescent is more likely to engage in risky sexual behavior, including unwanted, unintended, and unprotected sexual activity and sex with multiple partners, while drinking. Youth have an increased risk of encountering legal problems, such as being arrested for drunk driving or physically hurting someone while drunk, and being physically and sexually assaulted while drinking alcohol. Alcohol consumption among adolescents increases the risk for suicide and homicide, memory problems, and the use and misuse of other drugs. Alcohol use during adolescence is a risk factor for heavy drinking later in life, which can lead to other medical problems, such as but not limited to cancer, reproductive problems, cardiovascular disease, and diabetes. Youth who start drinking before age 15 are almost 5 times more likely to develop alcohol use disorders later in life than those who begin drinking at or after age 21 (SAMHSA, 2015b).

Other commonly used substances during the adolescent period include marijuana, cigarettes, and nonmedical use of over-the-counter pain relievers. In 2014, 7.4% of adolescents aged 12 to 17 were current users of marijuana; this means that approximately 1.8 million adolescents used marijuana in the past month (SAMHSA, 2014). Among adolescents aged 12 to 17 in 2014, 1.7 million reported using tobacco products in the past month, including 1.2 million, or 7.0% of adolescents, who identified themselves as current cigarette smokers (SAMHSA, 2014). In 2014, an estimated 467,000 adolescents aged 12 to 17 were current nonmedical users of over-the-counter pain relievers, which corresponds to 1.9% of adolescents (SAMHSA, 2014).

Risk and Protective Factors

Although adolescence brings an increased risk for alcohol use, some factors put teens at higher risk for misusing alcohol and other substances. These include high levels of impulsiveness, novelty seeking, and aggressive behavior; having conduct or behavior problems; and a tendency not to consider the possible negative consequences of one's actions. Other risk factors include the following:

- Having a family history of substance use or mood disorders

- Living with poor parental supervision and household disruption

- Having low academic achievement and/or academic aspirations

- Having untreated attention-deficit/hyperactivity disorder

- Living with perceived peer acceptance of substance use and substance use among peers

(NIDA, 2014b)

Protective factors include a stable and supportive home environment, involvement in one's school and community, and good academic performance (NIDA, 2014b).

Other protective factors include the following:

- Having parents who set clear rules and enforce them

- Eating meals together as a family

- Having parents who regularly talk with their children about the dangers of alcohol and drug use

- Having a parent in recovery

- Being involved in church, synagogue, or community programs

- Having opportunities for prosocial involvement in the community and adequate community resources

Screening

Adolescents are unique in that some substances that are legal for adults are illegal for them. It also may be difficult to differentiate between acting out and being affected by substance use. Further, they may be even less forthcoming than adults about their substance use. As with all patients, screening of adolescents should, at minimum, take place at all routine medical visits. However, many adolescents may not be seen regularly for such care; therefore, screening should occur whenever they present for care (AAP, 2011).

Because the number one cause of death among adolescents is accidents, with the largest subgroup being motor vehicle collisions (SAMHSA, 2015b), it is crucial that care providers screen for substance use, especially alcohol. Caution must be used regarding screening instruments designed for adults being used with adolescents. Such tools are usually developmentally inappropriate. The most commonly used screening tool used for the adolescent is the CRAFFT. The CRAFFT is an evidence-based screening tool that is commonly used to screen adolescents for alcohol and substance use. This tool has been recommended for use with adolescents by the AAP's Committee on Substance Abuse. CRAFFT is a mnemonic acronym for the first letters of the key words in the six screening questions: car, relax, alone, forget, friends, and trouble. The tool only takes a few minutes to administer and score.

There are two parts to the CRAFFT screen: part A and part B. There are three questions in part A, as follows:

In the past 12 months, did you

1. drink any alcohol (more than a few sips; do not count sips of alcohol taken during family or religious events),

2. smoke any marijuana or hashish, or

3. use anything else to get high ("anything else" includes illegal drugs, over-the-counter and prescription drugs, and things that you sniff or huff)?

A yes answer to any of these questions requires that part B be completed. Part B includes six questions related to the CRAFFT mnemonic acronym, and each "yes" response scores 1 point. A total score of 2 or higher in part B is considered a positive screen, indicating a need for additional assessment (Center for Adolescent Substance Abuse Research, n.d.). The six questions in part B are as follows:

C - Have you ever ridden in a CAR driven by someone (including yourself) who was "high" or had been using alcohol or drugs?

R - Do you ever use alcohol or drugs to RELAX, feel better about yourself, or fit in?

A - Do you ever use alcohol/drugs while you are by yourself, ALONE?

F - Do you ever FORGET things you did while using alcohol or drugs?

F - Do your family or FRIENDS ever tell you that you should cut down on your drinking or drug use?

T - Have you gotten into TROUBLE while you were using alcohol or drugs?

(The Center for Adolescent Substance Abuse Research, 2016)

Treatment

Screening, brief intervention, and referral to treatment (SBIRT) shows promise for those adolescents falling in the at-risk to moderate range of risk for substance use. For those adolescents with a substance use disorder needing more intensive treatment, group and family therapy, intensive outpatient programs, partial hospital programs, inpatient/residential facilities, and therapeutic boarding schools are referral options (AAP, 2011). In 2010, adolescents between the ages of 12 and 19 years constituted 13.6% of all admissions to publicly funded treatment facilities (SAMHSA, 2015b. Adolescents between the ages of 15 and 19 were

most commonly treated for using the following substances (in order of decreasing frequency): marijuana, hallucinogens, inhalants, and stimulants other than cocaine or methamphetamines (e.g., methylphenidate, which is prescribed for attention-deficit/hyperactivity disorder; SAMHSA, 2015b). The American Society of Addiction Medicine (2013) outlines six areas to consider when deciding the appropriate treatment approach for the adolescent patient.

Indicators for inpatient treatment of adolescents include the following:

1. Level of intoxication and potential for withdrawal

2. Presence of other medical conditions

3. Presence of other emotional, behavioral, or cognitive conditions

4. Readiness or motivation to change

5. Risk of relapse or continued drug use

6. Recovery environment (e.g., family, peers, school, legal system)

(American Society of Addiction Medicine, 2013)

Enrollment criteria for outpatient treatment include the following:

• Comorbid psychiatric disorders that do not require inpatient treatment

• Previous successful outpatient treatment with documented adherence to follow-up

• Agreement to a contingency contract that includes visit frequency, expected adherence to the curriculum with random urine drug screens, consequences of nonadherence, and participation in the community network program along with self-help groups

(NIDA, 2014b)

Behavioral treatments demonstrated to be successful with adolescents who report substance use include family therapy, cognitive-behavioral therapy, motivational interventions, contingency management, and 12-step programs. Research studies suggest that adolescents in residential treatment programs have better outcomes, such as reduced relapse, than those in outpatient programs (NIDA, 2014b).

Selected medications for adolescents should ideally have a low misuse potential. Regrettably, no research has comprehensively evaluated the safety and effectiveness of any psychotropic medication to treat adolescent substance misuse (Simkin & Grenoble, 2010). However, in the presence of comorbid psychiatric disorders, medications targeting other psychiatric disorders may be used indirectly to treat substance use disorders. Fortunately, clinically significant withdrawal symptoms have rarely been observed in this age group. Consequently, detoxification protocols for adolescents are not significantly different from those for adults (NIDA, 2014b).

Prevention

Prevention is the best strategy for addressing substance use and reducing the incidence of substance use disorders. Times of transition increase the risk of drug use for the adolescent. For example, at the move from elementary school to middle school, the early adolescent may be exposed to tobacco and alcohol for the first time. In high school, teens may have greater access to drugs by attending social activities where substances are present. Treatment programs that address substance use among all patients, including adolescents, can be found at SAMHSA's National Registry of Evidence-Based Programs and Practices (SAMHSA, n.d.). Examples of evidence-based programs include the Family Check-Up, Positive Parenting Prevents Drug Abuse, and the Strengthening Families Program for Youth 10 to 14 (NIDA, 2014a).

COLLEGE-AGE YOUNG ADULTS

More than one third of full-time college students aged 18 to 22 reported engaging in binge drinking in the past month; about one in five reported using an illicit drug in the past month (Lipari & Jean-Francois, 2016). In addition, daily use of marijuana is also on the increase among college-age students. Substance use is considered one of the most serious health problems facing young adults and can result in health, financial, and possible legal problems (Lipari & Jean-Francois, 2016).

Prevalence

The prevalence of alcohol use among college students is a serious concern (National Institute on Alcohol Abuse and Alcoholism, 2015). Of full-time college students aged 18 to 22, 1.2 million reported alcohol use, and 703,759 reported marijuana use (NIDA, 2015). In 2014, 18- to 25-year-olds had the highest rate of alcohol use disorders (16.3%) among all people aged 12 or older (Lipari & Jean-Francois, 2016). There has been an increase in marijuana use among college-age students, and one in four students who graduated from high school reported daily use of marijuana (Lipari & Jean-Francois, 2016).

Risk and Protective Factors

The risk and protective factors of college-age students for using substances are similar to those of adolescents. The greatest risk for substance use is when the college student leaves home for the first time. Planning for the transition and strengthening the protective factors, such as the perceived risk of harm associated with using drugs, perceived parental disapproval, and attitudes about their peers' substance use, will help to decrease substance use in this population (SAMHSA, 2016b).

Screening

Screening for substance use is important in identifying and reducing use among college students. College campuses are modeling SAMHSA's SBIRT initiative to implement screening programs for alcohol and drug use and help students with mental and/or substance use disorders (SAMHSA, 2016b). Identifying a patient's level of risk will inform the clinician of the level of treatment and intervention that is needed to reduce or eliminate use.

Treatment and Prevention

Prevention continues to be the best approach for reducing and eliminating substance use problems among college students. The National Institute on Alcohol Abuse and Alcoholism created the CollegeAim (Alcohol Intervention Matrix) guide and website. This toolkit, which was developed by college alcohol researchers, includes individual-level strategies and environmental-level strategies to address alcohol use on college campuses (NIDA, 2015). More information can be found at https://www.college drinkingprevention.gov/collegeaim/.

OLDER ADULTS

As individuals move through young adulthood and into middle adulthood, illicit drug use generally declines. Although there is a decline in substance use, studies have found that many older adults have a substance use disorder, which combined with chronic health problems places these individuals at a greater risk for physical, emotional, and social problems.

Prevalence

One million individuals age 65 or older had a substance use disorder in 2014. Of these individuals, 978,000 had an alcohol use disorder, and 161,000 had an illicit drug use disorder. These numbers are projected to increase as the baby boomers age (Mattson et al., 2017). The NSDUH, using combined data from 2007 to 2014, estimates that on an average day during the past month, 6 million older adults drank alcohol, 132,000 older adults used marijuana, and 4,300 older adults used cocaine (National Institutes of Health, 2015). The slowing metabolism and psychosocial changes associated with old age, including the loss of loved ones, can make the older adult more vulnerable to the effects of substances (Volkow, 2011). Alcohol can interact with other medications that the older adult may be taking, and the older adult can become more sensitive to the effects of alcohol, resulting in falls, strokes and memory issues (Mattson et al., 2017).

Risk and Protective Factors

At the individual level, risk factors for the older adult in developing a substance use disorder may include genetics, previous experience with substance use problems, relationship problems such as loss of loved ones, community violence, and poverty. Protective factors for older adults include engagement in the community, faith-based resources, and limited access to substances (SAMHSA, 2015a).

Screening

Screening the older adult for substance use is essential for early identification and treatment. CAGE-AID (i.e., a version of the CAGE questionnaire modified to include substance use) and the Drug Abuse Screening Test (DAST-10; Skinner, 1982) are two examples of evidence-based screening tools used in primary care to screen for substance use. CAGE-AID (Brown & Rounds, 1995) is a mnemonic acronym for the first letter of key words in the screening questions (Cut down, Annoyed, Guilty, and Eye-opener). Each question requires a yes or no response. The DAST-10 is a 10-item brief screening tool that can be administered by a clinician or self-administered. Each question requires a yes or no response, and the tool can be completed in less than 8 minutes. This tool assesses substance use, not including alcohol or tobacco use, in the past 12 months.

Treatment and Prevention

According to the 2012 CBHSQ Treatment Episode Data Set, there were 14,230 admissions of patients aged 65 or older to substance misuse treatment programs. Treating older adults with substance use disorders is no different from treating any other adult patient. Medications specific for substances used and therapies such as SBIRT and motivational interviewing have shown to be effective in this population (NIDA, 2012).

CASE STUDY 16-1

*A*lfred, a 68-year-old male patient, has reported to his primary care nurse practitioner (NP) that he experiences moderate to severe abdominal pains that radiate to his back. Alfred describes his pain as dull and constant; the pain becomes worse when he is supine. He also reports that for the last 3 days he has experienced anorexia and nausea.

Alfred's NP conducts a physical examination, which reveals abdominal distension and epigastric tenderness. Laboratory testing reveals a serum amylase level of 345 U/L (normal 23-85 U/L) and a serum lipase level of 850 (normal 160 U/L). Alfred tells his NP that he currently has five to six drinks (mostly bourbon and vodka) on most days of the week. He tells his NP that since he was let go from his job as a bank executive 8 years ago, he has been drinking alcohol heavily. Alfred explains that he was fired for making decisions that had a negative outcome for the company for which he worked. From Alfred's explanation, the NP suspects that he may have been drinking on the job when those decisions were made.

Alfred's social history includes a divorce 6 years ago. He currently lives alone and has two children who are both married and live out of town; he has infrequent contact with them. He relates that drinking helps him feel less worried and lonely and helps him to avoid ruminating on his failed marriage.

Alfred's medical history is positive for hypertension and hypocholesteremia. Alfred's current medications include the following:

- *Atorvastatin (Lipitor), 60 mg daily*
- *Aspirin, 81 mg daily*
- *Lisinopril (Zestril), 20 mg daily*
- *Metoprolol (Lopressor), 50 mg daily*

Alfred's current vital signs are as follows:

- *Blood pressure 154/92 mm Hg*
- *Pulse 128 beats/min*
- *Temperature 100.6°F*

Questions

1. What is a possible diagnosis for Alfred?

2. What are the priority treatment approaches for Alfred?

3. After stabilization of medical problems, what are the treatment priorities for Alfred, given his level of alcohol intake?

Answers

1. Alfred's laboratory test results and physical examination suggest acute and severe pancreatitis secondary to his high level of alcohol intake. He is also likely to be dehydrated due to anorexia and the nausea and vomiting associated with pancreatitis.

2. Severe acute pancreatitis is a medical emergency, and hospitalization is needed. Treatment needs to include restriction of oral food and fluid intake, restoration of electrolyte balance, oxygenation, intravenous hydration, and pain management. The healthcare

provider also needs to consider the possibility of alcohol withdrawal because his vital signs are elevated, which could be attributed to symptoms of alcohol withdrawal, the pain and inflammation associated with pancreatitis, or both. The NP needs to obtain information about the timing of Alfred's last drink, and the physical examination needs to assess for additional symptoms of alcohol withdrawal, including diaphoresis, tremors, anxiety, and restlessness. If symptoms of alcohol withdrawal are present, treatment needs to include benzodiazepines.

3. Alfred has been a heavy alcohol drinker for years. Upon medical stabilization, he should be referred for substance use counseling. Substance use counseling involves the use of motivational interviewing to help examine negative patterns in drinking. The healthcare provider can ask Alfred about the pros and cons of alcohol use by asking him to describe what he likes about drinking and what he does not like about drinking. The NP would also explore his perceptions about the importance of changing his drinking behaviors and his confidence and readiness to do so. The healthcare provider would assess Alfred's perception of the importance of changing his alcohol use by rating importance on a 0-to-10 scale, with 0 being "not at all important" and 10 being "extremely important." The level of confidence and readiness to change are also assessed on 0-to-10 scales. The healthcare provider would explore Alfred's rationale for his ratings of importance, confidence, and readiness to change, then discuss any ambivalence that Alfred may have about changing. A plan would be negotiated with measurable goals for reducing alcohol intake (e.g., dilute the drinks with water, have three drinks instead of five on the nights he

drinks). Alfred should also be assessed for major depressive disorder, given his job and family-related losses, guilt, self-blame, and social isolation. An additional treatment priority is suicide assessment. Suicidal ideation is a common feature of major depressive disorder with comorbid substance use. He is in a high-risk group for suicide due to his age and alcohol use.

SUMMARY

Substance use in reproductive-age women, adolescents, college-age adults, and older adults presents unique challenges and opportunities to nurses and clinicians in addressing this issue. Toxic exposure to substances in utero can have detrimental outcomes for the developing fetus. Prevention programs that target women during the reproductive years can reduce the incidence of substance use during pregnancy and improve outcomes for infants (Forray, 2016). Addressing underage drinking can reduce the number of motor vehicle accidents related to drinking and driving (CDC, 2016). Referral to SBIRT provides a promising intervention to reduce substance use, including the use of alcohol and illicit drugs, on college campuses (AAP, 2011). Substance use and chronic health problems place the older adult at greater risk for physical, emotional, family, and social problems (National Institutes of Health, 2015). Understanding the unique challenges contributing to substance use in each population will better prepare the nurse to intervene and ensure that patient-centered care and treatment are provided to promote optimal patient outcomes.

EXAM QUESTIONS

CHAPTER 16
Questions 89–93

Note: Choose the one option that BEST answers each question.

89. Fetal alcohol spectrum disorder is caused by exposure of the fetus to alcohol in

    a. breast milk.

    b. utero.

    c. medicine.

    d. conjunction with nicotine.

90. A protective factor during the adolescent period in delaying substance use is

    a. low academic achievement and/or academic aspirations.

    b. untreated attention-deficit/hyperactivity disorder.

    c. perceived peer acceptance of substance use and substance use in one's peers.

    d. parents who set clear rules and enforce them.

91. Daily use on college campuses is on the increase for which substance?

    a. Marijuana

    b. Cocaine

    c. Heroin

    d. Inhalants

92. The college-age young adult is more likely to use substances

    a. during the transition period from high school to college.

    b. while engaging in community service.

    c. while attending a faith-based organization on campus.

    d. when around peers who do not use substances.

93. A substance that is commonly used by older adults and likely to interact with other medications is

    a. marijuana.

    b. alcohol.

    c. tobacco.

    d. cocaine.

REFERENCES

American Academy of Pediatrics. (2011). *Policy statement: Subcommittee on Substance Abuse: Substance use screening, brief intervention, and referral to treatment for pediatricians.* Retrieved from http://pediatrics.aap publications.org/content/early/2011/10/26/ peds.2011-1754?rss=1

American Academy of Pediatrics. (2012). Clinical report: Neonatal drug withdrawal. Committee on Drugs and Committee on Fetus and Newborn. *Pediatrics, 129*(2), e540-e560.

American Academy of Pediatrics Division of Health Care Finance. (2015). Become familiar with ICD-10-CM guidelines for newborn, neonate care. *AAP News, 36*(5). Retrieved from http://www.aappublications. org/content/36/5/26

American College of Obstetricians and Gynecologists Committee on Health Care for Underserved Women & American Society of Addiction Medicine. (2012). *Opioid abuse, dependence, and addiction in pregnancy* (Committee Opinion No. 524). Washington, DC: American College of Obstetricians and Gynecologists.

American College of Obstetricians and Gynecologists. (2015). *Alcohol Abuse and Other Substance Use Disorders: Ethical Issues in Obstetric and Gynecologic Practice.* Retrieved from https://www.acog.org/-/media/ Committee-Opinions/Committee-on-Ethics/ co633.pdf?dmc=1

American Society of Addiction Medicine (2013). *The ASAM criteria: Treatment criteria for addictive, substance-related, and co-occurring conditions.* Retrieved from https://www.asam. org/resources/the-asam-criteria/about

Asato M. R., Terwilliger, R., Woo, J., & Luna, B. (2010). White matter development in adolescence: A DTI study. *Cerebral Cortex, 20*(9), 2122-2131.

Brown, R. L., & Rounds, L. A. (1995) Conjoint screening questionnaires for alcohol and other drug abuse: Criterion validity in a primary care practice. *Wisconsin Medical Journal, 945,* 135-140.

Center for Adolescent Substance Abuse Research. (n.d.). *The CRAFFT screening tool.* Retrieved from http://www.ceasar-boston.org/CRAFFT/

Center for Adolescent Substance Abuse Research. (2016). Children's Hospital Boston. *Screening Tool.* Retrieved from http://www. ceasar@childrens.harvard.edu

Center for Behavioral Health Statistics and Quality. (2015). *Behavioral health trends in the United States: Results from the 2014 National Survey on Drug Use and Health* (HHS Publication No. [SMA] 15-4927, NSDUH Series H-50). Rockville, MD: Substance Abuse and Mental Health Services Administration. Retrieved from http://www. samhsa.gov/data/

Center for Substance Abuse Treatment. (2009). *Substance abuse treatment: Addressing the specific needs of women* (Treatment Improvement Protocol [TIP] Series, No. 51, HHS Publication No. [SMA] 14-4426). Rockville, MD: Substance Abuse and Mental Health Services Administration.

Centers for Disease Control and Prevention. (2016). *Fact sheets: Underage drinking.* Retrieved from https://www.cdc.gov/alcohol/fact-sheets/underage-drinking.htm

Forray, A. (2016). Substance use during pregnancy. *F1000 Research, 5*(F1000 Faculty Rev.), 887. doi:/10.12688/f1000research.7645.1

Heikkinen, N., Niskanen, E., Könönen, M., Tolmunen, T., Kekkonen, V., Kivimäki, P., … Vanninen, R. (2017). Alcohol consumption during adolescence is associated with reduced grey matter volumes. *Addiction, 112*(4), 604-613. doi:10.1111/add.13697

Hudak, M. L., Tan, R. C., Committee on Drugs, & Committee on Fetus and Newborn. (2012). Neonatal drug withdrawal. *Pediatrics, 129*, e540-e560.

Lipari, R. N., & Jean-Francois, B. (2016). A day in the life of college students aged 18 to 22: Substance use facts. *CBHSQ Report.* Retrieved from https://www.samhsa.gov/data/sites/default/files/report_2361/ShortReport-2361.html

Mattson, M., Lipari, R. N., Hays, C., & Van Horn, S. L. (2017). A day in the life of older adults: Substance use facts. *CBHSQ Report.* Retrieved from https://www.samhsa.gov/data/sites/default/files/report_2792/ShortReport-2792.html

National Institute on Alcohol Abuse and Alcoholism. (2015). *Alcohol and Your Health: Older Adults.* Retrieved from https://www.niaaa.nih.gov/alcohol-health/special-populations-co-occurring-disorders/older-adults

National Institute on Alcohol Abuse and Alcoholism. (2015). *Alcohol and Your Health: College drinking.* Retrieved from https://pubs.niaaa.nih.gov/publications/collegefactsheet/Collegefactsheet.pdf

National Institute on Drug Abuse. (2012). *Principles of drug addiction treatment: A research-based guide* (3rd ed.). Retrieved from https://www.drugabuse.gov/publications/principles-drug-addiction-treatment-research-based-guide-third-edition

National Institute on Drug Abuse. (2014a, March 31). *Prevention.* Retrieved from https://www.drugabuse.gov/related-topics/prevention

National Institute on Drug Abuse. (2014b). *Principles of adolescent substance use disorder treatment: A research-based guide.* Retrieved from https://www.drugabuse.gov/publications/principles-adolescent-substance-use-disorder-treatment-research-based-guide

National Institute on Drug Abuse. (2015). *College-age & young adults.* Retrieved from https://www.drugabuse.gov/related-topics/college-age-young-adults

National Institute on Drug Abuse. (2017). *Health consequences of drug misuse.* Retrieved from https://www.drugabuse.gov/related-topics/health-consequences-drug-misuse

National Institutes of Health. (2015, August). *Alcohol use and older adults: How alcohol affects safety.* Bethesda, MD: National Institutes of Health, U. S. Department of Health and Human Services. Retrieved from http://nasadad.org/2015/06/nasadad-releases-fact-sheet-on-neonatal-abstinence-syndrome/#more-10836

Ross, E. J., Graham, D. L., Money, K. M., & Stanwood, G. D. (2015). Developmental consequences of fetal exposure to drugs: What we know and what we still must learn. *Neuropsychopharmacology, 40*(1), 61-87. http://doi.org/10.1038/npp.2014.147

Simkin, D. R., & Grenoble, S. (2010). Pharmacotherapies for adolescent substance use disorders. *Child and Adolescent Psychiatric Clinics of North America, 19,* 591-608. doi: 10.1016/j.chc.2010.03.010

Siu, A., & Robinson, C. A. (2014). Neonatal abstinence syndrome: Essentials for the practitioner. *Journal of Pediatric Pharmacology and Therapeutics, 19*(3), 147-155. doi:10.5863/1551-6776-19.3.147

Skinner, H. A. (1982). The drug abuse screening test. *Addictive Behaviors, 7*(4), 363-371.

Substance Abuse and Mental Health Services Administration. (n.d.). *NREPP: SAMHSA's national registry of evidence-based programs and practices.* Retrieved from http://nrepp.samhsa.gov/landing.aspx

Substance Abuse and Mental Health Services Administration. (2014). *Results from the 2013 National Survey on Drug Use and Health: Summary of national findings* (NSDUH Series H-48, DHHS Publication No. [SMA] 14-4863). Rockville, MD: Author.

Substance Abuse and Mental Health Services Administration. (2015a). *Risk and protective factors.* Retrieved from https://www.samhsa.gov/capt/practicing-effective-prevention/prevention-behavioral-health/risk-protective-factors

Substance Abuse and Mental Health Services Administration. (2015b). *Underage drinking.* Retrieved from https://www.samhsa.gov/underage-drinking-topic

Substance Abuse and Mental Health Services Administration. (2016a). *A collaborative approach to the treatment of pregnant women with opioid use disorders* (HHS Publication No. [SMA] 16-4978). Rockville, MD: Author. Retrieved from https://ncsacw.samhsa.gov/files/Collaborative_Approach_508.pdf

Substance Abuse and Mental Health Services Administration. (2016b). *SAMHSA's efforts in schools and on college campuses.* Retrieved from https://www.samhsa.gov/school-campus-health/samhsas-efforts

Volkow, N. D. (2011). *Substance abuse among older adults.* Retrieved from https://www.drugabuse.gov/news-events/nida-notes/2011/12/substance-abuse-among-older-adults

Williams, J. F., Smith, V. C., & Committee on Substance Abuse. (2015). Fetal alcohol spectrum disorders. *Pediatrics, 106*(2), 358. doi:10.1542/peds.2015-3113

Wu, C.-S., Jew, C. P., & Lu, H.-C. (2011). Lasting impacts of prenatal cannabis exposure and the role of endogenous cannabinoids in the developing brain. *Future Neurology, 6*(4), 459-480.

Yonkers, K. A., Gotman, N., Kershaw, T., Forray, A., Howell, H. B., & Rounsaville, B. J. (2010). Screening for prenatal substance use: Development of the substance use risk profile-pregnancy scale. *Obstetrics and Gynecology, 116*(4), 827-833. doi:10.1097/AOG.0b013e3181ed8290

CHAPTER 17

SUBSTANCE USE AND COMORBIDITY

LEARNING OUTCOME

After completing this chapter, the learner will be able to identify harmful effects of substance use on physical and mental health.

CHAPTER OBJECTIVES

After completing this chapter, the learner will be able to:

1. Review physical complications associated with intravenous drug use.

2. Describe the physical effects of substance use during pregnancy and early childhood developmental periods.

3. Discuss the relationship between mental illness and substance use.

INTRODUCTION

Many of the substances reviewed in this course have a profound effect on the physical and mental health of users. As discussed throughout the course, substances generally have unique characteristics associated with both acute intoxication and withdrawal, as well as long-term consequences. This chapter focuses on potential physical and psychological impairments that are associated with substance use. The harmful effects described are associated with injecting drugs of various types, fetal exposure to substances, impact on the developing brain, and the interplay between substance use and mental illness.

INTRAVENOUS DRUG USE

As substance users develop tolerance, injecting substances intravenously can become a way to get a desired effect more quickly with enhanced effectiveness. It is estimated that in 2011, over 6.6 million people in the United States had a lifetime history of intravenous drug use, or 2.6% of the population, with nearly 775,000 people injecting drugs within the past year (Lansky et al., 2014). Mortality rates in people who inject drugs (PWID) are significantly higher (up to 22%) than in the general population (Lavender & McCarron, 2013). The dangers of intravenous drug use include the risk of acute and chronic infection, either from autoinoculation or cross-contamination from using shared needles; the accidental introduction of contaminants into the bloodstream; and greater risk of acute overdose. Infections associated with intravenous drug use are a major cause of morbidity and mortality (Martin, Zweben, & Payte, 2014). Exposure to toxins in the misused substances can also have a variety of harmful effects depending on the variety of substances used.

Acute Infections

Acute Hepatitis

Hepatitis B virus (HBV) and hepatitis C virus (HCV) infections are most commonly associated with intravenous drug use in the United States (Centers for Disease Control and Prevention [CDC], 2014). Of particular concern is the significant and alarming rise in

HCV infections, particularly in people living in regions of the country where the prevalence of intravenous drug use is high (Zibbell et al., 2015). Both HBV and HCV infections can easily be undetected in the acute stages, suggesting that current estimates of prevalence are low (CDC, 2014). Symptoms of acute hepatitis often include malaise, fever, headache, and gastrointestinal maladies such as anorexia, diarrhea, nausea, and abdominal pain. Often these symptoms are indistinguishable from those experienced in withdrawal, particularly in relation to opioid dependence. In some instances, jaundice can develop. However, it is estimated that in 50% to 75% of the cases of acute infection, people are asymptomatic (Martin et al., 2014).

Although a vaccine currently exists for HBV, there is no vaccine for HCV. These factors make it particularly challenging to prevent the spread of HCV infection among PWID. It is estimated that the overall prevalence of HCV in PWID ranges between 66% and 88%, with an estimated 94% positive for those using intravenously for 10 years or more (Martin et al., 2014). Nearly 4 million people in the United States have been diagnosed with HCV, and chronic hepatitis C infection is a leading cause of advanced liver disease, hepatocellular carcinoma, and liver transplantation (Haber, Batey, & Mgaieth, 2014).

Human Immunodeficiency Virus

It is estimated that nearly one in five PWID is human immunodeficiency virus (HIV) positive (Martin et al., 2014). Needle sharing is the most common vehicle of transmission in PWID. Approximately one third of those who inject drugs report sharing needles. Nearly 50% of those injecting heroin were unaware of their HIV infection when tested (CDC, 2015). With the increased effectiveness of HIV treatment and no vaccine, needle exchange programs are an effective strategy for reducing the spread of

HIV infections in PWID. Additionally, HIV testing for PWID in treatment centers can aid in the early recognition and treatment of HIV infection, limiting the progression to AIDS (Martin et al., 2014).

Abscesses

Intravenous site infections are relatively common in PWID, particularly among those injecting drugs subcutaneously. Common pathogens include streptococci and staphylococci, although outbreaks of more unusual pathogens, such as wound botulism and anthrax, can also occur (Lavender & McCarron, 2013; Sulis, 2014). These infections can present as cellulitis or abscesses, and hospitalization can be necessary for treatment. In recent decades, there has also been an alarming increase in methicillin-resistant *Staphylococcus aureus* (MRSA) skin and soft tissue infections in PWID. The use of nonsterile needles also puts users at risk for polymicrobial infections, including both anaerobic and aerobic bacterial infections. An infection spreading to the deep tissues can result in necrotizing fasciitis, a potential limb- and life-threatening complication requiring emergent treatment and debridement (Sulis, 2014).

Endocarditis, Septic Emboli, and Sepsis

Infective endocarditis (IE) is a life-threatening complication of intravenous drug use caused by bacteria in the bloodstream. People with pre-existing cardiac problems, such as mitral valve prolapse or prosthetic heart valves, are at greatest risk. However, all PWID are at risk because bacteria in the bloodstream can lead to clot and fibrin formation (vegetation) in otherwise healthy heart valves. This vegetation can cause septic emboli, which can travel and lodge in the lungs, kidney, brain, bone, and other organs, resulting in heart, respiratory, or kidney failure and stroke, splenic infarcts, septic arthritis, and osteomyelitis (Lavender & McCarron, 2013; Sulis, 2014).

As with soft tissue infections, the causative organisms for IE in PWID are somewhat atypical from those found in noninjecting people with IE. The most prevalent are staphylococcal infections, with over a third of these being MRSA infections. People with alcoholism also have higher rates of IE. Generally, symptoms of IE include fever; cardiac symptoms, including murmurs and symptoms of congestive heart failure; and a variety of additional symptoms related to the organs affected by septic emboli. People may experience night sweats, myalgia, and arthralgia, and they may have signs of vasculitis, such as splinter hemorrhages. Because of the high risk of mortality from advancing infection, any unexplained fever in PWID should prompt an evaluation for IE (Sulis, 2014).

A recently published case study reviewing repeated hospitalizations and interventions for an intravenous substance user with IE illustrates the need for a comprehensive approach to treating these patients (Libertin, Camsari, Hellinger, Schneekloth, & Rummans, 2017). The case illustrates the challenges of providing intensive substance use treatment in the context of an all-too-common trajectory of repeated hospitalizations and surgeries for serious medical complications of persistent intravenous drug use. Both the patient and the healthcare system incur exorbitant costs when the system fails to intensively treat the underlying substance use disorder.

Tuberculosis

Tuberculosis (TB) has been less prevalent in the United States than in other regions of the world, where it remains a leading cause of morbidity and mortality. However, factors associated with substance use, particularly related to alcohol use disorder and PWID, such as higher-than-average rates of smoking, incarceration, homelessness, and HIV, have all contributed to sporadic surges of TB in the United States (Sulis, 2014).

Cotton Fever

Cotton fever is a condition that has been reported in case studies in the literature for decades but has limited empirical support. An Internet search reveals references to this condition from many nonscientific and nonclinical sources. The precipitating cause of cotton fever is described in the case-study literature as the use of a cotton ball to filter a heated, injectable drug (primarily heroin), resulting in a relatively rapid onset of fever, chills, headache, tachycardia, abdominal pain, and myalgias (Zerr, Ku, & Kara, 2016). The symptoms are generally self-limiting, and infectious disease studies are negative. The exact cause of the symptoms is not clear but includes suspicion of an immune-mediated response, a pyrogenic reaction to cotton, or the presence of an endotoxin (Torka & Gill, 2013).

Other Conditions

Cirrhosis, Liver Failure, and Chronic Hepatitis

Many substances are associated with toxic effects on the liver. These effects may be related to the toxic effects of the substance itself, such as alcohol, 3,4-methylenedioxy-N-methamphetamine (MDMA; Ecstasy), cocaine, or androgens, or related to the infectious or contaminant processes discussed in the previous sections. Regardless of the causative agent, liver disease and subsequent liver failure are major causes of morbidity and mortality among both PWID and those misusing other substances (Haber et al., 2014). For many who develop advanced liver disease, transplantation is the only viable treatment option. To be a candidate for transplantation, the individual must be abstinent from substance use for a clearly determined duration of time.

Renal Syndromes

The substances that primarily affect the kidney are alcohol (as a complication of liver failure), opioids, and cocaine. With opioid use, and particularly heroin use in PWID, many of the infectious conditions described previously can have a profound effect on renal function. Hypertension associated with cocaine use can lead to kidney infarction and failure. Rhabdomyolysis, a severe form of muscle ischemia related to the use of certain substances, such as cocaine, heroin, alcohol, MDMA, and methamphetamines, can also lead to acute renal failure (Crittendon & Silberzweig, 2014).

DEVELOPMENTAL IMPACT OF SUBSTANCE USE

Pregnancy

Exposure to substance use during pregnancy can have a profound effect on embryonic and fetal development. In 2015, the highest rates of illicit substance use were among people aged 18 to 25, the prime childbearing years (Center for Behavioral Health Statistics and Quality [CBHSQ], 2016). It has been reported that as many as 30% to 50% of pregnancies are unintended, and it is also thought to be the case that many women using substances experience unplanned pregnancies and are also more likely to be in abusive relationships than the general population (Weaver, Jones, & Wunsch, 2014). Substance use during pregnancy may also cause women to feel stigmatized, and this, in combination with an unintended pregnancy, can result in significantly delayed prenatal care, further jeopardizing the prenatal health of the mother and fetus. Use of substances early in pregnancy can also increase the risk of fetal loss (Weaver et al., 2014).

Multiple substances can have a deleterious effect on fetal development. Although much is still unknown about the specific fetal effects of many of the various misused substances, the most common and well-known effects are reviewed here. It is important to remember that polysubstance use is common, such as the use of alcohol and tobacco, both of which are known to have the most harmful effects on fetal development (Weaver et al., 2014).

Tobacco

Around 40% of women who smoke quit during pregnancy (Weaver et al., 2014). The primary tobacco-associated risks for the fetus include reduced oxygen supply from carbon monoxide exposure. Nicotine readily crosses the placenta and puts the fetus at risk for altered neurologic development. Generally, stimulant use in any form has been associated with premature labor, placental abruption, and intrauterine growth restriction.

Infants born to mothers who use tobacco in any form are more likely to be irritable, hypertonic, and difficult to calm. Infants with fetal exposure to tobacco are also more likely to die of sudden infant death syndrome (Weaver et al., 2014). Studies have also linked multiple behavioral disorders to prenatal and perinatal tobacco smoke exposure, but the correlations are not clearly understood. These include attention-deficit hyperactivity disorder (ADHD), oppositional defiant disorder, conduct disorder, anxiety, depression, Tourette's syndrome, schizophrenia, and intellectual disability (U.S. Department of Health and Human Services, 2014).

Alcohol

Around 60% of women who consume alcohol quit during pregnancy. Alcohol readily crosses the placenta and has a direct effect on the developing fetus. Additionally, due to immature liver development, there is a delay in the elimination of alcohol from the fetus that is slower than that experienced by the mother (Weaver et al., 2014). Numerous effects, both physiologic and cognitive, have been clearly associated with fetal alcohol exposure. These are categorized along a continuum of fetal alcohol spectrum disorders, with the most widely understood being fetal alcohol syndrome (FAS). Classically, FAS is defined as pre- and/or postnatal retardation of growth, including reduced head circumference, altered brain development, and physical facial anomalies (Weaver et al., 2014).

Opioids

Although there was a nearly fivefold increase in the use of opioids by women during pregnancy from 2000 to 2009 (1.19 to 5.63 per 1,000 hospital births per year), past-month use of opioids among pregnant women was less than use in nonpregnant women of the same age cohort (0.9% vs. 2.6%) in 2012. However, the incidence of neonatal abstinence syndrome (NAS), or fetal withdrawal from exposure to substances in utero, is estimated to be between 70% and 95% for those using opioids during pregnancy (Smith & Lipari, 2017).

Although any opioid use, including medication-assisted treatment, can lead to abstinence symptoms in the newborn, it is considered more harmful to subject the fetus to opioid withdrawal while in utero. Opioid withdrawal during the perinatal period can cause fetal distress and premature labor (Weaver et al., 2014). Perinatal exposure to opioids has been associated with congenital heart defects (Smith & Lipari, 2017) and intrauterine growth restriction (Weaver et al., 2014).

For the newborns of mothers who engage in opioid use during pregnancy, neonatal abstinence begins shortly after birth and causes the following effects in the newborn: central nervous system irritability, including tremors and feeding difficulties, and autonomic nervous system activation, including temperature instability via sweating and fevers (see Table 17-1). NAS-affected infants are more likely to experience respiratory distress, feeding difficulty, and low birth weight; are more prone to seizures; and

TABLE 17-1: SIGNS OF NEONATAL ABSTINENCE SYNDROME

Central nervous system irritability

High-pitched, continuous crying

Decreased sleep

Tremors

Increased muscle tone

Hyperactive Moro reflex

Seizures

Gastrointestinal dysfunction

Feeding difficulties

Vomiting

Loose/watery stools

Autonomic nervous system activation

Sweating

Fever

Frequent yawning and sneezing

Increased respiratory rate

Nasal stuffiness and flaring

Note. From Ko, J. Y., Wolicki, S., Barfield, W. D., Patrick, S. W., Broussard, C. S., Yonkers, K. A., ... Iskander, J. (2017). CDC grand rounds: Public health strategies to prevent neonatal abstinence syndrome. *Morbidity and Mortality Weekly Report,* *66*(9), 242-245.

have a significantly longer average length of stay (2.1 vs. 16.9 days) than nonaffected infants. Currently, there is no standardized approach to treating NAS in infants, although most recommendations include environmental measures such as rooming-in, swaddling, and breastfeeding, along with tapered doses of morphine or methadone based on NAS scales (Ko et al., 2017).

The long-term effects of opioid exposure in utero suggest there are cognitive and motor skill deficits that persist into school age, with increased risk for inattention, hyperactivity, and ADHD (Ross, Graham, Money, & Stanwood,

2015). The long-term effects of using opioids in the treatment of NAS are less clearly understood.

Long-Term Effects

Data are surprisingly sparse and conflicting related to both the long-term effects of perinatal exposure to misused substances and the effects of paternal use of substances. Those with developmental effects noted at birth or shortly after often catch up with their peers during the school-age years, although changes in brain structure and function have been well documented with exposure to many substances (Ross et al., 2015). Many confounders complicate the exploration of long-term effects, such as exposure to multiple substances, extent of exposure, brain plasticity, and the environment.

SUBSTANCE USE AND MENTAL ILLNESS

Risk Factors

Addictive substances affect the reward system of the brain and alter the chemistry related to the regulation of pleasurable emotions and the alleviation of stress. There are many potential precipitants for using substances, and many involve adverse childhood experiences, which increase the risk for substance use and other health problems (Substance Abuse and Mental Health Services Administration, 2016). These experiences can include the following:

- Physical abuse
- Sexual abuse
- Emotional abuse
- Physical neglect
- Emotional neglect
- Mother treated violently
- Substance misuse within household
- Household mental illness

- Parental separation or divorce
- Incarcerated household member

Genetics also plays a role; studies have demonstrated that genetic susceptibility to substance use is more clearly associated with progression to addiction than with substance initiation (Simkin, 2014). In addition, undiagnosed mental illness during any stage of development is also associated with an increased risk of substance misuse, possibly related to neurobiological vulnerability. As noted previously, several other disorders may result from perinatal exposure to substances and are considered risk factors for substance use:

- ADHD
- Mood disorders
- Conduct disorders
- Anxiety disorders
- Learning disorders
- Schizophrenia

(Simkin, 2014)

It is important to consider that no one risk factor is associated with the development of a substance use disorder. Family and peer exposures, school performance, and personality traits such as sensation seeking also play roles (Simkin, 2014). However, these risk factors are important to consider for the prevention and early detection of substance use disorders before they progress to problematic use and addiction.

Comorbid Mental Illness and Substance Use

In 2014, there were nearly 8 million adults with co-occurring mental illness and substance use disorders. People with mental illness are more likely to have a substance use disorder than those without mental illness (CBHSQ, 2015). Treatment for people with co-occurring disorders can be complex due to the overlapping of symptoms between the effects of specific substances and the underlying mental illness. As healthcare providers, it is critical to assess substance use in people with mental illness and, conversely, mental illness in people with substance use disorders. The risk of underdiagnosing and undertreating can have serious ramifications, such as increased incarceration and physical complications associated with addiction. Integrated treatment settings and strategies are recommended to meet the needs of this challenging population (Lipari, Park-Lee, & Van Horn, 2016).

SUMMARY

Substance misuse involves a complex array of physical and psychological effects. The physical complications of addiction, primarily those associated with intravenous drug use, can have long-lasting and life-threatening consequences. The cumulative effects of multiple substances on the various organ systems in the body can cause significant morbidity for the user. Substance use during pregnancy can have serious and long-lasting effects on the fetus and throughout early childhood development. These effects can influence the child's risk for developing a substance use disorder. There is also significant overlap between mental illness and substance use disorders. It is imperative that healthcare providers consistently and systematically screen for substance use and ensure people in need of treatment obtain care that is integrated and comprehensive to meet all their physical and mental health needs.

EXAM QUESTIONS

CHAPTER 17
Questions 94–96

Note: Choose the one option that BEST answers each question.

94. Advanced liver disease and liver failure are complications of intravenous substance use that are associated with the toxic effects of the substance, contaminated intravenous needles, and

    a. repeat hospitalizations.
    b. resulting infections.
    c. lack of vaccines.
    d. renal conditions.

95. The incidence of neonatal abstinence syndrome is very high after birth for infants of mothers using

    a. opioids.
    b. methamphetamine.
    c. nicotine.
    d. alcohol.

96. The underdiagnosis of mental health conditions in patients with substance use disorders can result in

    a. decreased physical complications.
    b. decreased addiction.
    c. increased incarceration.
    d. increased use of mental health services.

REFERENCES

Center for Behavioral Health Statistics and Quality. (2015). *Behavioral health trends in the United States: Results from the 2014 National Survey on Drug Use and Health* (HHS Publication No. [SMA] 15-4927, NSDUH Series H-50). Retrieved from http://www.samhsa.gov/data/

Center for Behavioral Health Statistics and Quality. (2016). *Key substance use and mental health indicators in the United States: Results from the 2015 National Survey on Drug Use and Health* (HHS Publication No. [SMA] 16-4984, NSDUH Series H-51). Retrieved from http://www.samhsa.gov/data/

Centers for Disease Control and Prevention. (2014). *Viral hepatitis surveillance – United States, 2014.* Retrieved from https://www.cdc.gov/hepatitis/statistics/2014surveillance/pdfs/2014hepsurveillancerpt.pdf

Centers for Disease Control and Prevention. (2015). *HIV infection, risk, prevention, and testing behaviors among persons who inject drugs – National HIV behavioral surveillance: Intravenous drug use, 20 U.S. cities, 2012* (HIV Surveillance Special Report 11, revised edition). Retrieved from http://www.cdc.gov/hiv/library/reports/surveillance/

Crittendon, S. D., & Silberzweig, J. I. (2014). Renal and metabolic disorders related to alcohol and other drug use. In R. K. Reis (Ed.), *The ASAM principles of addiction medicine* (5th ed., pp. 1133-1144). Philadelphia, PA: Wolters Kluwer.

Haber, P. S., Batey, R. G., & Mgaieth, S. E. (2014). Liver disorders related to alcohol and other drug use. In R. K. Reis (Ed.), *The ASAM principles of addiction medicine* (5th ed., pp. 1106-1132). Philadelphia, PA: Wolters Kluwer.

Ko, J. Y., Wolicki, S., Barfield, W. D., Patrick, S. W., Broussard, C. S., Yonkers, K. A., … Iskander, J. (2017). CDC grand rounds: Public health strategies to prevent neonatal abstinence syndrome. *Morbidity and Mortality Weekly Report, 66*(9), 242-245.

Lansky, A., Finlayson, T., Johnson, C., Holtzman, D., Wejnert, C., Mitsch, A., … Crepaz, N. (2014). Estimating the number of persons who inject drugs in the United States by meta-analysis to calculate national rates of HIV and hepatitis C virus infections. *PLoS One, 9*(5), e97596. doi:10.1371/journal.pone.0097596

Lavender, T. W., & McCarron, B. (2013). Acute infections in intravenous drug users. *Clinical Medicine, 13*(5), 511-513.

Libertin, C. R., Camsari, U. M., Hellinger, W. C., Schneekloth, T. D., & Rummans, T. A. (2017). The cost of a recalcitrant intravenous drug user with serial cases of endocarditis: Need for guidelines to improve the continuum of care. *IDCases, 8,* 3-5.

Lipari, R. N., Park-Lee, E., & Van Horn, S. (2016). *America's need for and receipt of substance use treatment in 2015.* The CBHSQ Report: September 29, 2016. Rockville, MD: Substance Abuse and Mental Health Services Administration, Center for Behavioral Health Statistics and Quality.

Martin, J., Zweben, J. E., & Payte, J. T. (2014). Opioid maintenance treatment. In R. K. Reis (Ed.), *The ASAM principles of addiction medicine* (5th ed., pp. 759-777). Philadelphia, PA: Wolters Kluwer.

Ross, E. J., Graham, D. L., Money, K. M., & Stanwood, G. D. (2015). Developmental consequences of fetal exposure to drugs: What we know and what we still must learn. *Neuropsychopharmacology, 40*(1), 61-87.

Simkin, D. R. (2014). Neurobiology of addiction from a developmental perspective. In R. K. Reis (Ed.), *The ASAM principles of addiction medicine* (5th ed., pp. 1580-1600). Philadelphia, PA: Wolters Kluwer.

Smith, K., & Lipari, R. N. (2017). *Women of childbearing age and opioids.* The CBHSQ Report: January 17, 2017. Rockville, MD: Substance Abuse and Mental Health Services Administration, Center for Behavioral Health Statistics and Quality.

Substance Abuse and Mental Health Services Administration. (2016). *Adverse childhood experiences.* Retrieved from https://www.samhsa.gov/capt/practicing-effective-prevention/prevention-behavioral-health/adverse-childhood-experiences

Sulis, C. A. (2014). Human immunodeficiency virus, tuberculosis, and other infectious diseases related to alcohol and other drug use. In R. K. Reis (Ed.), *The ASAM principles of addiction medicine* (5th ed., pp. 1195-1215). Philadelphia, PA: Wolters Kluwer.

Torka, P., & Gill, S. (2013). Cotton fever: An evanescent process mimicking sepsis in an intravenous drug abuser. *Journal of Emergency Medicine, 44*(6), e385-e387.

U.S. Department of Health and Human Services. (2014). *The health consequences of smoking: 50 years of progress. A report of the surgeon general.* Atlanta, GA: U.S. Department of Health and Human Services, Centers for Disease Control and Prevention, National Center for Chronic Disease Prevention and Health Promotion, Office on Smoking and Health.

Weaver, M. F., Jones, H. E., & Wunsch, M. J. (2014). Alcohol and other drug use during pregnancy: Management of the mother and child. In R. K. Reis (Ed.), *The ASAM principles of addiction medicine* (5th ed., pp. 1254-1271). Philadelphia, PA: Wolters Kluwer.

Zerr, A. M., Ku, K., & Kara, A. (2016). Cotton fever: A condition self-diagnosed by IV drug users. *Journal of the American Board of Family Medicine, 29*(2), 276-279.

Zibbell, J. E., Iqbal, K., Patel, R. C., Suryaprasad, A., Sanders, K. J., Moore-Moravian, L., ... Holtzman, D. (2015). Increases in hepatitis C virus infection related to intravenous drug use among persons aged ≤30 years – Kentucky, Tennessee, Virginia, and West Virginia, 2006-2012. *Morbidity and Mortality Weekly Report, 64,* 453-458.

CHAPTER 18

IMPAIRED PRACTICE IN HEALTHCARE PROFESSIONALS

LEARNING OUTCOME

After completing this chapter, the learner will be able to describe the ethical and legal implications of impaired practice and the role of healthcare professionals in identifying and reporting impaired practice.

CHAPTER OBJECTIVES

After completing this chapter, the learner will be able to:

1. Define impaired practice by a healthcare professional with a substance use disorder.

2. Identify the prevalence of substance use disorders in healthcare professionals.

3. Describe the clinical indicators of impaired practice in healthcare professionals.

4. Discuss the rationale for reporting a healthcare professional with impaired practice to the appropriate resource for treatment.

INTRODUCTION

Substance use disorders among healthcare professionals present special challenges to the profession. Alcohol and drug misuse in healthcare professionals exists but can be challenging to identify (Kunyk, 2015; Monroe, Kenaga, Dietrich, Carter, & Cowan, 2013).

Healthcare professionals are just as vulnerable to mental health and substance use disorders as the general public. Impaired practice encompasses an inability to provide care consistent with the legal and ethical standards of the profession. Impaired practice includes activities performed not only by clinicians with substance use disorders but also those performed by clinicians with any mental health or personal problem or distress that interferes with the quality and safety of patient care (Winland-Brown, Lachman, & O'Connor Swanson, 2015). In a broad sense, this can include fatigue secondary to sleep deprivation, poor communication among clinicians, and overwork (Earley, 2014). For the purposes of this chapter, impairment is narrowly defined as that caused by or related to a substance use disorder. The impact of impairment on the quality and safety of patient care is of great concern to all healthcare professionals; health consumers; boards of nursing, medicine, and social work; and policymakers.

HISTORY

The history of drug and alcohol misuse in health care has been documented since the 1800s. Jane Gibson, a young nurse who accompanied Florence Nightingale to the battlefields of the Crimean War, was fired from her postwar nursing position for coming to work under the influence of alcohol. The press vilified her, implying that she had ruined the image of the "Nightingale Nurses" – an image replete with behaviors described as angelic, pure, caring, and virginal (Monahan, 2003).

Additionally, Dr. William Oster described the addiction of a legendary 19th-century surgeon, Dr. William Halstad. Oster states, "I saw him in severe chills, and this was the first information I had that he was still taking morphia. Subsequently, I had many talks about it and gained his full confidence. He had never been able to reduce the amount to less than three grains daily; on this, he could do his work comfortably and maintain his excellent physical vigor. I do not think that anyone suspected him" (Noland & Halstad, 1991, p. 17).

Dr. Halstad continued in his surgical practice; however, Ms. Gibson's fate was more reflective of the public and professional response to healthcare professionals with impaired practice. Historically, the response was usually overwhelmingly punitive and resulted in devastating personal and professional losses (Monahan, 2003). Since the 1980s, the healthcare professions have worked to develop a more measured response that focuses on protecting public safety while providing a nonpunitive opportunity for treatment and rehabilitation. Each health discipline has developed a code of ethics that addresses the issue of impaired practice associated with a substance use disorder. These codes of ethics are developed by such organizations as the American Nurses Association, the American Medical Association (ANA), and the National Association of Social Workers. The codes of ethics are unique to each organization, but they are consistent in their mandates that require healthcare professionals report all instances of impaired practice of a colleague to the appropriate resource. These resources vary by state law and include administrators, licensing boards, and professional organizations. The codes of ethics require that the professional must not only report unsafe or incompetent practice (again, for the purposes of this chapter, incompetent practice is defined as "impaired practice associated with substance misuse") but also all reasonable suspicions of impaired practice.

Additional issues surrounding impairment have been raised in recent years with the legalization of both medical and recreational marijuana use (Phillips et al., 2015). Although alcohol levels can be measured, and standards exist for legal levels of impairment, this is not the case for other drugs, particularly those with a longer half-life, such as marijuana. The actual use of a substance that can potentially affect practice may be challenging to identify unless it results in impairment in judgment or clinical effectiveness. Therefore, the focus in the workplace is on both identifying impairment when it occurs and working to reduce the risk of impairment through early identification and assistance for those using substances in a manner that can impact the quality and safety of their work performance. For many, workplace policies regarding these issues continue to evolve (Phillips et al., 2015).

Impaired nursing practice may be defined as the inability of a registered nurse to perform his or her roles and responsibilities because of a chemical dependency on drugs, alcohol, or both. ANA Code of Ethics (2015), this also includes impairment due to "mental or physical illness, fatigue, substance use, or personal circumstances" (p. 13). Codes of ethics espoused by professional organizations are considered an ethical mandate. However, licensing boards, specifically the Board of Nursing, Board of Medical Examiners, and Board of Social Work, exist in each state to protect the public and regulate and license the profession. Licensing boards carry the force of law (for additional information, see http://www.deadiversion.usdoj.gov). Therefore, it is both an ethical and legal responsibility to report a colleague whose practice is impaired.

EPIDEMIOLOGY

The key risk factors for alcohol and drug use disorders among healthcare professionals involve personal, genetic, environmental, and occupational risks. Healthcare professionals commonly consider themselves to be at low risk by virtue of their extensive education and training in human physiology and pathophysiology; however, these professionals are no different from the general population in terms of their risk factors (e.g., availability of drugs, history of unstable family relationships) for developing substance use disorders (Earley, 2014; Merlo, Singhakant, Cummings, & Cottler, 2013).

The American Association of Nurse Anesthetists (AANA) has developed a comprehensive website addressing the problem of substance use in anesthesia professionals (http://www.aana.com/resources2/health-wellness/Pages/Substance%20Use%20Disorder.aspx). The AANA identifies risk factors that are similar to those associated with the general population, such as depression and other mental health concerns, pain, genetic factors, social instability, risk-taking behaviors, and stress. Risks associated with healthcare anesthesia settings are also identified, such as ready availability of substances, including propofol, which is unregulated.

Occupational and environmental risks factors include work in a stressful and demanding environment; variable shift work and sleep patterns, which can result in sleep deprivation and self-medication with stimulants and sedatives; increased access to and familiarity with drugs and controlled substances; and self-medicating behaviors. A qualitative study of physicians in treatment for substance use disorders found that most used prescription medications not only for the purposes of treating physical pain and managing stress and emotional distress but also for recreational use and to prevent withdrawal (Merlo et al., 2013).

Healthcare professionals working in the same specialty area tend to misuse similar substances. This is particularly true with nurses and doctors. Nurses in emergency departments, intensive care units, and operating rooms report easier access to controlled substances and more prescription-type substance misuse than do nurses who do not work in critical care (Dunn, 2005). Psychiatrists, anesthesiologists, and emergency medicine clinicians are the specialists most likely to misuse substances, with pediatricians and pathologists having the lowest prevalence (Earley, 2014).

Nurses and clinicians in general are more likely to misuse prescription drugs over other substances. The foundation for alcohol and drug misuse commonly begins in college, with at-risk behaviors and heavy drinking occurring in nursing, medical, or social work school. It is thought that substance misuse most frequently begins in training and early practice, but this has not been a consistent finding (Earley, 2014). Marijuana is the most frequently reported substance used by medical residents, whereas benzodiazepines are misused by psychiatrists at nearly double the rate of misuse by other clinicians. Propofol is the most frequently misused substance among anesthesia providers (Earley, 2014).

PREVALENCE

Although the overall prevalence of addiction in clinicians and nurses is thought to be similar to that of the general population, the substances used by various types of clinicians differ from the substances used by the general population (Bush & Lipari, 2015; Earley,

2014). For example, clinicians tend to use more alcohol, opioids, and sedatives than the general population, but the prevalence of tobacco use is lower in clinicians (Cottler et al., 2013; Earley, 2014). Nurses have a slightly higher prevalence of alcohol and drug misuse than the general population when controlling for education (some college) and gender (women), with those nurses misusing substances also having higher rates of tobacco use (Kunyk, 2015). The National Institute on Drug Abuse (NIDA, 2015) reports that healthcare professionals have higher rates of alcoholism than the general population. Physicians, dentists, and nurses also misuse controlled substances at higher rates than other professionals due to having easy access to these substances (NIDA, 2015).

Another report found that healthcare professionals have a higher prevalence of illicit drug use than that of alcohol misuse (5.5% versus 4.4%), with rates staying relatively stable over the past decade (Bush & Lipari, 2015). Illicit drugs in this survey were defined as marijuana or hashish, cocaine (including crack), inhalants, hallucinogens, heroin, and prescription-type drugs used nonmedically. Many nurses with substance use disorders go unreported and untreated (National Council of State Boards of Nursing [NCSBN], 2014).

CLINICAL FINDINGS

Early identification of impaired practice and substance use disorders in nurses and other clinicians is critical to the safety and quality of patient care and crucial to the long-term recovery of the professional. The importance of early identification of impairment cannot be overstated. Physical and behavioral symptoms of misuse are generally no different in healthcare providers than in the general population and are related to the specific substance or substances being used

(Angres, Bologeorges, & Chou, 2013). Concerns regarding impairment can be raised by patients, colleagues, and supervisors. Recognition and reporting of unsafe or incompetent practice protects the safety and quality of patient care, improves treatment outcomes, and is considered to be an ethical and legal responsibility of all healthcare professionals (Winland-Brown et al., 2015). Early identification is challenging because job performance can be one of the last areas of life affected for a healthcare professional with a substance use disorder. However, it is important to suspect impairment when certain activities in the workplace become evident, such as frequent narcotic count errors, poor pain control in patients for whom narcotics are ordered, and frequent absences from work. A pattern of behavior with resulting negative consequences provides cues for early identification of impaired practice (see Table 18-1).

TREATMENT

The ANA Code of Ethics states, "Nurses must protect the patient, the public, and the profession from potential harm when practice appears to be impaired. The nurse's duty is to take action to protect patients and to ensure that the impaired individual receives assistance" (ANA, 2015, p. 13). The Code further states, "if impaired practice poses a threat or danger to patients, self or others, regardless of whether the individual has sought help, the nurse must report the practice to persons authorized to address the problem" (ANA, 2015, p. 13). It is clear and unequivocal that patient safety is paramount and that it is the responsibility of the nurse to report questionable practice. The Code is also quite clear that compassion, treatment, and rehabilitation are the goals of care for the impaired healthcare professional.

It is not uncommon for the colleagues of the professional with a substance use disorder to be

TABLE 18-1: CUES FOR EARLY IDENTIFICATION OF IMPAIRMENT

Area of Life	Cues
Family life	• Withdrawal from family activities • Marital conflict • Acting out by children • Sexual problems
Community life	• Withdrawal from community activities • Embarrassing behaviors at community functions
Financial and legal well-being	• Legal problems • Driving under the influence • Financial difficulties
Spiritual and emotional well-being	• Changes in emotional health • Mood swings • Anger • Denial and rationalization • Depression, anxiety, and panic disorders • Forgetfulness
Physical health	• Poor personal hygiene • Weight loss • Sniffing, sneezing, and watery eyes • Cough • Unexplained bruises • Frequent visits for health care • Multiple prescriptions • Chronic pain
Job performance	• Deteriorating job performance • Excessive use of sick time • Calling in sick on Fridays and/or Mondays • Poor judgment • Disorganization • Withdrawal from coworkers

Note. Western Schools, 2017.

suspicious. However, many choose not to document or communicate these concerns, allowing the impaired practice to continue. The literature suggests barriers that healthcare professionals encounter when considering reporting impaired colleagues, including concerns regarding direct confrontation, feeling already overburdened with patient care, and assuming it is a supervisor's responsibility to take action (Bettinardi-Angres & Bologeorges, 2011). The professional may choose to take no action because of fear of repercussions, lack of awareness of a policy that addresses the process of reporting impairment, or concerns about personal liability. The healthcare professional may choose to perform the duties or cover the mistakes of an impaired colleague in an attempt to protect the colleague's job or to act as a counselor. These professionals enable the continued impaired practice of their colleague. In any case, a professional who is aware of a colleague with a substance use disorder and willfully does not report this colleague is jeopardizing patient safety and could face disciplinary action. If a healthcare professional has a reasonable suspicion of impairment, is concerned about patient safety, is reporting this suspicion in good faith, and has documented his or her concerns, successful litigation by the professional with impaired practice is highly unlikely. This is true even in the event that the professional may benefit personally from reporting the individual (Berge, Seppala, & Schipper, 2009).

Historically, medical and nursing boards have taken a punitive approach to addressing impaired practice. As addiction is increasingly recognized as a treatable condition rather than a moral failing, more care has gone into providing access to treatment for healthcare professionals with substance use disorders. Additionally, healthcare professionals have been noted to have a better response to treatment than the general population (Earley, 2014). In the United States, there are programs specifically tailored to treating addicted healthcare providers. Yet the political climate can vary from state to state and among professional regulatory boards, resulting in recent swings back to a more punitive approach (Earley, 2014). However, in the case of nurses specifically, punitive approaches have been seen as counterproductive decisions that promote biases, such as moral failure, which are inconsistent with our current understanding of addiction (Kunyk, 2015; Kunyk, Milner, & Overend, 2016).

The NCSBN (2011) has provided guidance for reporting and addressing impairment in nurses. The NCSBN lists state regulations that specifically include certain acts or events that are cause for disciplinary action against the nurse, such as the following:

- Drug diversion
- A positive screen for a drug for which there is no lawful prescription
- Violation of a state or federal narcotics or controlled substances law
- Criminal convictions
- Addiction to or dependency on a habit-forming drug or controlled substance
- Illegal use of a drug or controlled substance
- Use of a habit-forming drug or controlled substance to the extent that the use impairs the nurse physically or mentally
- Failure to comply with the contract provisions of the state nursing board's nurses assistance program

A healthcare professional who chooses to report the suspected impaired practice should document his or her concerns and address these concerns in terms of facts to the appropriate resource. This resource is defined by state law and may be an administrator, a licensing board, or a professional organization. The healthcare professional should carefully consider the ramifications of confronting the colleague with his or her suspicions. If he or she chooses to discuss suspicions of impaired practice with this colleague, it is important to address the facts, the effect on patient safety, and the opportunity for treatment. This should not be a punitive discussion but a discussion that is both factual and hopeful. An approach similar to motivational interviewing may be used. The healthcare professional should state that compassion, treatment, and rehabilitation are the goals of care for the colleague and that treatment is available. These events are often windows of opportunity to engage in treatment (Kunyk, Inness, Reisdorfer, Morris, & Chambers, 2016; Monroe et al., 2013). If the colleague is unwilling to seek care and denies impaired practice, the professional must report his or her concerns to the appropriate resource.

Patient safety and colleague treatment are the goals of the intervention, and it is important to balance the privacy of the healthcare professional who is in treatment for a substance use disorder with public safety. The healthcare professional's information and the intervention are considered confidential, which is a key element of enhancing treatment engagement (Earley, 2014; Kunyk, Inness, et al., 2016).

Many states offer nondisciplinary, confidential, and voluntary programs for healthcare professionals with substance use disorders that do not automatically result in loss of licensure. The success of these treatment programs relies on defined intervention processes, such as contracts related to treatment expectations. In some instances, healthcare professionals using medication-assisted treatment for opioid use disorders may return to work, but these policies are complicated and controversial (Earley, 2014). The recovering healthcare professional typically participates in monitored treatment and recovery programs for indefinite periods.

INTERNET RESOURCES FOR INFORMATION ON IMPAIRED PRACTICE IN THE HEALTHCARE PROFESSIONS

Internet resources that focus on identifying information for the treatment of healthcare professionals with impaired practice include the following:

American Society of Addiction Medicine (ASAM), http://www.asam.org

Federation of State Physician Health Programs, http://www.fsphp.org

Hazelden Betty Ford Foundation, http://www.hazelden.org

International Nurses Society on Addictions, http://www.intnsa.org

National Association of Social Workers, http://www.socialworkers.org

National Institute on Alcohol Abuse and Alcoholism (NIAAA), http://www.niaaa.nih.gov

National Organization of Alternative Programs, http://www.alternativeprograms.org

After the recovering professional returns to work, safeguards are put in place to protect the individual and the institution. The recovering professional should be assigned to areas with limited drug availability and should not dispense opioids or hold keys that allow access to opioids. He or she should not be floating or working in relatively unstructured clinical areas and should be on a predictable schedule, allowing for the opportunity to participate in meetings and rehabilitation (Earley, 2014).

The Emergency Nurses Association (ENA) and the International Nurses Society on Addictions (IntNSA) have developed a joint position paper that encourages workplaces to view substance misuse as a "serious and treatable disease," provide education, develop policies that "promote safe, supportive, drug-free workplaces" (p. 105), and encourage access to nonpunitive treatment (Strobbe & Crowley, 2017). Physician health programs are widespread in the United States, but a lack of national standards and oversight has raised concerns (Boyd, 2015).

CASE STUDY 18-1

Ann is a 27-year-old registered nurse who has been working in a busy trauma center of a large metropolitan hospital for the past 12 months. Ann has also recently returned to school to obtain a Master's in Nursing degree, as her goal is to become a manager of nursing staff in an emergency care setting. Ann is single, with no children, and she lives several hundred miles away from any family members. Ann has increasingly found it challenging to socialize with the few friends she has met in her new environment due to her demanding work and school schedules.

Two months ago, Ann slipped on an icy hospital sidewalk while reporting for work and injured her left arm and wrist. Ann sought care at the employee health center of the hospital. A radiograph confirmed that Ann had a distal radial fracture. After proper stabilization, the nurse practitioner in the employee health center prescribed acetaminophen with oxycodone (Percocet) to Ann, instructing her to follow up with her primary care practitioner in a couple of days and to stay home during this time period.

One week later, Ann was able to return to work with some duty modifications. Ann continued to take the remainder of her Percocet prescription as ordered; she liked the way it made her feel, giving her more energy and helping her to focus better at work. However, Ann ran out of Percocet shortly after returning to her job, and she began to experience symptoms of feeling depressed and exhausted. Having access to narcotics in the trauma center, Ann began stealing the waste of opioid pain medication that she administered to patients. She then began self-medicating the pain medication to avoid the negative withdrawal symptoms she was experiencing. Eventually Ann began taking greater risks by using some of the prescribed dose of pain medication for patients for her own use.

The nurse manager of the trauma center soon realized what Ann was doing and confronted Ann with her suspicions. Ann is devastated by her actions and confided to her manager that she needs help.

Questions

1. Which cues may have alerted the nurse manager that Ann was stealing opioid pain medication?

2. What are the recommended actions of the nurse manager after confirming that Ann is stealing opioid pain medication?

3. What are resources for Ann to prevent further misuse of narcotics?

Answers

1. The nurse manager most likely became aware of a pattern of frequent narcotic count errors and poor pain control in patients for whom Ann was caring. Ann may have also begun to have more frequent absences from work due to her increasing physical dependence on narcotic pain medication. When Ann began experiencing early withdrawal, the nurse manager may have noted symptoms of agitation and anxiety (e.g., restlessness, difficulty concentrating, irritability) in Ann while she was working.

2. The ANA Code of Ethics states that nurses who become aware of impaired practice in another nurse must put patient safety first by reporting the impaired practice to persons authorized to address the problem. The nurse manager can confront Ann with her suspicions and let her know that she is supportive of finding help and medical treatment for Ann. The nurse manager will most likely report Ann's substance use problem to her own nursing manager, and she will assist with investigating and reporting the incident to the appropriate State Board of Nursing. The hospital nursing personnel

can also consult the NSBN for information about reporting and addressing issues of nurse practice impairment.

Upon confirmation of Ann's substance use, it is imperative that the nurse manager immediately and thoroughly document her suspicions and any follow-up actions. The nurse manager reinforces to Ann that she is there to help her in seeking treatment and rehabilitation so that she can return to work safely. She advises Ann that there are programs (e.g., nurse assistance programs) to help nurses with substance use issues to abstain from using drugs and continue to practice nursing.

3. In addition to entering a specialized substance use treatment and rehabilitation program, Ann can prevent misuse of future substances by seeking additional resources. These include the following:

    -   Monitored treatment and recovery programs implemented within the hospital after completion of a specialized treatment program

    -   Internet resources (e.g., ASAM, IntNSA, NIAAA, etc.) for more information on treatment for impaired nursing practice

    -   Safeguards that other institutions have developed to protect the nurse and the hospital from further risk of impaired practice after the nurse returns to work

    -   The ENA and INSA joint position paper advocating for policies and practices on nonpunitive treatment of nurses with impaired practice

SUMMARY

In summary, the importance of early identification of an impaired colleague with timely reporting to an appropriate administrator is critical to the rehabilitation of the healthcare professional. Taking action to protect the patient from an impaired colleague is also considered an ethical, and often legal, responsibility of all healthcare professionals. Impaired practice puts everyone at risk, including the patient, the healthcare facility, and the healthcare professional. Disciplinary actions against impaired professionals can result in loss of licensure and potential incarceration, resulting in lifelong consequences. Although progress has been made to reduce stigma and improve access to care for healthcare professionals, a concerted effort on the part of clinicians, workplaces, and licensing boards is still needed to get impaired nurses and other professionals the treatment they need.

EXAM QUESTIONS

CHAPTER 18
Questions 97–100

Note: Choose the one option that BEST answers each question.

97. The nurse with impaired practice due to a substance use disorder finds it difficult to

    a. have a positive response to treatment.

    b. find appropriate care and treatment.

    c. make the best of a very difficult situation.

    d. perform his or her roles and responsibilities.

98. The overall prevalence of substance use disorders among healthcare workers is

    a. significantly lower than in the general public.

    b. very similar to the general public.

    c. significantly higher than in the general public.

    d. unknown because the risks of disclosing substance misuse are too great.

99. A "red flag" raising suspicion of a substance use disorder in a healthcare professional is

    a. making frequent phone calls at work.

    b. displaying emotional stress due to marital problems.

    c. having one unreconciled narcotic count.

    d. having a pattern of caring for patients with poor pain control from narcotics.

100. An impaired healthcare professional has been referred to an employee assistance program for recovery from a substance use disorder. This referral and subsequent treatment are most likely to result in the clinician's

    a. loss of licensure for a 2- to 3-year period.

    b. return to work with safeguards to protect him or her and the institution.

    c. disclosure of his or her impairment to colleagues and request for forgiveness.

    d. inability to work in a healthcare institution for at least 2 years.

This concludes the final examination.

Please answer the evaluation questions found on page v of this course book.

REFERENCES

American Nurses Association. (2015). *Code of ethics for nurses.* Washington, DC: American Nurses Publishing. Retrieved from http://nursingworld.org/DocumentVault/Ethics-1/Code-of-Ethics-for-nurses.html

Angres, D., Bologeorges, S., & Chou, J. (2013). A two year longitudinal outcome study of addicted health care professionals: An investigation of the role of personality variables. *Substance Abuse: Research and Treatment, 7,* 49-60.

Berge, K. H., Seppala, M. D., & Schipper, A. M. (2009). Chemical dependency and the physician. *Mayo Clinic Proceedings, 84*(7), 625-631.

Bettinardi-Angres, K., & Bologeorges, S. (2011). Addressing chemically dependent colleagues. *Journal of Nursing Regulation, 2*(2), 10-17.

Boyd, J. W. (2015). A call for national standards and oversight of state physician health programs. *Journal of Addiction Medicine, 9*(6), 431-432.

Bush, D. M. & Lipari, R. N. (2015). *The CBHSQ report: Substance use and substance use disorder, by industry.* Rockville, MD: Substance Abuse and Mental Health Services Administration, Center for Behavioral Health Statistics and Quality.

Cottler, L., Ajinkya, S., Merlo, L. J., Nixon, S. J., Ben Abdallah, A., & Gold, M. (2013). Lifetime psychiatric and substance use disorders among impaired physicians in a physicians health program: Comparison to a general treatment population: Psychopathology of impaired physicians. *Journal of Addiction Medicine, 7*(2), 108-112.

Dunn, D. (2005). Substance use among nurses – Defining the issues. *AORN Journal, 82*(4), 573-82, 585-588, 592-596.

Earley, P. H. (2014). Physician health programs and addiction among physicians. In R. K. Reis (Ed.), *The ASAM principles of addiction medicine* (5th ed., pp. 602-621). Philadelphia, PA: Wolters Kluwer.

Kunyk, D. (2015). Substance use disorders among registered nurses: Prevalence, risks and perceptions in a disciplinary jurisdiction. *Journal of Nursing Management, 23*(1), 54-64.

Kunyk, D., Inness, M., Reisdorfer, E., Morris, H., & Chambers, T. (2016). Help seeking by health professionals for addiction: A mixed studies review. *International Journal of Nursing Studies, 60,* 200-215.

Kunyk, D., Milner, M., & Overend, A. (2016). Disciplining virtue: Investigating the discourses of opioid addiction in nursing. *Nursing Inquiry, 23,* 315-326.

Merlo, L. J., Singhakant, S., Cummings, S. M., & Cottler, L. B. (2013). Reasons for misuse of prescription medication among physicians undergoing monitoring by a physician health program. *Journal of Addiction Medicine, 7*(5), 349-353.

Monahan, G. (2003). Drug use/misuse among health professionals. *Substance Use and Misuse, 38*(11-13), 1877-1881.

Monroe, T. B., Kenaga, H., Dietrich, M. S., Carter, M. A., & Cowan, R. L. (2013). The prevalence of employed nurses identified or enrolled in substance use monitoring programs. *Nursing Research, 62*(1), 10-15.

National Council of State Boards of Nursing. (2011). *Substance use disorder in nursing: A resource manual and guidelines for alternative and disciplinary monitoring programs.* Chicago, IL: Author.

National Council of State Boards of Nursing. (2014). *What you need to know about substance use disorder in nursing.* Retrieved from https://www.ncsbn.org/SUD_Brochure_2014.pdf

National Institute on Drug Abuse. (2015). *Drug facts.* Retrieved from https://www.drugabuse.gov/publications/drugfacts/nationwide-trends

Noland, S., & Halstad, W. S. (1991). Idiosyncrasies of a surgical legend. *Harvard Medical Alumni Bulletin, 65,* 17-23.

Phillips, J. A., Holland, M. G., Baldwin, D. D., Gifford-Meuleveld, L., Mueller, K. L., Perkison, B., ... Dreger, M. (2015). Marijuana in the workplace: Guidance for occupational health professionals and employers: Joint guidance statement of the American Association of Occupational Health Nurses and the American College of Occupational and Environmental Medicine. *Workplace Health and Safety, 63*(4), 139-164.

Strobbe, S., & Crowley, M. (2017). Substance use among nurses and nursing students: A joint position statement of the Emergency Nurses Association and the International Nurses Society on Addictions. *Journal of Addictions Nursing, 28*(2), 104-106.

Winland-Brown, J., Lachman, V. D., & O'Connor Swanson, E. (2015). The new code of ethics for nurses with interpretive statements: Practical clinical application, part I. *MedSurg Nursing, 24*(4), 268-271.

RESOURCES

GENERAL

Caffeine Awareness Alliance:
    http://www.caffeineawareness.org/calcu.php

Truth Tobacco Industry Documents:
    https://www.industrydocumentslibrary.ucsf.edu/tobacco/

SCREENING INSTRUMENTS: ALCOHOL

Alcohol Use Disorders Identification Test (AUDIT):
    http://www.integration.samhsa.gov/AUDIT_screener_for_alcohol.pdf

AUDIT Alcohol Consumption Questions (AUDIT-C):
    http://www.integration.samhsa.gov/images/res/tool_auditc.pdf

CAGE-AID (cut down, annoyed, guilty, eye opener – adapted to include drugs):
    http://www.integration.samhsa.gov/images/res/CAGEAID.pdf

CRAFFT (car, relax, alone, forget, friends, trouble):
    http://www.ceasar-boston.org/CRAFFT/index.php

Michigan Alcoholism Screening Test:
    http://adai.washington.edu/instruments/pdf/Michigan_Alcoholism_Screening_Test_156.pdf

National Institute on Alcohol Abuse and Alcoholism Materials Order Form:
    http://pubs.niaaa.nih.gov/OrderForm/EncForm/Youth_Guide_Order_Form

TWEAK (tolerance, worried, eye opener, amnesia, cut down) Test:
    http://adai.washington.edu/instruments/pdf/TWEAK_252.pdf

SCREENING INSTRUMENTS: OTHER DRUGS

Addiction Severity Index:
    http://adai.washington.edu/instruments/pdf/Addiction_Severity_Index_Baseline_Followup_4.pdf

Alcohol, Smoking, and Substance Involvement Screening Test*:
    http://www.who.int/substance_abuse/activities/en/ASSIST%20V.3-%20Guidelines%20for%20
    use%20in%20primary%20care_TEST.pdf

*An online modified version with support resources for clinicians is available at
    https://www.drugabuse.gov/nmassist/

Drug Abuse Screening Tool:
    https://www.drugabuse.gov/sites/default/files/dast-10.pdf

Substance Abuse and Mental Health Services Administration: Screening, Brief Intervention,
    and Referral to Treatment and evidence-based screening tools:
    http://www.integration.samhsa.gov/clinical-practice/sbirt

WITHDRAWAL

Clinical Institute Withdrawal Assessment for Alcohol – Revised:
    http://www.ci2i.research.va.gov/paws/content/7.htm

Clinical Opiate Withdrawal Scale:
    https://www.drugabuse.gov/sites/default/files/files/ClinicalOpiateWithdrawalScale.pdf

GLOSSARY

addiction: The most severe form of substance use disorder, associated with compulsive or uncontrolled use of one or more substances; a chronic brain disease that has the potential for both recurrence (relapse) and recovery.

aerosols: Sprays that contain propellants and solvents, such as hairsprays, spray paints, and deodorants.

agonist: A substance that binds to a receptor and initiates or facilitates a physiologic response.

alcohol use disorder (AUD): A medical condition that a qualified licensed healthcare provider diagnoses when a patient's drinking causes distress or harm. This disorder has mild, moderate, and severe specifiers.

anabolic: Muscle-building activity or substance.

androgenic: Substance that increases male characteristics.

antagonist: A substance that inhibits or interferes with a physiologic response.

autoinoculation: The spread of infection or bacteria from one part to other parts of the same body.

barbiturate: Pharmacologic agent used to promote sedation in anesthesia and outpatient surgical procedures.

benzodiazepine: An anxiolytic pharmacologic agent that promotes sedation, amnesia, and respiratory depression; acts on gamma-aminobutyric acid-A ($GABA_A$), receptor subtypes alpha 1 (α1), alpha 2 (α2), alpha 3 (α3), and alpha 5 (α5).

binge drinking: Having five or more alcoholic drinks for males or four or more alcoholic drinks for females on the same occasion (i.e., at the same time or within a couple of hours of one another) on at least 1 day in the past month.

cannabinoid: One of the chemical compounds found in marijuana, including cannabidiol, cannabinol, and delta-9-tetrahydrocannabinol (THC).

cannabis: The name for the marijuana or hemp plant and the products coming from that plant material.

comorbid substance use disorder: A substance use disorder in individuals with psychotic or mood disorders.

comorbidity: The occurrence of two or more disorders or disease states in a single individual, occurring either simultaneously or sequentially.

compulsive use: Continued use of a substance despite harmful or negative consequences.

cycling: Taking doses of anabolic steroids for a period, stopping for a time, and then restarting.

delta-9-tetrahydrocannabinol (THC): A cannabinoid that is the primary psychoactive agent in the marijuana plant.

delusion: A fixed false belief that is not supported by reality.

designer drug: An illegal synthetic chemical that is manufactured in a laboratory and mimics the action of a naturally occurring drug.

detoxification: Withdrawing patients from substances safely and effectively.

diversion: The transfer of a legally prescribed substance to someone for whom it was not prescribed with the intent of illicit drug use.

D-lysergic acid diethylamide: A synthetic hallucinogen manufactured from lysergic acid. Found in ergot, a fungus that grows on grains. Common street names include LSD, acid, blotter acid, and window pane.

dopamine: A neurotransmitter present in several brain regions involved in movement, emotion, motivation, reinforcement, and feelings of pleasure.

drug addiction: A chronic, relapsing brain disease characterized by compulsive drug seeking and use, despite harmful consequences.

fetal alcohol syndrome (FAS): A condition resulting from alcohol exposure during the mother's pregnancy that develops in the fetus and causes brain damage and growth problems that vary from child to child; defects caused by FAS are not reversible.

flashback: The recurrence of a previous drug experience, which may consist of hallucinations or visual disturbances. Flashbacks occur without warning and can occur a few days or more than a year after drug use.

GABA$_A$ agonist: A pharmacologic agent used in the treatment of insomnia; acts on GABA$_A$ α1 receptors.

gamma-aminobutyric acid (GABA): An inhibitory neurotransmitter in the brain.

gas: A substance in a physical state that can expand to occupy any container; used as anesthetics in medical procedures (e.g., nitrous oxide, isoflurane, and halothane) and in household products (e.g., butane lighters and propane tanks).

hallucination: A sensory perception that is not supported by reality; hallucinations can be auditory, visual, tactile, olfactory, or gustatory.

hallucinogens: Drugs that alter the perceptions of one's surroundings, thoughts, and feelings.

healthcare professional: Person with advanced training to work in the medical or dental fields, including nurses, social workers, physicians, and dentists.

heavy alcohol use: Binge drinking on 5 or more days in the past month.

hypertension: Elevated blood pressure.

impaired practice: The use of a substance such as alcohol or drugs in a manner that impacts professional competence, resulting in unsafe care of patients.

indicated prevention: A strategy designed for patients who are identified as having minimal but detectable signs, symptoms, or precursors of some illness or condition but whose condition is below the threshold of a formal diagnosis of the condition.

indolylalkylamine: A hallucinogen derived from mushrooms; includes psilocybin. Common street names include little smoke, magic mushrooms, purple passion, and shrooms.

NBOMe drugs: Synthetic hallucinogens that are similar to phenylethylamines. Common street names include N-bomb and smiles.

negative reinforcement: The negative emotions occurring in the absence of substance use that drive continued use.

neonatal abstinence syndrome (NAS): A constellation of problems affecting an infant soon after delivery resulting from the withdrawal of a substance (usually an opioid) used by the birth mother.

neurotransmitters: Chemical substances that transmit signals between neurons and that modulate neuronal activity.

nitrite: A chemical or drug that does not cross the blood-brain barrier but acts directly on blood vessels and muscles.

phenylethylamine: A substance with both hallucinogenic and stimulant properties, such as MDMA (Ecstasy).

physical dependence: The occurrence of an abstinence syndrome after abrupt total withdrawal from or substantial reduction in the use of a substance.

piperidine: A dissociative anesthetic that has hallucinogenic properties; includes ketamine and phencyclidine.

positive reinforcement: A pleasurable sensation serving as a reward for using a substance and establishing a pattern of use or habit.

prevention: Interventions that take place before the onset of a disorder.

protective factors: Individual resilience and other circumstances that reduce the likelihood of initiating substance use.

psychosis: A condition affecting the mind in which there is gross impairment in the understanding of reality that is manifested as hallucinations or delusions.

pyramiding: Slowly increasing the dose or frequency of anabolic steroid misuse, reaching a peak amount, and then gradually tapering off it.

rave: An all-night gathering or party that features loud electronic music; dancing; electronic visual effects, such as bright flashing lights; and illicit drugs, especially psychedelic substances.

recovery: A process of change through which individuals with substance use disorders improve their health and wellness, live a self-directed life, and strive to reach their full potential.

relapse: The return to drug use after a significant period of abstinence.

resilience: The ability to quickly recover from stressful life events and other difficulties.

risk factors: Those influences that contribute to increased vulnerability to the initiation, continuation, or escalation of substance use.

selective prevention: A strategy designed for individuals who are members of population subgroups whose risk of developing an imminent or lifetime disease or disability is significantly above average.

serotonin: A neurotransmitter that has been implicated as having a role in states of consciousness, mood, depression, and anxiety.

stacking: Combining two or more different types of anabolic steroids.

substance: A psychoactive compound with the potential to cause health and social problems.

substance dependence: A maladaptive pattern of substance use leading to clinically significant impairment or distress.

substance misuse: The use of any substance in a manner, situation, amount, or frequency that can cause harm to users or to those around them. For some substances or individuals, any use would constitute misuse (e.g., underage drinking, injection drug use).

tobacco products: Items used to deliver nicotine from tobacco leaves or extract. These include conventionally manufactured cigarettes, roll-your-own cigarettes, smokeless tobacco (chew, dip, snus, or snuff), pipe tobacco, cigars and cigarillos, hookahs, bidis, electronic cigarettes, heat-not-burn cigarettes, and vaping devices containing nicotine.

tolerance: A condition in which higher doses of a drug are required to produce the same effect as experienced initially; often leads to physical dependence.

universal prevention: A strategy designed for everyone in the eligible population, both the public and all members of specific eligible groups.

volatile solvent: A liquid that vaporizes at room temperature, such as toluene, gasoline, or paint thinner.

withdrawal: A psychological and/or physical syndrome caused by the abrupt cessation of the use of a drug in a habituated individual.

INDEX

Page numbers followed by an italicized *f* indicate figures; *t*, tables.